Clinical Challenges in Psychiatry

Clinical Challenges in Psychiatry

Edited by

William H. Sledge, M.D.
Professor of Psychiatry and Associate Chair for Education
Yale University School of Medicine;
Clinical Director
Connecticut Mental Health Center
New Haven, Connecticut

Allan Tasman, M.D.
Professor and Chairman
Department of Psychiatry and Behavioral Sciences
University of Louisville School of Medicine
Louisville, Kentucky

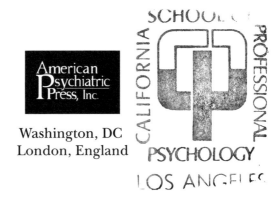

American Psychiatric Press, Inc.

Washington, DC
London, England

Copyright © 1993 American Psychiatric Press, Inc.
ALL RIGHTS RESERVED
Manufactured in the United States of America on acid-free paper
96 95 94 93 4 3 2 1
First Edition

American Psychiatric Press, Inc.
1400 K Street, N.W., Washington, DC 20005

Library of Congress Cataloging-in-Publication Data
Clinical challenges in psychiatry / edited by William H. Sledge,
 Allan Tasman. — 1st ed.
    p. cm.
  Includes bibliographical references and index.
  ISBN 0-88048-510-8
  1. Psychotherapy—Complications. 2. Countertransference
(Psychology). 3. Psychotherapist and patient. I. Sledge, William
H., 1945– . II. Tasman, Allan, 1947– .
  [DNLM: 1. Countertransference (Psychology). 2. Psychotherapy
—methods. WM 420 C6413]
RC480.5.C5535 1993
616.8914—dc20
DNLM/DLC   92-49970
for Library of Congress   CIP

British Library Cataloguing in Publication Data
A CIP record is available from the British Library.

Contents

Contributors

Victor A. Altshul, M.D.
Associate Clinical Professor of Psychiatry
Yale University School of Medicine;
Private Practice
New Haven, Connecticut

Claudia Bemis, M.D.
Assistant Professor of Psychiatry
Yale University School of Medicine;
Director, Psychiatric Emergency Services and Outpatient Clinic
Psychiatric Geriatric Consultant to the Adler Geriatric
  Assessment Center
Yale–New Haven Hospital
New Haven, Connecticut

Howard C. Blue, M.D.
Assistant Professor of Psychiatry
Yale University School of Medicine;
Director, Entry and Crisis Services
Connecticut Mental Health Center
New Haven, Connecticut

Sara C. Charles, M.D.
Professor of Clinical Psychiatry
Department of Psychiatry
University of Illinois at Chicago
Chicago, Illinois

Arnold M. Cooper, M.D.
Stephen P. Tobin and Arnold M. Cooper Professor
  in Consultation Liaison Psychiatry
New York Hospital–Cornell Medical Center
Payne Whitney Psychiatric Clinic
New York, New York

John A. Grimaldi, M.D.
Assistant Clinical Professor of Psychiatry
New York Hospital–Cornell Medical Center—
    Westchester Division;
Director, Long-Term Inpatient Unit
White Plains, New York

Dianna E. Hartley, Ph.D.
Assistant Adjunct Professor
Graduate Program in Clinical Psychology
University of Kentucky;
Private Practice
Lexington, Kentucky

Gerald L. Klerman, M.D.[*]
Professor and Associate Chairman for Research
New York Hospital–Cornell Medical Center
Payne Whitney Psychiatric Clinic
New York, New York

Gary J. Maier, M.D.
Director of Psychiatric Services for the Forensic Center
Mendota Mental Health Institute
Madison, Wisconsin

John C. Markowitz, M.D.
Assistant Professor of Psychiatry
New York Hospital–Cornell Medical Center
Payne Whitney Psychiatric Clinic
New York, New York

Richard L. Munich, M.D.
Professor of Clinical Psychiatry
New York Hospital–Cornell Medical Center—
    Westchester Division; Director, Division of Extended
Treatment Services, White Plains, New York;
Training and Supervising Analyst
Center for Psychoanalytic Training and Research
Columbia University
New York, New York

---

[*]Deceased

Michael A. Norko, M.D.
Assistant Clinical Professor of Psychiatry
Yale University School of Medicine;
Unit Chief
Whiting Forensic Institute
Middletown, Connecticut

Samuel W. Perry, M.D.
Professor of Psychiatry
New York Hospital–Cornell Medical Center
Payne Whitney Psychiatric Clinic
New York, New York

Eric M. Plakun, M.D.
Clinical Instructor in Psychiatry
Harvard Medical School;
Director of Admissions
Austen Riggs Center
Stockbridge, Massachusetts

Douglas A. Puryear, M.D.
Associate Professor of Psychiatry
University of Texas Southwestern Medical School;
Associate Director of Emergency Psychiatric Services
Parkland Memorial Hospital
Dallas, Texas

Richard S. Schottenfeld, M.D.
Associate Professor of Psychiatry
Yale University School of Medicine;
Director, Substance Abuse Treatment Unit
Connecticut Mental Health Center
New Haven, Connecticut

Michael A. Selzer, M.D.
Associate Professor of Clinical Psychiatry
New York Hospital–Cornell Medical Center—
   Westchester Division
White Plains, New York

William H. Sledge, M.D.
Professor of Psychiatry and Associate Chair for Education
Yale University School of Medicine;
Clinical Director
Connecticut Mental Health Center
New Haven, Connecticut

Stuart Sugarman, M.D.
Clinical Director, Associate Chairman, and Associate
  Professor of Psychiatry
Department of Psychiatry
University of Connecticut
Farmington, Connecticut

Allan Tasman, M.D.
Professor and Chairman
Department of Psychiatry and Behavioral Sciences
University of Louisville School of Medicine
Louisville, Kentucky

Howard Zonana, M.D.
Professor of Psychiatry
Yale University School of Medicine;
Director, Law and Psychiatry Division
Connecticut Mental Health Center
New Haven, Connecticut

Introduction

The idea for this book grew out of our experience in preparing a section for the 1989 *American Psychiatric Press Review of Psychiatry*. The response to that section on difficult clinical situations was extremely gratifying for all involved and suggested that there may be a need for and an interest in more attention to the difficult clinical challenges confronting practitioners. Thus, we chose to produce this volume. We have tried to identify difficult clinical problems that are common enough to bear examination and comment, yet unusual enough to be vexatious and problematic. The primary aim of the book is to explore in depth relatively common clinical situations that pose problems for the practitioner.

We chose leading experts to develop these topics into 14 chapters, roughly organized into patient factors, situational factors, and therapist factors. There is a substantial emphasis on borderline personality psychopathology in the first section because of the variety of problems that often arise in the care of patients with this disorder. The book, however, is by no means a comprehensive approach to borderline personality disorder and its varied presentations and treatments. Also included are chapters that address the conceptual understanding of borderline pathology as it relates to psychotherapeutic technique and treatment approaches for self-destructive and acting-out patients, as well as a clinical formulation of self-injurious behavior. There are chapters that address dual diagnosis, aggression, HIV-seropositivity, noncompliance, and management of the suicidal patient. In each chapter the author(s) addresses themes related to the need for both specific knowledge (technical as well as attitudinal) and the understanding and mastery of countertransference feelings specifically related to each situation.

For the section on therapist factors we have selected chapters that address countertransference issues with psychotic patients and with those who pose characteristic resistance. There is, in addition, a chapter on therapists' contribution to negative therapeutic reactions.

While the challenging situations selected for this volume have been diverse, we do not claim that we have been exhaustive in our choices. For instance, we have not dealt with the problems of psychopharmacology. Our emphasis is primarily on a psychodynamic perspective as a psychological treatment approach. Further, we have not addressed some of the major psychopathological states in any comprehensive fashion, nor do we discuss some of the problems involved in providing high-quality care in the face of diminishing resources to support that care in both the private and the public sectors. By not addressing these issues, we make no implied statement of their importance or value. We are confident that other investigators will take them up or that we will come back to them in subsequent volumes.

We have assembled a group of authors whose work we know and who have demonstrated not only expertise in the particular clinical area but also an active interest in teaching. The authors, who are all outstanding communicators, have a facility for solving the information transfer problems that one encounters when dealing with clinical challenges.

One of the main goals of this volume is to teach. We want to engage the reader in an endeavor in which we convey not only specific information but something of the values and the attitudes necessary to successfully engage and resolve clinical difficulty. We have encouraged our authors to develop a practical, problem-solving approach. Many of the authors are psychoanalytic or psychodynamic in their orientation. This is a reflection of our conviction of the value and utility of a psychodynamic perspective. Having indicated this slant toward psychodynamic thinking, however, we must point out that this is not a book on psychoanalysis or psychodynamic psychotherapy. Indeed, a substantial number of the authors have no direct connection to psychoanalysis or a psychodynamic orientation.

We have tried to ensure that the chapters are practical and useful. We have aimed for a harmonious balance between theory and abstract principles and specific concrete advice. This harmony varies from chapter to chapter, as does the placement of the fulcrum to achieve balance. In all chapters there is a mixture of technical detail and advice, the explication of an approach that includes something of a particular attitude, and the exposition of a philosophy based on clinical science as the author(s) knows it. Most chapters contain substantial clinical illustrations.

The creation of this volume has forced us to think more precisely about what we mean by a difficult clinical challenge. Certainly one definition of difficulty entails the notion of great technical, intellectual, or emotional effort. A situation may be difficult because there is not enough knowledge within the field to determine the most efficacious approach. The solution to these kinds of problems is the development of new knowledge through research. Situations may also be difficult because the practitioner simply does not have the skill and knowledge appropriate to the situation, in which case the solution is one of education and training.

Much psychiatric practice is difficult and ambiguous because of the complex relationship between interventions and outcomes. This complexity may at times lead to magical thinking, in which case causality is ascribed to chance or noncausal events. This phenomenon can lead to behaviors and actions becoming rigid and inflexible, largely because of the anxiety-reducing function of certain behavior and beliefs for the practitioners. This rigidity can create increasing difficulty when practitioners adhere to nonrational practices. In this volume we hope to address these uncertain relationships between means and ends through the importation of knowledge and emotional attitudes.

Another aspect of difficulty has to do with the uncontrollable and unpredictable nature of many phenomena. These include self-destructive acts, problems with compliance, and co-occurrence of other illnesses that create harmonics of an uncontrollable and unpredictable nature in the expression of disorder and disease.

Psychiatry is a difficult profession in that the work frequently (but, of course, not always) involves making a professional relationship intimate. This kind of work involves the use of the personality as a therapeutic instrument and can lead to a variety of role strains and difficulties. Hence, countertransference or the emotional reaction that a therapist has toward a patient's particular psychology can become a major part of the definition of what comprises a clinical challenge.

Other emotional components of the work are also difficult. Here we refer to clinical work that generates unpleasant affect, stimulates strong emotions and intrapsychic conflict, and in some cases puts the therapist at risk for litigation or violence. Broadly speaking, these emotional reactions can be considered countertransference. We have tried to ensure that the subjective side of the clinician's work is given appropriate emphasis in these chapters.

Running throughout the book are certain common themes. In addition to the theme of difficulty—its definition, management, organization, and treatment—is the theme of accountability and responsibility. Indeed, in the face of clinical difficulty it is impressive how the problems, those that hurt and cause pain, frequently evolve around issues of who is in charge and who is responsible. On the negative side, this may come down to issues of blame, that is, who is at fault. In a more positive direction, accountability and responsibility, when clearly delineated, provide a structure for the conduct of demanding and arduous work. Indeed, it is quite debatable whether this work can ever be carried out appropriately without clear lines of accountability, responsibility, and authority. This holds true especially in circumstances that are troubling and, by definition, difficult.

It is with pride that we present these 14 chapters. We have divided the volume into sections, each of which has a brief introduction that orients the reader to the contents of the section. As editors, we hope that the book will be useful, both as a stimulus for thought and reflection and as a reference whenever a difficult clinical challenge arises.

William H. Sledge, M.D.
Allan Tasman, M.D.

Section I:

Patient Factors

Introduction to Section I

The eight chapters in this section focus on medical and biologically based problems and aggressive and self-destructive behaviors, as well as with themes of control and compliance.

Richard Schottenfeld, in Chapter 1, discusses patients with dual diagnosis. For years, clinicians have cared for patients with this particular constellation of disorders; however, it is only recently that these patients have received attention in the psychiatric literature commensurate with the difficulty in treating their condition. Another group of patients whom psychiatrists have increasingly worked with are those patients who are seropositive for human immunodeficiency virus (HIV). In Chapter 2, John Markowitz and colleagues address a psychotherapeutic approach to these patients. Perhaps no group of psychiatric patients are as difficult to manage and treat as those with borderline personality problems. Richard Munich, in Chapter 3, provides an innovative conceptual framework for understanding a variety of issues in the psychopathology of these patients.

The issue of self-destructiveness is addressed in the next three chapters, which provide a different perspective on working with patients who threaten self-destruction. In Chapter 4, Howard Blue and colleagues present a comprehensive approach to the evaluation of the suicidal patient, particularly when the clinician is meeting this patient for the first time. The authors emphasize the work being carried out in an emergency or crisis setting. Eric Plakun, in Chapter 5, gives us a fine account of the psychotherapy of an acting-out, self-destructive patient and develops several principles that can be generalized to other patients and settings. In Chapter 6, Arnold Cooper provides a masterful psychoanalytically oriented overview of masochism and self-defeating personality disorder. Cooper does not, however, exclusively orient his discussion toward self-destruction, which is a subcategory of behavior related to self-defeating behaviors in general.

In Chapter 7, Gary Maier provides us with an approach to the management of the repetitively aggressive patient, primarily from an inpatient perspective. His conceptualizations can, however, readily be applied to any setting. Maier emphasizes the anticipation of aggression and the understanding of the aggressive behavior from an adaptive perspective. Douglas Puryear, in his chapter on compliance problems, provides us with clinical wisdom concerning the art of negotiation and the avoidance of unconscious or conscious manipulation on the part of the patient.

Chapter 1

Psychotherapeutic Approaches to Dual-Diagnosis Patients

Richard S. Schottenfeld, M.D.

Prevalence of Comorbid Psychiatric and Substance-Use Disorders

The high prevalence of substance-use disorders among patients with schizophrenia, affective disorders, and personality disorders, as well as the increased severity of illness of these patients, underscores the need for specialized psychotherapeutic strategies that can be used to treat those patients with substance abuse and psychiatric comorbidity.

Substance abuse or dependence is a problem for between 20% and 50% of young, chronically mentally ill patients suffering from schizophrenia, schizoaffective, or bipolar disorders (Ananth et al. 1989; Dixon et al. 1990; Mueser et al. 1990; Negrete et al. 1986; Richard et al. 1985; Siris 1990; Siris et al. 1988). These patients are particularly likely to abuse stimulants, such as cocaine or amphetamine, or to abuse marijuana, hallucinogens, or alcohol (Dixon et al. 1990; Richard et al. 1985). Data from the National Institute of Mental Health (NIMH) Epidemiologic Catchment Area (ECA) study suggest that schizophrenic patients have a threefold increased lifetime risk for alcohol abuse or dependence, and more than a sixfold increased risk for drug abuse or dependence (Regier et al. 1991).

Substance-use disorders are also prevalent among patients with depressive or anxiety disorders. The ECA data document about a twofold increased risk for alcohol abuse or dependence and a fourfold increased risk for drug abuse or dependence in patients with any affective disorder. The lifetime prevalence of any substance-use disorder in patients with bipolar disorder exceeds 60%; these patients have more than a fivefold increased risk for an alcohol disorder and are at an elevenfold increased risk for drug abuse or dependence (Anthony and Trinkoff 1989). Consistent with these findings, depressive and anxiety disorders as well as severe personality disorders are present in 25% to 60% of patients seeking treatment for substance-use disorders (Rounsaville et al. 1982, 1991; Schottenfeld et al., in press).

Prognostic Significance of Comorbidity

With the possible exception of depression in alcoholic women, who appear to do better in treatment than alcoholic women without any other psychiatric disorder (Rounsaville et al. 1987; Schuckit and Winslow 1972), comorbid psychiatric and substance-use disorders appear to have a poorer prognosis than either disorder alone. Substance abuse in the chronically mentally ill is associated with more frequent and severe relapse, higher rates of rehospitalization, and greater difficulty engaging or retaining in treatment (Barbee et al. 1989; Crowley et al. 1974; Hall et al. 1977). Similarly, measures of psychopathology are inversely correlated with measures of sustained abstinence or improved outcome in follow-up studies of patients treated for substance abuse (McLellan et al. 1983; Rounsaville and Kleber 1987; Rounsaville et al. 1986).

Integration of Treatment Approaches

Although substance abuse treatments and psychodynamic psychotherapies utilize very different approaches, they can be integrated successfully. Adjunctive supportive and expressive psychotherapies have been shown to lead to significant improvement in opiate addicts with midrange or high psychiatric severity concurrently treated in a methadone maintenance program (Kranzler and Liebowitz 1988; Rounsaville and Kleber 1987; Woody et al. 1983). Successful treatment involves striking a balance between traditional substance abuse treatment approaches—which emphasize therapist activity, confrontation, behavioral modification, and the importance of peer interactions and involvement in self-help groups—and a psychodynamic approach, with its emphasis on exploration of psychological conflict and of the meaning of symptoms, and therapist inactivity (Table 1–1) (Brown 1985; Kaufman 1989).

In the treatment of patients with comorbid psychiatric and substance-use disorders, an eclectic approach is essential. Therapists need to be able to utilize cognitive, behavioral, and psychodynamic therapies, as well as to include family members and significant social supports in the treatment. The sequence and timing of interventions, however, are often the critical factors. Too early exploration of some psychodynamic issues may lead to intolerable anxiety, depression, and relapse, while the failure to address other issues early in treatment (e.g., intense negative transference) may lead to increased resistance, relapse, and premature termination of treatment (Brown 1985; Kaufman 1989). Similarly, for particularly fragile patients who are unable to sustain abstinence or tolerate group interactions, insistence on these goals from the outset of treatment may lead to lowered self-esteem, increased resistance, relapse, or premature termination of treatment.

In this chapter I describe the special treatment approaches that

Table 1–1. Substance-abuse and psychodynamic treatment approaches

Substance-abuse treatment approaches	Psychodynamic approaches
Therapist activity	Therapist inactivity
Confrontation	Exploration of psychological conflict
Behavioral modification	Meaning of symptoms
Peer interactions, self-help groups	

can be utilized with dual-diagnosis patients and that can be integrated into psychotherapeutic practice. These special approaches include 1) motivational strategies; 2) family interventions; 3) pharmacological treatments; 4) derivatives of cognitive and behavioral treatments, such as behavioral monitoring, contingency contracting, relapse prevention training, and social skills training; and 5) encouragement of involvement in peer-oriented recovery and fellowship activities, such as Alcoholics Anonymous (AA), Narcotics Anonymous (NA), and Cocaine Anonymous (CA).

In the main, the special approaches discussed in this chapter can be utilized for patients with alcohol, stimulant (e.g., cocaine), sedative, opiate, marijuana, hallucinogen, or polydrug disorders. Because there are differences among the different types of substance abusers, however, and these differences have important therapeutic implications, I address this issue first. Because countertransference issues may play a critical role in the treatment of dual-diagnosis patients, special attention is paid to these issues in the final section of this chapter. Fictionalized clinical examples, based on actual cases, will be used throughout the chapter to illustrate the problems that are likely to arise in the treatment of patients with comorbid psychiatric and substance-use disorders.

Substances of Abuse

Although generalizations can be misleading in specific cases, it is important to recognize that there are major sociodemographic and cultural differences associated with the different substances of abuse. By and large, alcohol and sedative abuse is considerably more likely in substance-abusing patients over age 40, while cocaine, marijuana, and polydrug abuse (including alcohol) are more likely in younger patients. Similarly, because intravenous drug abuse and heroin abuse have remained quite rare in the general population, patients who abuse these types of drugs are considerably more often involved in extremely deviant subcultures and in antisocial behaviors than are patients who abuse alcohol, sedatives, or marijuana. Cocaine appears to occupy a middle position in this regard—its widespread use and relative social acceptability up until the mid-1980s indicate that many users are not otherwise particularly deviant. The more recent overall decline in the use and acceptability of cocaine suggests that cocaine-using patients will be increasingly involved in more deviant subcultures.

Self-Medication Hypothesis

Different classes of psychoactive drugs may be preferentially self-administered or more likely to be abused depending on the person's specific underlying psychopathology (i.e., self-medication hypothesis; see Khantzian 1985). Thus, for example, stimulants may be preferred by those persons with depression; alcohol, benzodiazepines, and other sedatives by those with anxiety or phobias; and opiates by those attempting to control violent or aggressive tendencies. Additionally, alcohol, sedatives, and marijuana are used by many bipolar patients to self-medicate hypomania or mania. Although specific treatment of an underlying psychiatric disorder may be necessary, treatment must usually also be directed at the substance-use disorder once it has developed.

Because it is often not known whether the symptoms that purportedly led to substance abuse (according to the self-medication hypothesis) actually preceded use of the substance, there is controversy about the hypothesis as an etiological theory. It has been clearly demonstrated, however, that prolonged use of and dependence on different types of substances lead to specific patterns of psychiatric symptomatology (McLellan et al. 1979), and that many of these symptoms can be expected to resolve spontaneously within a few days to several weeks following withdrawal and without specific treatment. During the first weeks following alcohol detoxification, for example, patients often experience severe depressive symptoms and cognitive dysfunctions (impaired memory, abstraction, and problem-solving ability) indicative of an organic affective disorder (Jaffe and Ciraulo 1986; Schottenfeld and O'Malley 1989). Protracted abstinence symptomatology from cocaine includes most prominently anhedonia (Gawin and Kleber 1986) and, in some recent reports, cognitive dysfunctions (O'Malley et al.

1992). Unlike alcohol use, prolonged opiate use has not been associated with significant cognitive dysfunction; protracted abstinence symptoms, however, may contribute to relapse.

Treatment Implications of Different Substances of Abuse

Differences in the substances of abuse have important treatment implications. It is usually advisable, for example, to delay pharmacological treatments for depression following alcohol withdrawal for at least 2 to 4 weeks, because most symptoms of depression will resolve spontaneously during this period. Some protracted abstinence symptoms (e.g., disturbances of sleep, appetite, or sexual function and libido) may persist for 6 to 12 months following last use of alcohol. Pharmacological treatment for these symptoms may not be necessary or advisable unless abstinence is threatened. Because reversible cognitive dysfunction associated with alcoholism may persist for more than a month, insight-oriented therapies, requiring intact intellectual functioning and problem-solving abilities, may need to be delayed until neuropsychological deficits have abated.

Just as there are differences regarding the acute and long-term neuropsychiatric effects of the various classes of drugs, different pharmacological treatments are available for these drugs. Methadone maintenance, which can be used only in a licensed methadone program, reduces craving for opiates and leads to substantial reductions in opiate use and high rates of treatment retention for opiate-dependent patients. Methadone maintenance programs may provide an optimal "holding environment" for psychiatrically impaired opiate-dependent patients. The opiate antagonist naltrexone, for example, is used to block euphoria from opiates; patients maintained on naltrexone cannot get "high" from heroin and, when compliant with taking the medication, almost invariably stop using heroin. Although naltrexone does not directly antagonize ethanol, recent studies suggest that naltrexone may be beneficial for recently abstinent alcoholic individuals (O'Malley et al. 1992; Volpicelli et al. 1990).

Pure blocking agents are not, however, available for the other drug abuse classes. Disulfiram, which is used in alcohol treatment, causes a severe physiological reaction following alcohol consumption. The reaction consists of flushing, headache, vomiting, and palpitations, and can lead to arrhythmias, hypotension, circulatory failure, or myocardial infarction. Alcoholic patients maintained on disulfiram will often experience reductions in craving, because alcohol is effectively "not available" (Meyer and Mirin 1981). Use of disulfiram is problematic in extremely impulsive and self-destructive patients or in patients who intermittently become severely disorganized and psychotic, because they may drink alcohol while on disulfiram and experience severe reactions. This is not a problem for naltrexone.

Desipramine, which has been shown to have some efficacy in facilitating initial abstinence from cocaine, may also be particularly beneficial for persistently depressed cocaine-abusing patients and for cocaine-abusing schizophrenic patients with depressive symptoms, but these uses have not yet been clearly established in controlled clinical trials.

Motivational Strategies: Developing a Commitment to Abstinence

Numerous motivational strategies, as described below and summarized in Table 1–2, are used to develop the patient's commitment to abstinence.

Shifting the Focus From Psychiatric Symptoms to Substance Abuse

Because psychiatric symptoms, such as hallucinations, psychotic disorganization, or severe depression, are often so prominent and even life-threatening, the significance of substance-use disorders may often be overlooked or minimized by both patient and therapist. One common problem results from the temptation to believe that substance abuse will remit once the underlying psychiatric disorder is treated. It is more likely, however, that persistent substance abuse will preclude successful treatment of psychiatric symptomatology or the underlying psychiatric disorder. In the following vignette, the importance of shifting from a focus on the patient's psychiatric difficulties to the significance of continued substance abuse is illustrated:

Case 1

Mr. K., a 19-year-old single white male who lives with his widowed mother, was referred for a possible trial of antidepressant medications by his psychotherapist. He had been treated as an outpatient for chronic depression for the past 4 years, following a 3-week hospitalization for severe depression at age 15.

Therapy had focused on Mr. K.'s characterological difficulties, especially his passive-aggressive and avoidant traits, and his loneliness and difficulty in finding a suitable peer group. Although clearly bright and a gifted athlete, he had never lived up to his academic potential, nor had he followed through on any projects or activities. His self-esteem seemed to have been shattered by his frequent failures. He did not, however, have any significant problems with the law or with truancy.

Following his hospitalization, Mr. K. had fallen in with a crowd of boys his own age who were involved in keg parties and heavy drinking. Initially, his drinking was restricted to the weekends, but eventually it occurred on weeknights as well. Mr. K. and his

---

Table 1–2.   Motivational strategies in developing a patient's commitment to abstinence

◆ Shift focus from psychiatric symptoms to substance abuse.

◆ Evaluate substance-use patterns and their temporal relationship to patient's problems and symptoms.

◆ Educate patient about effects of substance use on psychiatric symptoms.

◆ Confront patient about special problems that have resulted from substance use.

◆ Involve family to support recognition of problems resulting from patient's substance use and implementation of contingencies for abstinence or continued use.

therapist understood that Mr. K. joined in the drinking to fit in with the crowd. He felt he had little to offer anyone and thought he would be excluded if he did not drink.

Evaluating Substance Use and Dependence

Although Mr. K., his mother, and his therapist were all aware that alcohol was a problem for him, the focus of their concerns was Mr. K.'s depression, loneliness, low self-esteem, and difficulty finding appropriate friends. Alcohol problems were seen in the periphery, were believed to be secondary to psychiatric problems, and were considered likely to remit once the underlying psychiatric problems were resolved.

In the initial psychiatric consultation, however, the extent of Mr. K.'s alcohol problems became apparent. In addition to helping him fit in with peers, Mr. K. also enjoyed the emotional release associated with drinking. Usually quiet and compliant, he became boisterous and more assertive when he drank, ultimately to the point of becoming verbally abusive and engaging in reckless and dangerous behavior, including driving while intoxicated and fighting. He felt considerable remorse about his behavior, but he had been unable to control his drinking, abusiveness, or violence, despite repeated attempts.

When Mr. K.'s mother came into the evaluation session, she reported additional confirmation of the severity of Mr. K.'s drinking problems. She noted that he often had difficulty getting to school in the morning after being out with friends the night before. She had been aware that Mr. K. had driven home intoxicated on many occasions, but she had not confronted him because of her fear that this would only intensify his drinking or lead him to become resistant in therapy or more depressed. She also reported a strong family history of alcoholism on both sides of Mr. K.'s family.

Education About the Effects of Substance Use

Although Mr. K. fulfilled all the criteria for a diagnosis of major depression, rather than begin a trial of antidepressant medication, the consultant focused the initial intervention on Mr. K.'s alcoholism. A straightforward educational approach was employed in the first consultation session. Mr. K. and his mother were informed that his alcoholism was contributing to his depression, and that it would not be safe to use antidepressant medications until he had achieved abstinence. Because Mr. K.'s first episode of depression had preceded heavy drinking, Mr. K. and his mother were skeptical that his depression would resolve simply as a result of stopping drinking. They seemed to accept the explanation, however, that cessation of drinking might lead to some improvement of his mood, and that medication for depression might be warranted if he remained depressed after he became abstinent.

Consciousness-Raising Interventions

Denial is considered one of the hallmarks of substance-use disorders and an impediment to behavior change. Denial, or the minimization of the significance of problems related to alcohol, constituted a shared belief of Mr. K., his mother, and his therapist that Mr. K.'s primary problems were his depression and low self-esteem. Everyone involved seemed to believe that his alcohol use would diminish once the primary problems were resolved. Denial thus needed to be the focus of the initial intervention.

Viewed from a perspective of understanding behavioral change as a process with discrete stages, denial is characteristic of the earliest stage of change, *precontemplation* (Prochaska and DiClemente 1986). In this phase, persons who abuse substances do not perceive or are unaware of the significance of any problems associated with their alcohol or other drug use. Thus, they are not yet thinking about or contemplating changing their behavior. The primary task at this stage is to focus attention on problematic substance use and raise consciousness about its harmful effects.

Movement into the *contemplation* stage usually requires a combination of coercion and individual choice. Many approaches can be used to lead the patient to begin thinking about changing behavior. These approaches include confrontation and family interventions. To be maximally effective, a positive therapeutic alliance needs to be maintained during these interventions.

Confrontation

Although Mr. K. was not aware of the severity of his alcohol-related problems, a detailed assessment of his substance-abuse history revealed a number of adverse consequences of alcohol use:

1. Increasingly severe depression caused or exacerbated by the direct pharmacological effects of heavy alcohol consumption
2. Behavioral changes, including becoming angry and violent and driving while intoxicated, which increased his feelings of shame, guilt, and remorse
3. An inability to refrain from drinking or to control how much he drank on any given occasion, which exacerbated his low self-esteem and sense of being a failure

Beginning with the summary given to Mr. K. at the end of the initial consultation, these adverse consequences of alcohol use were highlighted. The consultant stated quite simply that while depression and low self-esteem were major problems for Mr. K., alcohol was making things worse, and he needed to stop drinking. In addition, the consultant pointed out that while Mr. K. had utilized alcohol to allay his initial awkwardness in socializing, awkwardness was common at his age, and alcohol prevented him from developing and practicing additional social skills.

In confronting substance abuse, it is essential to avoid moralizing or engaging in theoretical arguments, such as whether or not drug use or underage drinking is bad, which is a common pitfall especially in working with adolescent patients. It is also essential to align the intervention with the patient's views of and hopes for himself or herself. In the example of Mr. K., the consultant made use of information reported by the patient to reframe Mr. K.'s problems as resulting from alcohol, holding out the possibility that Mr. K. could successfully address his other problems after achieving abstinence. Although still skeptical, Mr. K. seemed relieved about the possibility that this reformulation was accurate.

Family Involvement and the Use of Significant Others in Treatment

Because the movement from precontemplation to contemplation usually requires some external motivating factor or changed circumstances, family interventions may be critical at the outset of treatment. The family members' previous collusion with the patient's hiding and minimization or denial of substance abuse, or even their covert encouragement of substance use (such as by supplying money that is then used to buy drugs), does not necessarily mean that family members will be unwilling or unable to shift into a useful role. Collusion and enabling usually develop insidiously over time and represent failed attempts of family members to respond helpfully to their addicted relative. Therefore, it is as much a mistake to adopt a moralizing or blaming stance with family members as it is to blame the patient for his or her substance or alcohol dependence.

In the case of Mr. K., the consultant attempted to enlist the mother's support by acknowledging her difficult position: Although Mr. K.'s alcohol problems were evident to her, she was concerned that confrontation would lead Mr. K. to dig in his heels and drink more heavily. Mr. K.'s mother added to this formulation that she did not want to take away Mr. K.'s only source of satisfaction, his socializing with his drinking buddies, or make him more depressed. When confronted with the reality that he could die from drunk driving and that his condition would only deteriorate further if he continued drinking, she agreed to take an active role in helping Mr. K. curtail his drinking.

At the outset of treatment, family members often need help in developing and implementing effective interventions to facilitate initial abstinence. While blaming the family members for enabling substance abuse is never helpful, articulating clearly the ways that their previous efforts have backfired is critical in bringing about a change in their behavior. Families need to be educated that change is more likely to occur if the addicted person suffers the consequences of his or her addiction and actions. By reframing family collusion or enabling as a failed attempt to protect the substance-abusing family member from harm, the therapist can assist the family to adopt a more constructive approach.

Family Interventions

Families often need to learn about effective family interventions, such as developing clear rules about behaviors that need to occur (e.g., working full-time, attending school, taking supervised disulfiram or naltrexone, attending AA, NA, or CA meetings) or that will not be tolerated (e.g., any drug or alcohol use, returning home after the agreed-upon time). Clear contingencies related to these behaviors must be specified. The family can obtain support for implementing these interventions by participating in Alanon or Naranon groups, self-help groups for family members of alcohol- or drug-dependent persons that serve as the counterparts to AA and NA. Through participation in these groups, family members may gain sufficient support as to their own feelings of guilt and enough encouragement to follow through on reasonable limit setting.

Families are frequently reluctant to implement negative contingencies if the contingencies chosen are felt to be too harsh or severe—for example, having the substance-abusing individual arrested for drug possession or forcing him or her out on the street. Rather than begin with such extreme contingencies, families can be helped to develop a range of less severe contingencies, such as prohibiting use of the car, withholding an allowance, or grounding the substance-abusing family member for defined periods of time. Families can also be counseled not to cover up or provide excuses for the substance-abusing family member's actions or errors. For example, frequent absences or lateness should be attributed to bingeing, hangovers, drug use, or drinking rather than illness. Likewise, exacerbations of psychotic symptoms or angry or violent outbursts should be attributed to cocaine or other drug use and not excused merely as symptoms of an underlying psychiatric disorder. Positive contingencies, such as use of the stereo or television or permission to attend a special event, can also be incorporated to reward compliance with the treatment plan.

In the case of Mr. K., the evaluation had revealed that Mr. K.'s mother had previously been successful in setting firm limits on her husband's drinking. This approach by Mr. K.'s mother was held up as an example *par excellence* of an appropriate response to a family member's problematic drinking. Because she clearly had acted so effectively in the past, the obvious question was what had stopped her from acting similarly with her son? Rather than exploring at this time the complicated issues in her relationship with her son that had interfered with confronting him about his alcoholism and setting firm limits, however, the immediate task was to develop a clear plan that she would implement to stop enabling Mr. K.'s continued drinking. By the end of the second session, which took place after Mr. K. had gone out drinking and had driven home intoxicated over the weekend, she decided that Mr. K. would not be allowed access to the family car unless he was taking disulfiram under careful supervision.

Maintaining the Therapeutic Alliance and the Patient's Sense of Autonomy

Even when the therapist recruits family members or significant others to set limits on the patient's behavior or to use coercive measures, it is important that the therapist be seen as helping to process events in a friendly and supportive manner and as not undermining the patient's sense of autonomy (Prochaska and DiClemente 1986). Reasonable limitations set by family members are supportive of the substance-abusing patient's growth, development, and eventual autonomy, and they do not negate the importance of the patient's own choice to become abstinent.

In the case of Mr. K., for example, his mother's decision to bar him from using the family car unless he was taking disulfiram under supervision was clearly tied to concerns about his safety and linked to a positive contingency for abstinence (i.e., access to the car). In addition, although access to the car was clearly up to the mother to decide, it was still Mr. K.'s decision whether or not he would stop drinking.

Because it is often difficult to gain agreement about lifelong abstinence at the outset of treatment, it may be useful to suggest a trial period of abstinence. Mr K. was asked to agree to a 3-month period of initial abstinence in order to see whether abstinence made any positive difference in his mood. Thus, while his decision to stop was facilitated by the action of his mother, it was important that Mr. K. gave his explicit agreement to a trial of abstinence. Considering Mr. K.'s long history of losing interest in his own initiatives as soon as he perceived any loss of autonomy, it was to be anticipated that this pattern would reoccur with regard to his decision to stop drinking. As expected, he went through recurrent cycles of owning and disowning his abstinence, and it was essential throughout treatment to encourage his recognition that abstinence was beneficial to him and truly *his* decision.

Achieving and Maintaining Abstinence

Keys to long-term abstinence identified in studies of successfully recovering substance-abusing individuals include 1) commitment to complete abstinence, 2) involvement in productive social roles and leisure activities, 3) development of alternative sources of satisfaction, 4) spiritual or religious conversion, and 5) repair of medical or social damage and restoration of self-esteem (Vaillant 1988). Effective treatment is directed at helping patients achieve these goals.

Structuring the Initial Treatment

After obtaining agreement to at least a trial of abstinence, the therapist needs to help the patient and family develop a comprehensive plan for achieving and maintaining abstinence (Kaufman 1989). Based on a thorough evaluation of the patient's substance abuse history, the treatment plan needs to address structural, pharmacological, and cognitive and behavioral interventions, and it must specify what the patient, family members, and therapist will do to facilitate treatment.

The initial treatment plan needs to take into consideration whether a medical withdrawal is necessary, whether hospitalization is necessary to safeguard the patient, and whether there are sufficient social supports and drug-free activities to foster abstinence outside a structured setting, such as a residential or partial hospital program. Patients with the most severe dependence syndromes and the fewest resources to become or remain drug-free, and especially those with other comorbid psychiatric disorders, however, often either do not have access to hospital or residential treatment or refuse hospitalization. Even when it seems doubtful that treatment can succeed outside a hospital, unless it is not safe to do so (e.g., if the patient is severely suicidal, homicidal, or grossly psychotic), these patients can be offered a trial ambulatory treatment program. Repeated failure to achieve or maintain abstinence outside a residential setting can be used to demonstrate their need for a structured environment.

Pharmacological Treatment

Pharmacological treatments for dual-diagnosis patients can be targeted to one or more of the following:

◆ Preventing the patient from getting "high" from drug or alcohol use (i.e., disulfiram to prevent alcohol intake; naltrexone to block opioid euphoria)
◆ Diminishing craving or ameliorating symptoms associated with protracted abstinence (e.g., desipramine for protracted cocaine abstinence symptomatology)
◆ Treating underlying psychiatric disorders or minimizing medication side effects

Compliance with disulfiram or naltrexone is a major problem, but one that can often be addressed through family interventions or as a result of the therapist's insistence that supervised intake is a necessary precondition for continuing the treatment.

Careful assessment of the causes and consequences of substance use may point to the appropriate pharmacological treatment. Some patients with schizophrenia, for example, turn to cocaine or amphetamine use to relieve anhedonia and other negative symptoms of schizophrenia or to relieve neuroleptic side effects. These patients may benefit from a trial of adjunctive antidepressant medication or neuroleptic dose reduction. Persistent cocaine use in these patients may be indicative of neuroleptic failure, and a trial of clozapine might be indicated. Other patients may use alcohol or, paradoxically, cocaine to reduce hallucinations. These patients may benefit from an increased dose of neuroleptic medication or from a change in neuroleptic.

Behavioral Monitoring of Patient's Drug and Alcohol Use

Monitoring of drug and alcohol use is an essential component of substance-abuse treatment that is often neglected by therapists who do not have specialized training in the addictions. Monitoring is essential because persons who abuse substances so often fail to disclose a slip or return to use. After making a commitment to abstinence, patients experience a profound sense of shame and failure following a slip or relapse. They may simply "forget" to mention a slip or minimize to themselves its importance and deny to the therapist its occurrence.

Without behavioral monitoring, patients may continue to use a substance for prolonged periods without their therapist knowing, often with disastrous consequences for the therapy, as is illustrated by the following clinical vignette:

Case 2

Ms. L. is a 24-year-old with a history of schizoaffective disorder and alcohol and cocaine dependence. She was treated in a twice-weekly psychotherapy for 5 months following her third hospitalization for a psychotic decompensation and depression. Although initially she had made a good connection with her therapist and talked about current problems in her relationship with her boyfriend and her family, after several months she began to devalue her therapist and to miss sessions. Despite her therapist's attempts to understand her negative transference and to reengage her in therapy, she persisted in seeing him as a cold, distant, and uncaring person, and as someone who, much like her mother, was too caught up in his own career and rigid ways to recognize her needs. She abruptly terminated treatment at the end of 5 months.

Following her fourth hospitalization, 1 year later, Ms. L. disclosed to her new therapist that she had resumed cocaine and alcohol about 2 months after her previous hospitalization. She had denied returning to drug or alcohol use to her therapist at the time, and she did not see any connection between the deterioration of her previous treatment and her covert cocaine and alcohol use.

Behavioral monitoring consists of frequent, random urine testing for drugs of abuse and determination of breath alcohol concentrations. It is also important to monitor reports about the patient's drug and alcohol use from collaterals, including family members, friends, or roommates of the patient (see Table 1–3).

Patients are often reluctant to agree to behavioral monitoring, claiming it signifies a lack of trust or is overly intrusive. Therapists too may resist utilizing behavioral monitoring because of concerns that it disrupts the boundaries of psychotherapy, places the therapist in too active a role, distorts the transference, and interferes with the therapeutic alliance. The case example of Ms. L., however, demonstrates how much the *failure* to monitor her drug and alcohol use disrupted the therapy. Her complaints about the therapist as cold, uncaring, distant, and caught up in a rigid professionalism may have reflected her frustration about his failure to insist on measures to detect her return to cocaine and alcohol use. She begrudgingly accepted her second therapist's comment that her crit-

---

Table 1–3.   Behavioral monitoring of patient's drug and alcohol use

◆ Random urine testing
◆ Random breathalizer results
◆ Reports from collaterals about patient's alcohol or drug use
◆ Patient's self-monitoring of craving or use

---

icism of her previous therapist was a result of cocaine- and alcohol-related thinking (i.e., rationalizing her behavior and finding fault with others), and reluctantly agreed to urine monitoring.

Patients with substance-use disorders may also benefit from self-monitoring of their craving for or use of drugs and alcohol. For the alcohol- or drug-dependent person, substance use has become an automatic or habitual behavior. To gain control over this automatic behavior, patients may find it useful to keep an hourly or daily log of their activities, mood, craving, and drug use. Keeping the log may help them recognize high-risk situations for drug or alcohol use (see discussion of relapse-prevention training that follows) and the harmful effects of use. It may also give them some added control over their behavior by interposing a thinking and decision-making process into their otherwise automatic actions.

Family Involvement and Contingency Contracting

The importance of structuring family involvement in the evaluation and initial phases of treatment has been discussed above. Continuing contact with the family is necessary to encourage utilization of contingencies and to serve as an aid in monitoring the patient's return to drug or alcohol use. If family members have contracted to implement negative contingencies for the patient's failure to remain abstinent, it is essential that communication be maintained with the family to track whether these contingencies are applied and with what effect. Without such tracking, there is a tendency for slippage to occur on the part of the family as well as the patient.

In traditional psychodynamic therapies, contact with the family is often regarded as an unwanted intrusion and consequently is discouraged. In the treatment of substance-abusing patients, however, family members should routinely be invited, at a minimum, to contact the therapist whenever they suspect or become aware of the patient's return to drug or alcohol use. Therapists have very limited windows into their patient's drug and alcohol use, and family members are often in the best position to detect a slip or relapse. If they believe that the therapist is reluctant to hear from them, they will often refrain from contacting the therapist until a crisis has occurred.

Family members who have had difficulty setting and sticking to reasonable limitations on the patient's behavior, who are "codependent," or who enable continued dysfunctional behavior in particular may benefit from referral to Alanon or Naranon meetings. Family therapy, including working on a family genogram to identify multiple generations of substance abuse and the origins of dysfunctional relationship patterns, may also be of benefit.

Although there are situations in which it is best to have separate individual and family therapists, in many cases family therapy alone may be advisable, and in others the individual therapist can take on the role of working with the family too. Structuring relatively straightforward family interventions, such as clarifying family expectations about abstinence and defining contingencies for behaviors, may facilitate rather than disrupt the formation of a therapeutic alliance with the patient. Patients will often come to respect the therapist for taking a straightforward and direct position about something as dangerous and damaging to them as substance abuse. Including structured family interventions as part of the psychotherapy can also prevent the formation of unhealthy alliances. Otherwise, family members may undercut the individual therapy because they feel the therapist is blaming them for the patient's difficulties or because they misperceive the therapist's focus on drugs or alcohol as a lack of concern about the patient's other problems. Similarly, unless contact with the family is maintained, therapists may unwittingly undercut appropriate responses of family members because, out of context, they seem too severe.

There are situations, however, when the therapeutic alliance is disrupted by contact between the therapist and the family. Patients with severe borderline personality features, for example, may not be able to maintain an image of the "good" therapist while the therapist is making contact with a "bad" relative. Similarly, some family members may become too intrusive in the individual work and not respond to the therapist's attempts to protect the privacy of the individual therapy. Longer-term family therapy may also best be undertaken by a separate therapist. If the patient cannot tolerate even the most transient empathic contact between the therapist and a family member, or if a family member cannot tolerate the therapist's more sustained alliance with the patient, referral of the family to a separate family therapist and coordination of the individual and family therapies may be necessary.

Relapse Prevention Training

Relapse prevention (RP) refers to a systematic cognitive and behavioral approach to the treatment of addictive disorders (Marlatt and Gordon 1985). In RP, patients are taught to identify high-risk situations for relapse and to develop strategies and coping skills to minimize the likelihood of relapse. Potential precipitants of relapse include

◆ Availability of or exposure to drugs or alcohol
◆ Social pressures to use
◆ Positive and negative emotional states
◆ Conditioning factors

In the early stages of treatment, the safest coping strategies usually involve avoidance of exposure to drug availability or to reminders of substance use. Patients are instructed to throw away all substances and drug paraphernalia (e.g., pipes used for smoking cocaine, cigarette rolling papers, etc.) and to cut off contact with substance-using friends, acquaintances, or dealers. They are instructed that craving for drugs or alcohol may be evoked by situations, places, things, or emotional states that have previously been linked to substance use. Keeping a daily log of craving may be useful for the patient to learn to recognize and anticipate precipitants of craving.

In RP, patients are also taught ways to cope with craving, including, for example, removing themselves from the situation evoking craving, reminding themselves that craving will pass after a short period if they do not use, reminding themselves of the harmful consequences of use, or making contact with a non–drug-using support person. Some patients find it useful to make and keep with them at all times on an index card a list of ways that they can handle a high-risk situation or intense craving (i.e., an emergency card). Because there is a natural tendency over time for persons who abuse substances to forget the harmful consequences of drug or alcohol use and to remember the pleasurable aspects only (i.e., *euphoric recall*), it may also be useful for patients to make a list of the harmful consequences that they have experienced and refer to this list several times a day and whenever they find themselves remembering the "good times" they had while using. Some patients may also find it useful to practice in therapy ways of responding to high-risk situations, such as how to say "No" when acquaintances or friends offer a drink or drugs.

Finally, because slips are so common despite all precautions, one emphasis in RP is on the importance of discussing, in advance of a slip, strategies to minimize the damage of a slip. Patients tend to experience a slip as further indication of their helplessness and inability to change, and they may resort to increased drug or alcohol use to cope with their intense guilt, shame, and humiliation about their failure to maintain abstinence (i.e., *abstinence violation effect*). Therapists can warn patients about the abstinence violation effect and suggest that, rather than succumbing to a full-blown relapse following a slip, patients will do better if they make immediate contact with their therapist and cease further use. It is essential, however, that in discussing the potential for slips the therapist not undercut the patient's commitment to abstinence.

Development of Drug- and Alcohol-Free Social Opportunities and Supports

Patients with severe, chronic mental illness often turn to drugs and alcohol to counter feelings of loneliness and social isolation. The pharmacological effects of chemicals can provide limited temporary relief of these feelings and thus contribute to addiction and relapse. Of additional importance, bars, clubs, and drug hangouts may provide the only comfortable opportunities for socializing. A crowded neighborhood bar may be the only place where a person with schizophrenia feels accepted and part of the crowd. Paranoia and hallucinations may not seem out of place in a group of drug-using individuals. Instant respect can be gained simply by paying for lines of cocaine or a round of drinks for the group. Drug and alcohol use thus comes to be highly reinforced by these social interactions, and for treatment to be successful, patients will need to develop alternative opportunities for socialization.

The following vignette illustrates the importance of social interactions in leading to substance abuse and the need to develop alternative social networks in treating the abuse:

Case 3

Mr. M., a 26-year-old single male with paranoid schizophrenia since age 20, lives at home with his parents and three younger siblings. His psychotic symptoms had been under relatively good control with perphenazine 12 to 24 mg daily. Despite occasional exacerbations of paranoid symptomatology, he has worked steadily and successfully as a cashier and assistant manager in a local restaurant. Eventually he began to make some efforts to socialize with co-workers and started to formulate plans to move out of home. During this period, however, "car troubles" occasionally prevented him from attending his weekly meeting with his psychiatrist, and, finally, he reported that he had squandered several thousand dollars in savings on cocaine and that he could no longer afford even to repair his car or continue with treatment. After further evaluation of his cocaine use, it became clear that Mr. M. had started to use cocaine to fit in with his co-workers who would go out to party after work. Cocaine was his ticket of admission to their social gathering, and Mr. M. also enhanced his esteem in their eyes by buying cocaine for them. His increasing anxiety as he anticipated his isolation, loneliness, and distress about moving out on his own had led him to make a desperate effort to establish friends. It also resulted in his sabotaging his efforts to move out, because he was no longer able to support himself on his own.

Mr. M.'s disclosure of his cocaine use brought about a crisis in his therapy: without a functioning car he could not get to his sessions, and without money he could not pay for treatment. Mr. M.

felt that he had failed badly, and his therapist experienced strong countertransference feelings of disappointment and anger. Rather than terminate treatment, however, the therapist worked with Mr. M. to postpone moving out on his own and to negotiate a loan from Mr. M.'s family to allow him to continue in treatment. Because it was not clear that Mr. M. could continue to work at his restaurant job without continuing drug use, the therapist began a urine drug-monitoring program for Mr. M. Subsequently, therapy focused on helping Mr. M. establish drug-free social activities, including fostering his participation in a sports program at the local YMCA and encouraging him to attend AA meetings and a local young-persons' group at his church.

Facilitating healthy social interactions in a patient with severe, chronic mental illness requires 1) alertness to the patient's fears, fantasies, and concerns about coming into contact with others and a concrete understanding of the basis for the fears, 2) practical training and encouragement in the development of social skills, and 3) considerable patience.

Although attendance at AA or NA meetings can provide an invaluable opportunity to foster healthy social interactions, actively psychotic or extremely fragile patients may find regular meetings too stressful, or they may feel out of place. Therapists can remind patients of the advantages of AA and NA:

◆ Membership is free.
◆ Meetings are usually held every day and evening.
◆ Newcomers are usually welcomed without questioning them or making demands on them to do more than come to the meetings sober.
◆ After-meeting get-togethers and drug-free picnics and dances are an enjoyable alternative to staying home alone or to going out to bars or drug parties.

Therapists must also be prepared to accompany patients to meetings to help facilitate their adjustment. Finally, in many communities, special AA and NA meetings are held for dual-diagnosis patients; these meetings are often ideal for psychotic or extremely fragile patients who might experience some sense of rejection or feel out of place in regular meetings. Mr. M.'s therapist accompanied him to an AA meeting for dual-diagnosis patients rather than a CA meeting because the local CA groups were too new to have a core of stable, abstinent participants and the AA meeting was known to be a good group for psychotic patients.

Psychotherapy and Adjunctive Substance-Abuse Treatment

Although my primary focus in this chapter has been on ways of integrating substance-abuse treatment and psychotherapy, dual-diagnosis patients may be successfully treated by a combination of separate but simultaneous individual therapy and substance-abuse treatment. Adjunctive substance-abuse treatment for a patient in individual therapy can consist of a family, group, or individual approach, depending on the circumstances of the patient and the available treatment resources. As in all joint treatments, it is essential, however, that the therapists conducting the separate components maintain sufficient contact to ensure a coordinated, consistent approach and message, as is demonstrated in the following case example:

Case 4

Mr. N. is a 34-year-old married white salesman who initially sought treatment for persistent dysthymia. Characteristic features of a narcissistic personality disorder were readily apparent, including pronounced grandiosity, entitlement, envy, and history of exploiting others, as well as a profound sense of shame and humiliation when criticized.

Mr. N. initially reported a past history of drug experimentation but denied any other problems associated with alcohol or drug abuse or dependence. During the course of twice-weekly psychodynamic psychotherapy, he eventually reported with considerable shame that he had become dependent on intramuscularly administered Demerol and that he had previous problems with prescription opiate abuse. Mr. N. claimed that he had successfully "kicked" his habit by locking himself in a hotel room over the weekend. Several months later, however, Mr. N. reported that he had started on Demerol again. Because Mr. N.'s therapist was not experienced in the treatment of opiate dependence, Mr. N. was referred for evaluation and treatment of addiction.

Referral of a patient for adjunctive substance-abuse treatment is indicated in the following circumstances: 1) the patient requires a multipronged approach, such as family or group treatment, that is best conducted separately from the individual therapy; or 2) the individual therapist lacks the expertise to treat addictions. Adjunctive therapy can include all of the elements of substance-abuse treatment discussed above, including behavioral monitoring, pharmacological treatments, contingency contracting, RP training, and fostering drug-free social and vocational opportunities (Nigam et al., in press).

In the case of Mr. N., pharmacological interventions included opiate detoxification using clonidine and naltrexone followed by supervised maintenance on three-times-per-week naltrexone. During the initial evaluation and detoxification period, Mr. N. was seen in conjunction with his wife, who reported being entirely "oblivious" to Mr. N.'s addiction. Although numerous marital problems were evident to the couple and therapist, Mr. N.'s wife agreed to see whether the marriage improved after Mr. N. had achieved a period of sustained abstinence.

To help keep the focus on his drug problems, which Mr. N. tended to minimize, Mr. N. was enrolled in a naltrexone induction group in the drug program, and he and his wife attended a multiple family group, which helped his wife end her enabling. The induction group provided RP training, behavioral monitoring, and encouragement to attend NA (including helping Mr. N. find a sponsor). Over time, group members confronted Mr. N. about behaviors and attitudes that seemed likely to lead him to relapse (such as missing doses of naltrexone and failing to attend NA meetings). Telephone contact between the group therapist and the individual therapist enabled the latter to feel secure that Mr. N. did not return to drug use at times of stress. Telephone contact also provided an opportunity to confront the individual therapist about his covert disparagement of NA as being "too religious" and to educate him about the value of NA.

12-Step Programs

Psychotherapists without training in the treatment of addictions often tend to devalue 12-step programs. In some respects, the ideology of 12-step programs, with its emphasis on the importance of acknowledging the centrality of addiction and a belief in a higher power, seems to conflict with the implicit values accorded to autonomy and individual choice and freedom in individual psychodynamically oriented psychotherapy. Involvement in self-help groups and establishment of an intense relationship with a sponsor may also detract, at least temporarily, from the establishment of a therapeutic alliance with the therapist (Brown 1985). Until abstinence has been securely established, however, intense transference to a therapist, often associated with strong affective arousal, may actually be counterproductive (cf. Brown 1985). Attendance at different AA meetings and establishment of supportive relationships with many other members of these groups can diffuse this type of powerful transference arousal and thus protect the patient's continued sobriety.

During the initial months (and often years) of treatment, one of the most valuable therapeutic approaches is often simply the encouragement of patients' affiliation with the fellowship activities of 12-step programs. During this period, patients may discuss little with their therapist other than their attempts to maintain abstinence and their involvement in AA, NA, or CA. Although therapists may feel bored by this nose-to-the-grindstone, one-day-at-a-time approach, and may even regard the patient's near obsessional focus on the ideology of the 12-step program as a resistance to the therapy, it is essential not to undercut the patient's tenuous abstinence. In-depth psychotherapeutic work may need to be delayed for a substantial period of time, at least until the patient can begin to focus on issues other than addiction without relapsing to drug use.

Countertransference

Addicted patients, and especially those with co-existing severe psychiatric disorders, often evoke powerful countertransference reactions in therapists. Ausubel (1948) described "disinterest, dread, and despair" as typical reactions, and the tendency for these patients to evoke disgust, disapproval, or hostility is often most evident (Imhof 1991; Perry 1985). Less intense countertransference reactions are perhaps even more common and may also interfere with diagnosis and treatment. Clinicians' personal history or current problematic use of alcohol or other drugs may impede recognition of the problems related to substance use in patients.

Disinterest, dread, and despair tend to reflect in large measure a view of addiction as an incurable disorder. This view can be countered by education, training, and experience. Clinicians whose primary contacts with addicted persons have been in emergency-room settings may never have had the opportunity to witness the profound changes that can occur in recovery or even to talk with a recovering addict who is leading a satisfactory and productive life. (A turning point in my own attitude came when I shared a panel with a recovering opiate-addicted physician who eloquently described his recovery.)

Empathic, nonjudgmental responses to addictions are also impeded by the common belief that drug or alcohol dependence is unlike other Axis I disorders in being deliberately self-induced. Impulsivity and continued substance abuse are perceived as motivated by self-destructive tendencies or conscious hostility, and this tends to evoke disapproval. Recognition that impulsivity as well as continued substance abuse often results from deficits in self-care functions is both a more accurate understanding of the nature of these disturbances and more likely to lead to useful interventions (Khantzian 1985).

Clinicians trained in dynamic psychotherapies may experience difficulties taking on the more active primary care role needed to treat patients with addictive disorders. Again, focusing on the patient's deficiencies in self-care functions provides the theoretical rationale for the more active therapeutic role.

Because the shame, guilt, and helplessness so often experienced by addicted patients at the outset of treatment are best countered by the clinician's understanding, acceptance, and recognition that out of such pain great gains may be made and great good may come, the experience of encountering successful persons in recovery or of successfully treating an addicted patient can lead to attitudes and beliefs in the clinician that foster successful treatment.

Conclusions

In this chapter I have described the special treatment approaches that can be utilized with dual-diagnosis patients and have suggested ways of integrating these approaches into psychotherapeutic practice. In the treatment of patients with substance-use disorders, including those patients with coexisting major psychiatric disorders, it is essential to maintain a sustained focus on the patients' drug and alcohol use or dependence. A primary focus on achieving and maintaining behavioral change can be facilitated by recognition of each patient's personality organization, vulnerability, and other psychiatric problems. Exploration and evaluation of these latter problems, however, cannot replace the importance of achieving and maintaining abstinence.

Although the discussion and case examples may make it seem that treatment of dual diagnosis is simple, easy, and always successful, nothing could be farther from the truth. Major psychiatric disorders and substance-use disorders tend to be severe, chronic disorders; relapse and exacerbation of psychiatric symptomatology are to be expected. At its best, treatment is not curative but palliative. Success needs to be measured in comparison with the outcomes that would be expected in the absence of treatment. If patients suffer fewer or less severe relapses and psychiatric symptoms, if social and occupational functioning is improved, or if some of the worst consequences of addiction and psychiatric disorders (e.g., suicide, overdose, HIV infection) are prevented or minimized, then our treatments can be considered a success.

References

Ananth J, Vandewater S, Kamal M, et al: Missed diagnosis of substance abuse in psychiatric patients. Hosp Community Psychiatry 40:297–299, 1989

Anthony JC, Trinkoff AM: United States epidemiologic data on drug use and abuse: how are they relevant to testing abuse liability of drugs? in Testing for Abuse Liability of Drugs in Humans. Edited by Fischman MW, Mello NK. NIDA Res Monogr No 92 (DHHS Publ No [ADM]89-1613). Rockville, MD, National Institute on Drug Abuse, 1989, pp 241–266

Ausubel DP: The psychopathology and treatment of drug addiction in relation to the mental hygiene movement. Psychiatr Q 22(suppl):219–250, 1948

Barbee JG, Clark PD, Crapanzano MS, et al: Alcohol and substance abuse among schizophrenic patients presenting to an emergency psychiatric service. J Nerv Ment Dis 177:400–407, 1989

Brown S: Treating the Alcoholic. New York, Wiley, 1985

Crowley TJ, Chesluk D, Dilts S, et al: Drug and alcohol abuse among psychiatric admissions: a multidrug clinical-toxicologic study. Arch Gen Psychiatry 30:13–20, 1974

Dixon L, Haas G, Weiden P, et al: Acute effects of drug abuse in schizophrenic patients: clinical observations and patients' self-reports. Schizophr Bull 16:69–79, 1990

Gawin FH, Kleber HD: Abstinence symptomatology and psychiatric diagnosis in cocaine abusers. Arch Gen Psychiatry 43:107–113, 1986

Hall RCW, Popkin MK, Devaul R, et al: The effects of unrecognized drug abuse on diagnosis and therapeutic outcome. Am J Drug Alcohol Abuse 4:455–465, 1977

Imhof JE: Countertransference issues in alcoholism and drug addiction. Psychiatric Annals 21:292–306, 1991

Jaffe JH, Ciraulo DA: Alcoholism and depression, in Psychopathology and Addictive Disorders. Edited by Meyer R. New York, Guilford, 1986, pp 293–320

Kaufman E: The psychotherapy of dually diagnosed patients. J Subst Abuse Treat 6:9–18, 1989

Khantzian EJ: The self-medication hypothesis of addictive disorders: focus on heroin and cocaine dependence. Am J Psychiatry 142:1259–1264, 1985

Kranzler HR, Liebowitz NR: Anxiety and depression in substance abuse: clinical implications. Med Clin North Am 72:867–885, 1988

Marlatt GA, Gordon JR (eds): Relapse Prevention: Maintenance Strategies in the Treatment of Addictive Behaviors. New York, Guilford, 1985

McLellan AT, Woody GE, O'Brien CP: Development of psychiatric illness in drug abusers: possible role of drug preference. N Engl J Med 301:1310–1314, 1979

McLellan AT, Luborsky L, Woody GE, et al: Predicting response to alcohol and drug abuse treatments: role of psychiatric severity. Arch Gen Psychiatry 40:620–625, 1983

Meyer RE, Mirin SM: A psychology of craving: implications of behavioral research, in Substance Abuse: Clinical Problems and Perspectives. Edited by Lowinson JH, Ruiz P. Baltimore, MD, Williams & Wilkins, 1981, pp 57–62

Mueser KT, Yarnold PR, Levinson DF, et al: Prevalence of substance abuse in schizophrenia: demographic and clinical correlates. Schizophr Bull 16:31–56, 1990

Negrete JC, Knapp WP, Douglas DE, et al: Cannabis affects the severity of schizophrenic symptoms: results of a clinical survey. Psychol Med 16:515–520, 1986

Nigam R, Schottenfeld RS, Kosten TR: Treatment of dual diagnosis patients: a relapse prevention group approach. J Subst Abuse Treat (in press)

O'Malley SM, Adamse M, Heaton RK, et al: Neuropsychological impairment in chronic cocaine abusers. Am J Drug Alcohol Abuse 18:131–144, 1992

Perry SW: Irrational attitudes toward addicts. Bull N Y Acad Sci 61:706–727, 1985

Prochaska JO, DiClemente CC: Toward a comprehensive model of change, in Treating Addictive Behaviors. Edited by Miller WR, Heather N. New York, Plenum, 1986, pp 3–27

Regier DA, Goodwin FK, Rae DS, et al: Comorbidity of mental and addictive disorders: implications for the futures of children. Paper presented at the American Enterprise Institute Conference, Williamsburg, VA, July 1991

Richard ML, Liskow BI, Perry PJ: Recent psychostimulant use in hospitalized schizophrenics. J Clin Psychiatry 46:79–83, 1985

Rounsaville BJ, Kleber HD: Psychotherapy/counseling for opiate addicts: strategies for use in different treatment settings. Int J Addict 175:641–650, 1987

Rounsaville BJ, Weissman MM, Kleber HD, et al: Heterogeneity of psychiatric diagnosis in treated opiate addicts. Arch Gen Psychiatry 39:161–166, 1982

Rounsaville BJ, Kosten TR, Weissman MM, et al: Prognostic significance of psychopathology in treated opiate addicts. Arch Gen Psychiatry 43:739–745, 1986

Rounsaville BJ, Dolinsky ZS, Babor TF, et al: Psychopathology as a predictor of treatment outcome in alcoholics. Arch Gen Psychiatry 44:505–513, 1987

Rounsaville BJ, Anton SF, Carroll K, et al: Psychiatric diagnoses of treatment-seeking cocaine abusers. Arch Gen Psychiatry 48:43–51, 1991

Schottenfeld RS, O'Malley SS: Clinical note: limitation and potential hazards of MAOI's for the treatment of depressive symptoms in abstinent alcoholics. Am J Drug Alcohol Abuse 15:339–344, 1989

Schottenfeld RS, Carroll K, Rounsaville B: Comorbid psychiatric disorders and cocaine abuse, in Advances in Cocaine Treatment. NIDA Res Monogr. Rockville, MD, National Institute on Drug Abuse (in press)

Schuckit MA, Winslow G: A short term follow up of women alcoholics. Diseases of the Nervous System 33:672–678, 1972

Siris SG: Pharmacological treatment of substance-abusing schizophrenic patients. Schizophr Bull 16:111–122, 1990

Siris SG, Kane JM, Frechen K, et al: Histories of substance abuse in patients with postpsychotic depressions. Compr Psychiatry 29:550–557, 1988

Vaillant GE: What can long-term follow-up teach us about relapse and prevention of relapse in addiction? Br J Addict 83:1147–1157, 1988

Volpicelli JR, O'Brien CP, Alterman AI, et al: Naltrexone and the treatment of alcohol dependence: initial observation, in Opioids, Bulimia, Alcohol Abuse and Alcoholism. Edited by Reid LD. New York, Springer, 1990, pp 195–214

Woody GE, Luborsky L, McLellan AT, et al: Psychotherapy for opiate addicts: does it help? Arch Gen Psychiatry 40:639–645, 1983

Chapter 2

An Interpersonal Psychotherapeutic Approach to Depressed HIV-Seropositive Patients

John C. Markowitz, M.D.
Gerald L. Klerman, M.D.
Samuel W. Perry, M.D.

Case 1

Mr. A., a 32-year-old gay photographer, reported having become depressed 4 years before. He had learned that he was infected with human immunodeficiency virus (HIV) upon developing a severe case of shingles. He had increasing difficulty concentrating and paid less attention to his work, and his promising career collapsed. Putting his savings into a country house, which he saw as a refuge for himself and his HIV-seronegative lover, Mr. A. soon found himself socially isolated and heavily in debt.

Mr. A. had attended an HIV support group, but found this more depressing, as over the years more than half of its members died. In fact, more than 100 people he knew had died of acquired immunodeficiency syndrome (AIDS), including most of his business contacts and close friends. In the year prior to his seeking psychiatric treatment, his T-cell count fell to 400, then stabilized around 500 per mm^3 with zidovudine (AZT). He felt

Supported in part by National Institute of Mental Health Grant MH-19069.
We dedicate this chapter to the late Gerald L. Klerman, M.D.

depressed, anxious, unmotivated, suicidal, helpless, hopeless, worthless, and guilty that he had not attended all of his friends' funerals. He reported decreased sleep and appetite, diurnal mood variation, derealization, and preoccupation with his health. His Hamilton Depression Rating Scale (Ham-D) score was 34. He saw no possibility of regaining a meaningful life: "It's like a B movie, a nightmare happening."

Case 2

Ms. B., a 35-year-old separated Roman Catholic Hispanic diabetic mother of two, was on methadone maintenance and had been depressed for a year and a half. A former intravenous heroin user, she had been maintained on methadone for 15 years, but 3 years earlier had tried intravenous cocaine a few times. Testing positive for HIV 2 years before, she had tried to suppress this knowledge, but gradually found that this terrible secret isolated her from her close relationships with her sisters. Her depression seemed clearly linked to this social withdrawal from her family.

This obese, overtly depressed woman presented in tears, with guilt, passive suicidal ideation, loss of interest and concentration, decreased energy, sleep and appetite loss, and high levels of anxiety accompanied by somatic panic symptoms. Her initial Ham-D score was 34.

These patients are clearly depressed—the temptation is to add, "with good reason." Not only do they lack hope, but their medical, social, and psychic stressors of living with HIV may daunt the therapist as well. Yet with proper preparation, the psychiatrist may disarm his or her own fear and the patient's fears and help the patient through the crisis of infection.

This chapter is based on the authors' clinical experience as psychiatrists in a New York City tertiary care hospital, on *pro bono* consultations undertaken as part of the American Psychiatric Association (APA) New York County District Branch Committee on AIDS, and on research in *interpersonal therapy* (IPT; Klerman et al. 1984; Markowitz et al. 1992). We are studying the comparative efficacy of IPT, cognitive-behavior therapy (Beck et al. 1979), supportive psychotherapy, and tricyclic antidepressants in the treatment of depressed HIV-seropositive patients. This chapter thus reflects general hospital, private practice, volunteer, and research modes. Because most of our psychotherapeutic experience in treating HIV-positive patients has been with IPT, we shall focus on that modality. Other psychotherapeutic approaches may prove equally effective with this treatment population—a possibility our research will test.

The reader should look elsewhere for reviews of the psychiatric and medical literature on AIDS (Markowitz and Perry 1990, 1992; Perry 1990; Perry and Markowitz 1986); here we shall offer our experiences in what can be difficult, draining, but also extremely rewarding work. To help such patients, the psychiatrist must be aware of countertransferential responses. He or she needs skills from consultation liaison, psychopharmacology, and psychotherapy. There are also benefits to having a structured psychotherapeutic framework such as IPT. Examining each in turn, we will provide case vignettes—clinical pearls and pointers—and attempt to demonstrate what makes working with these patients unique.

Defining the Patient

HIV seropositivity is diagnosed by blood tests. At least a million Americans are estimated to be seropositive for this virus (Centers for Disease Control 1987a). It is important to remind oneself and the patient that this is not a "test for AIDS," but rather for presence of a virus of usually long latency. HIV infection is chronic, and for much of its course it is likely to be asymptomatic. Psychiatric diagnosis is complex. As HIV has myriad physical expressions, ranging from a protracted asymptomatic state to mild symptoms to full-blown AIDS, psychiatric symptoms in HIV-seropositve patients similarly cover a spectrum from successful coping to adjustment disorders, to severe depression and organic mental syndromes (Faulstich 1987; Perry et al. 1990a). The AIDS Dementia Complex (Navia and Price 1987) is an end-stage extreme.

Most patients whom psychiatrists see as outpatients will probably be physically asymptomatic (i.e., Centers for Disease Control

[CDC] stage II) or nearly so (chronic lymphadenopathy; CDC stage III) (Centers for Disease Control 1987b). HIV-seropositve patients can die, and the death of such young patients can be a wrenching experience for the therapist. Psychotherapy with moribund patients entails a less ambitious, more palliative and supportive approach than the one we shall outline for relatively asymptomatic individuals. Psychotherapy of the dying patient would require a separate chapter, albeit one that might well fit into this volume.

Generalizations about "seropositive patients" should be made with circumspection; these patients are richly individual. In this chapter we focus on recurrent themes arising in the treatment of depressed patients who are infected with HIV; it would be unfortunate, however, if the reader here left with the impression that a single treatment formula exists for seropositive patients, depressed or otherwise.

Facing the Patient: Patient/Therapist Issues

It is without doubt difficult working with patients who face severe illness and early death. Our irrational fears were easily identified. We more than occasionally found ourselves dreading appointments with patients whom we liked and who were doing quite well. We worried about contamination: we knew it was important to shake hands with these patients, to "normalize" and destigmatize them, and that such contact carries no risk of HIV transmission. Yet we several times feared we were putting ourselves at risk for seroconversion, noting imagined pains, ill-defined itchiness, and the pressure of expanding skin tumors during and after sessions with patients who had visible lesions of Kaposi's sarcoma. We wondered (and occasionally heard) about the effect upon other patients of seeing skeletally gaunt patients with advanced AIDS leave our offices. Treating a largely gay patient group also made us question what hospital colleagues might think of our motivations and sexual orientation. One might easily envision HIV-seropositive patients evoking other irrational fears, inappropriate anxiety about patient suicide risk, or emotional distancing.

Worst, it was easy to collude in the patients' despair. What, indeed, could we offer an obese, diabetic, methadone-dependent, isolated, unemployed, HIV-infected woman with a lifelong history of poor social and occupational functioning? or a chronically isolated gay man whose one relationship had gone sour, and whose mourning of that loss had been compounded by an episode of *Pneumocystis carinii* pneumonia (PCP) infection? Were they right to despair of reassembling what was left of their lives?

Yet collaboration with seropositive patients can have extremely positive outcomes, rather than shared hopelessness. Like many patients on consultation-liaison services, these HIV-seropositive patients were able to use the crisis of infection and acute or potential illness as motivation to work hard and effectively in therapy and to make impressive changes in their lives (Viederman 1983). Once sessions began, countertransferential fears largely vanished. The patients were likeable, sympathetic, courageous, and in great need of help. Even patients with long-standing interpersonal deficits were galvanized by their medical crises to engage in therapy, often to make dramatic, unprecedented improvements in their quality of life. The IPT framework was often helpful in providing therapist and patient with hope and direction (Markowitz et al. 1992).

The psychiatrist must also contend with negative expectations about doctors that HIV-seropositive patients frequently bring to therapy. Many patients were angry at the medical establishment for ignoring the plight of HIV-seropositive individuals. They raged that insufficient research was being done, that effective medications were being withheld, and that some physicians refuse outright to see such "risky" patients. They also criticized those doctors with large HIV-related practices who had seen them: for exploiting patients as "guinea pigs" in research protocols, or for a fatalism born of overwork, repeated patient deaths, and burnout. (Mr. A., whose case was described at the beginning of this chapter, was understandably upset when his generally sympathetic internist, congratulating him on maintaining his health, confided how many of his other seropositive patients were dying.)

Doctors may be perceived as unavailable and uncaring, as more interested in testing a drug than in listening to patient needs, and/or as either too eager to ply these patients with medications or, conversely, not aggressive enough. The doctors are frequently too busy or uncomfortable to stop to discuss patients' fears of illness and dying. Some patients reported having been abandoned by physicians when they, the patients, no longer fit research protocols. In our experience, HIV-seropositive patients are further angered by lack of medical certainty: despite the real advances being made in the treatment of HIV-spectrum diseases, doctors cannot promise a cure, guarantee survival, or even state with assurance the optimal dosage of key HIV drugs. Depressed patients, already feeling helpless and hopeless, are further irritated by the need to become HIV experts themselves when medical authorities fail to provide definitive answers. They often fear expressing this anger, feeling that being "uncool" may further damage their frail immune systems.

Psychiatrists may draw fire not simply as physicians, but as members of a specialty with an unsympathetic history in treating the stigmatized patients at risk for HIV. Gay men may fear treatment from a profession that long considered their sexual orientation a perversion. Intravenous drug users also may have had unhappy encounters with psychiatrists, or have developed distrust in self-help groups suspicious of medical intervention.

Nonetheless, in our experience, these prejudices were easily overcome. As is always true in psychotherapy, affective engagement and the building of mutual understanding and alliance were crucial to induction into therapy. This achieved, some apparent liabilities that HIV-seropositive patients brought to therapy became advantages:

1. **Mistrust:** Once the irrational fears that patients (and therapists) brought to treatment were addressed, HIV-seropositive patients—depressed and otherwise—proved highly motivated and compliant with treatment. Our initial, irrational dismay gave way to the considerable satisfaction of finding that patients could be helped and usually responded well to treat-

ment. Perhaps because the challenge first seems so disheartening, the gratification of working with HIV-seropositive patients is immense. Here is an opportunity for the psychiatrist to assume the physician's traditional role: to listen to and help a patient in crisis.

2. **Time pressure:** Facing shortened longevity, HIV-seropositive patients understandably seek quick results. Time is running out, careers and relationships are amputated, every second counts. One patient stated, "If you're going to eat a meal or see a movie, it had better be good." Although this demand might disconcert a practitioner uncertain of how to help a depressed, HIV-seropositive patient, the urgency behind the demand also provides a motivational fulcrum. Once anxiety and hopelessness were addressed, the subjective urgency engendered by HIV seemed to promote active engagement in therapy. The severity of the danger posed by HIV to health is such that patients are often willing to undertake unprecedented risks in changing career trajectories or relationships:

Case 3

For Mr. C., an artist who developed and recovered from PCP during treatment in IPT, the medical episode confirmed his depressed sense that HIV had ruined his life. In IPT, however, he decided to pursue a lifelong fantasy of relocating to Europe. During therapy he took several transatlantic trips to prepare for his move, his mood lifted, and subsequently he set up a successful, gratifying practice there.

3. **Medical illness:** Time pressure especially affects physically sicker patients, who may correctly judge their lifespan to be shortened. Paradoxically, development of HIV-related physical illness may unavoidably interrupt therapy. As the case of Mr. C. demonstrates, life-threatening illness is not simply a fear, but a realized worst fear. The development of physical illness in seropositive patients is no occasion for therapeutic withdrawal but, on the contrary, an ideal opportunity to help the patient address his or her fears and deal with the illness. Therapy re-

quires flexibility about time, appropriate hiatuses for physical recovery, and the willingness to defer other focuses of therapy in order to recognize and adjust to medical decline. Calling or visiting physically incapacitated patients at home or in the hospital may assuage the perception of precious time being wasted, maintain momentum and continuity of psychiatric care, and cement the treatment alliance.

Differential Diagnosis

HIV-seropositive patients present with a variety of symptoms that may reflect multiple etiologies. The reader is referred elsewhere for more exhaustive consideration of the neuropsychiatric differential (Beckett 1990; Fernandez and Levy 1990; Markowitz and Perry 1990). Symptoms of depression and anxiety are common (Faulstich 1987; Perry et al. 1990a). Depression may be "functional," responding to or exacerbated by the threat of HIV; yet the same symptoms may result from organic mental syndromes: direct effects of HIV on the central nervous system, secondary infections or tumors consequent to immune failure, or iatrogenic side effects of medications such as zidovudine.

Fatigue, anorexia, and weight loss, as well as difficulty concentrating and other cognitive disturbances, may be symptoms of HIV rather than depression per se, although such patients may be less likely to feel guilty, worthless, and so forth. Substance abuse (particularly cocaine abuse), a risk factor for HIV infection, presents another confounding factor to depression. Patients also frequently explore regimens of megadoses of multivitamins, extreme health food diets, and other home remedies that might affect mood.

The great majority of HIV-seropositive patients will have no gross neuropsychological deficits. Neuropsychological evaluation is sometimes helpful, but there are no pathognomonic tests for mild HIV-related cognitive dysfunction, and the significance of such dysfunction in otherwise asymptomatic seropositive patients is controversial (Perry 1990). The psychiatrist treating seropositive patients will do well to learn about sequelae of HIV and to polish skills gained from consultation-liaison work. HIV has unique aspects—for example, it can produce a "subcortical" dementia marked by social withdrawal, apathy, lethargy, forgetfulness, and a subjective impression of mental slowing—but for the most part it raises issues similar to those of other somatopsychic illnesses (Markowitz and Perry 1992; Perry 1990). An empirical approach is sometimes necessary, with a tolerance for leaving definitive diagnosis an open, ongoing question. This yields some anxiety but also an intellectual, diagnostic challenge for the therapist. *Most important to keep in mind is that you can be fooled: what looks "organic" may be "functional," and vice versa.* Mild cognitive dysfunction secondary to HIV did not impede our therapy of depression.

Approaches to Treatment

To answer questions and counter distortions, therapists need to understand medical aspects of HIV (Markowitz and Perry 1990); like their patients, they must acquire expertise about the virus. Because HIV-seropositive individuals are at risk for neuropsychiatric sequelae (Marotta and Perry 1989), therapists must watch for subtle changes in mental status. Depressed HIV-seropositive patients also may be at significant risk for suicide (Marzuk et al. 1988; Perry et al. 1990b), although in our experience what has been more prominent is a despairing desire to live. Finally, the psychiatrist should address persisting behaviors that put the patient at high risk for being reinfected with HIV or transmitting it to others (Kelly et al. 1989).

Psychiatric literature on the treatment of HIV-seropositive patients has been largely anecdotal. Psychotherapy and psychopharmacology seem to benefit depressed patients irrespective of serostatus, although HIV adds nuances to both forms of treatment. Patient preference may be the most important factor in planning the initial treatment of nonpsychotic major depression or dysthymia for an outpatient. The patients often have previously attended HIV support groups, but many prefer individual psychotherapy to group therapy, where they feel they might receive less attention and confidentiality might be compromised.

Psychopharmacology

Several studies now testify to the effectiveness of antidepressants in treating depressed HIV-seropositive patients (Fernandez and Levy 1990; Manning et al. 1990; Rabkin and Harrison 1990). Most antidepressants have equivalent efficacy but differ in their spectrum of side effects. Because HIV-seropositive patients may have subtle compromise of the nervous system or blood-brain barrier, and hence greater sensitivity to medication side effects, it is prudent to begin with low dosages of antidepressants and to avoid tricyclic antidepressants with strong anticholinergic side effects (e.g., amitriptyline) that could contribute to delirium. Fernandez has advocated the use of psychostimulants in depressed patients with cognitive dysfunction due to HIV (Fernandez and Levy 1990).

Combining pharmacotherapy with psychotherapy is probably the treatment of choice for patients with severe or refractory depression (Manning and Frances 1990). Combining these modalities presents no theoretical or practical obstacle to psychotherapy using IPT (Klerman et al. 1984).

Interpersonal Psychotherapy

We began to treat depressed HIV-seropositive patients using IPT seeking pilot data for its effectiveness, but with no assurance that the treatment would work. To date there have been only two trials of a psychoeducational intervention or psychotherapy with this patient population (Kelly et al. 1989; Perry et al. 1991). We discovered that IPT fit the problems that depressed seropositive patients faced, and that it provided a helpful structure for both patient and therapist in addressing the patient's crisis. Readers not trained in IPT may nonetheless benefit from the treatment principles illustrated in this approach.

We do not suggest that IPT is the sole or most effective psychotherapy for depression in HIV-seropositive patients, but it is the approach with which we are most experienced. Our ongoing study will compare the efficacy of a variety of treatments.

What is IPT?

Interpersonal therapy is a focused, short-term psychotherapy of depression, first codified in a treatment manual by Klerman et al. (1984) and subsequently modified for depressed HIV-seropositive patients (J. C. Markowitz, G. L. Klerman, K. F. Clougherty, et al., unpublished manuscript, 1991). Numerous studies have established the effectiveness of IPT in treating HIV-seronegative depression (Elkin et al. 1989; Frank et al. 1990; Klerman and Weissman 1992). Treatment links depressive symptoms to interpersonal difficulties in one of four problem areas: 1) grief, 2) interpersonal role transitions, 3) role disputes, and 4) interpersonal deficits. In roughly 16 weekly sessions, patients learn to associate depressive symptoms with maladaptive patterns of interpersonal behavior in this problem area. By recognizing and correcting the behaviors, they achieve both symptom relief and a framework for understanding the depression.

The IPT therapist encourages a focus on dysfunctional interpersonal behaviors in the "here and now," as opposed to the genetic developmental interpretations and transferential, intrapsychic emphases of psychoanalytically oriented psychotherapy. The IPT therapist's stance is active and non-neutral, and may include making direct suggestions. The IPT therapist affectively engages the patient around an interpersonal focus, encouraging socialization and activity that yield symptomatic improvement and material for IPT discussion. An important IPT strategy is to facilitate exploration of options—a crucial issue for depressed, infected patients who feel they have none.

Why is IPT helpful?

Learning one is HIV-seropositive is a devastating life event with medical, personal, and interpersonal consequences. For many patients, including Mr. A. (see Case 1 above), the discovery of HIV infection brings life to a virtual halt despite the absence of physical symptoms. The brief term of treatment used in IPT is attractive to patients feeling time pressure, and it has conceptual value in providing patient and therapist with effective therapeutic strategies.

The "here and now" framework of IPT helps preserve a hopeful focus in the face of a lethal infection, from which depressed subjects can infer that life has not ended. It interrupts depressive ruminations on the "there and then," including self-blame for having contracted HIV. While always acknowledging the reality of HIV infection, the IPT therapist mobilizes internal resources through building a sense of mastery of the situation, and external supports by enhancing interpersonal relationships. This confident, pragmatic, and effective approach to depression underscores that HIV, too, can be confronted and treated. IPT offers a focused, organized, problem-oriented approach that keeps the clinical situation from being overwhelming.

Several interventions appear particularly helpful in mobilizing these depressed patients.

The sick role.   The IPT therapist explicitly inducts the patient into the "sick role" (Parsons 1951), offering exemption from certain social obligations and pressures while entailing the responsibility to work in therapy toward improved health. After appropriate psychiatric evaluation, we told each patient that he or she had *two* medical illnesses, depression and HIV infection, both of which were treatable, although depression might cause him or her to doubt this. *A crucial role transition for the seropositive patient, indeed, is acceptance of an ongoing patient role,* including medical follow-up, the anxious periodic wait for T-cell counts, trials of zidovudine, and so forth. Depressed patients benefit from understanding that their disturbances of sleep, appetite, and concentration may be due to depression rather than—as they generally assumed—HIV, and that their overly grim view of the future is distorted and treatable.

The interpersonal formulation.   The therapist collects an *interpersonal inventory:* a detailed anamnesis of the nature, quality, and expectations of important relationships, and of the patient's perceived role with other people. This process assists the therapist in determining the interpersonal problem area, which becomes the focus of treatment.

The therapist then molds diagnoses and interpersonal issues into an interpersonal formulation:

> Your symptoms are part of depression, and that depression is related to what's been happening in your life. Although your situation *feels* hopeless and untreatable, it isn't: that feeling is just a paradoxical symptom of depression, which is a common, highly treatable disorder. More than 8% of Americans develop significant depression in their lifetime. Depression nearly always improves with treatment. Depression affects and is affected by interpersonal relationships . . . [Here it is helpful to interject examples of social withdrawal, losses, and altered relationships in the patient's own case.] . . . and *interpersonal therapy*, a brief treatment based on this connection, has been proven effective in treating the kind of depression you have. We'll try to understand the stresses and relationships in your life that may be contributing to depression.

The patient must explicitly agree to this formulation before therapy can proceed.

Exploring options.   Hopelessness is frequently a symptom of depression, and HIV infection reinforces the patient's sense of impotence. IPT encourages exploring options, emphasizing that the stress of infection provides an opportunity to rethink unsatisfying aspects of relationship and career trajectories (Viederman 1983). Patients not only recovered from depression but frequently improved the quality of their lives. At the end of therapy, several patients commented that among the most helpful aspects of treatment had been the recognition that depressive symptoms were in fact aspects of mood disorder, and the hopeful realization that options always exist.

Psychoeducation.   In our experience, patients generally needed education about medical aspects of both major depression and HIV infection. Despite relative sophistication about HIV, patients nonetheless often held irrational beliefs and misconceptions. For many, therapy was a catalyst for seeking information and gaining expertise about HIV. One patient became active in a community HIV self-help movement; another relieved his anxieties about zidovudine by combing the medical literature, contacting agencies, and exploring research protocols. Calm, supportive discussion of these issues helped to reduce anxiety and instill hope.

How does IPT work?

For a fuller description of IPT, the reader is referred to the original text (Klerman et al. 1984). Here we review the adaptation of the four IPT problem areas to the treatment of depressed HIV-seropositive patients. For many HIV-seropositive patients the social consequences of HIV made several of the problem areas applicable, and choosing among them was a matter of clinical judgment. In general, the idea of recognizing HIV infection itself as a kind of role transition proved a useful concept.

Grief.   Uncomplicated grief is not a mental disorder: most mourners do not require psychiatric help, particularly if bolstered by interpersonal supports. Because the gay community has successfully mobilized support networks and self-help groups for HIV-infected individuals, we anticipated less complicated bereavement among HIV-seropositive gay men than would otherwise have been expected. It was the focal problem area in 7 (29%) of 24 cases.

Social stigma associated with homosexuality and intravenous drug use can magnify depressive shame and guilt, particularly when public acknowledgment of the stigmatized behavior coincides with discovery of a lethal disease. Moreover, having already seen sexual partners and others in their social network die from AIDS, most HIV-seropositive individuals experience *anticipatory mourning* for their own lost future well-being and foreshortened longevity. Like Mr. A., they may enter limbo upon discovering their HIV-seropositive status, even in the absence of physical symptoms. Therapists should confront this lassitude:

> You're acting as if you're mourning your own death, as if your life is over. Yet you have [almost] no symptoms of physical illness, and may have none for years. What you're suffering from is depres-

sion, which makes your life *seem* hopeless and ended. But in fact you do have options, and depression is treatable. Let's talk about what you can do with your life.

The majority of patients had friends who had died of AIDS. Some discovered their own seropositivity more or less simultaneously with their sexual partners. This knowledge complicated their quandary.

Case 4

Mr. D., a 42-year-old gay businessman, had been depressed since his lover's death from AIDS 3 years before. Mr. D. had nursed this man, 14 years older than he, for 3 years prior to his death, and had known of his own HIV infection for 4 years. His depressive symptoms intensified after the end of a relationship with a second, exploitative lover, who also had AIDS, 45 days before seeking treatment. Mr. D. felt helpless and hopeless, avoided his friends, and reported insomnia, weight loss, and compulsive behaviors. His HIV infection was asymptomatic, albeit he had been hospitalized a year earlier with PCP and had not complied with subsequent medical treatment.

The case was formulated as unresolved grief as well as a role transition. Sessions focused on complicated bereavement, identifying his more recent breakup as exacerbating his sense of loss of his first lover, and on the role transition to accepting and appropriately addressing his HIV infection. Initial sessions helped him to mourn his first lover while reviewing strengths and weaknesses of that relationship. As he reestablished contacts with friends, symptoms rapidly improved. He voiced newly recognized anger at his second, manipulative lover. At termination he understood the limitations of both relationships and how much he had grown: "If by chance I could go back [to either relationship], I wouldn't." Although still wary of prescribed medication, he did seek appropriate medical follow-up and was no longer depressed.

IPT facilitated mourning and then mobilized the patient to increase interpersonal contacts and plan appropriate responses to HIV infection.

Role transitions.   Because mourning one's anticipated death is inevitably an issue, even if not the focus of therapy, HIV-seropositive patients always undergo role transitions. They may change key social patterns—for example, some gay men who had previously relied on sexual encounters to meet others may find themselves without a method of introduction. HIV-seropositive individuals commonly respond not simply by restricting previous high-risk activities, but by carrying "safe sex" to the extreme of celibacy, even before depressive loss of libido. Goals of IPT are to help the patient restore safe activities and acknowledge the loss of pleasurable aspects of past activities, even when they were maladaptive. Role transitions were the focus of treatment in eight (33%) of our pilot cases.

Although the characteristics of seropositive individuals vary widely, clinical experience suggests that aspects of their *interpersonal environment* overlap. This environment has important implications for IPT. HIV-seronegative patients often become depressed following a single psychosocial stressor: complicated bereavement, job loss, or the onset of serious illness. In contrast, the HIV-seropositive patient often encounters all of the above simultaneously. In our experience, they may have learned of their HIV infection through a lover's illness or death, or lost their relationship when the lover learned the patient was seropositive. Friends and colleagues around them had died of AIDS; mourning was frequently hampered by the family's denial that the death was HIV related, and by the sheer number of such deaths. Physical and mood symptoms then compromised their work function. It was clinically useful to point out this concatenation of events to the patient to emphasize the stress he or she was undergoing.

The most common, most difficult role transition associated with HIV infection is accepting being seropositive and the potential or actual sick role. An anticipated further role transition is the onset of AIDS. The social imagery of HIV and AIDS, like other sexually transmitted diseases, often associates a fantasied punishment for sexual transgressions. There may be realistic fears of discrimination by employers, insurance companies, landlords, and others. In relationships, these patients feel contaminated, less attractive, and likely to be rejected because of their serostatus. Like Ms. B. (see above), they tend to withdraw from friends and family rather than reveal their secret.

Case 3 (continued from p. 43)

Mr. C., the 32-year-old gay artist referred to earlier in this chapter, became depressed after his only relationship ended. Previously physically healthy, he developed PCP during IPT treatment. Despite recovering, he felt that the ongoing threat of illness "destroyed everything," precluding opportunities for occupational advancement or finding another lover.

IPT addressed Mr. C.'s feelings about rejection by his ex-lover, an older man with whom he remained in contact, but also considered the gains he had achieved in that relationship. Treatment facilitated mourning the relationship and addressed his fears of having to depend on anyone for either emotional or—given his HIV status and PCP—physical support. He then enumerated future options, including risking future rejections and opportunities. Having acknowledged his fears of dependency, he found that his depression rapidly improved. His friendship with his former lover deepened, and he developed a transatlantic career and initiated involvement opportunities and involvement with men his own age. His Ham-D score fell from 20 at admission to 5.

Interpersonal disputes.   Both HIV seropositivity and depression increase tension in relationships, ending some altogether. Rejection by family or friends may precipitate or exacerbate depression. The interpersonal therapist addresses these interpersonal problems, often by relating depressive symptoms to a dispute in a key intimate relationship that has reached an impasse. Resolving the dispute may lead to reconciliation of lovers who had believed their disagreement insuperable, or to helping a patient leave and mourn the relationship. This framework, used with six (25%) of our subjects, may be useful for treating sexual partners, seropositive and seronegative, of HIV antibody-positive individuals.

Case 5

Mr. E., a 47-year-old gay male, had considered himself infected since the early 1980s and tested seropositive in 1988. He had been depressed for a year while sharing a studio with F., his intermittent partner of 13 years. He resented the latter, distrusting his commitment, but felt abandoned when they were apart. He supported his HIV-seropositive lover financially and worried more about F.'s medical status than his own.

Mr. E.'s depression was formulated as a role dispute that had reached an impasse. In sessions he acknowledged both his anger at F. and the anxiety, guilt, and loneliness he felt without him. After weighing available options, he arranged to have F. leave for 2-month intervals, allowing Mr. E. to test other relationships without feeling entirely abandoned. Having explored alternative contacts despite worries of rejection due to HIV, he ultimately reconciled with F. in a more satisfying relationship. Symptoms of depression entirely resolved.

Interpersonal deficits. Some HIV-seropositive individuals suffer from chronic interpersonal difficulties that socially isolate them prior to HIV infection. Some of our patients met criteria for schizoid, borderline, histrionic, narcissistic, avoidant, or obsessive-compulsive personality disorders. For patients who had had only transient, anonymous relationships, HIV infection confirmed underlying feelings of inadequacy and isolation. For example, a man with Kaposi's sarcoma saw himself as "a half-squashed roach with two legs still moving."

Interpersonal deficits, which may predispose to depression and impede recovery, are generally the most difficult to treat. Moreover, this IPT problem area has been the least conceptually developed. Therapists therefore employ the other three problem areas where possible, while using the crisis of HIV infection as an opportunity to challenge the patient to conquer interpersonal barriers. The ubiquitous role transition provides a convenient substitute focus. Mr. C. (see Case 3) is an example of a patient with significant interpersonal deficits whose depression was successfully managed in this way. The therapeutic relationship has particular importance in treating patients who have interpersonal deficits.

In four patients who had major interpersonal deficits, we focused on their current situation and depression rather than exploring characterological themes per se. Neither HIV seropositivity nor characterological issues prevented resolution of depression and interpersonal gains when IPT strategies framed issues in the "here and now."

Ending Treatment

Most psychiatrists probably would not seek to end treatment with a medically ill patient. Our practices include several HIV-seropositive patients in long-term psychotherapy and/or undergoing pharmacological maintenance. In the IPT study, however, we defined at the outset that the duration of therapy would be brief: roughly 4 months. Although this was an impetus to active therapy, many patients were pleased by its brevity, and almost all terminated without significant difficulty. The termination process included a summary of gains made in treatment, a review of the symptoms of depression and how the patient might counter a recurrence, and the option for psychotherapeutic referral to work on nonaffective, characterological issues when the patient sought this.

Pilot Results

We treated 24 depressed patients using IPT. Mean age was 37 (range 17–68). They were predominantly white, gay or bisexual, male, and reported a variety of HIV risk factors. All were HIV-seropositive except for one woman who tested negative 6 months after repeated unprotected intercourse with a lover who had AIDS. All but one patient showed clinical improvement, and 22 of 24 ultimately recovered from depression with IPT, although the case of Ms. B. must be called a failure based on research criteria (see below). The one other patient whose treatment was considered a failure left therapy after 5 sessions. Completers received a mean of 16 sessions (range 7–27). Six patients assessed serially showed a decrease in Ham-D score from 25.5 ± 6.8 initially, to 11.8 ± 6.5 in session 7, to 6.2 ± 5.0 at termination. These results are promising but clearly require replication.

Conclusions

What became of Mr. A. and Ms. B.? Their situations proved not to be as hopeless as they had feared.

Case 1 (continued from p. 38)

Mr. A., having recognized that his symptoms derived from a DSM-III-R (American Psychiatric Association 1987) diagnosis, used the sick role as a role transition to regain euthymia. He brought his parents to his house for support and improved his strained relationship with his lover. He mourned the late members of his support group and other friends while increasing his contacts with the survivors. After considering alternative options, he resurrected his career, reducing his debts and confronting creditors who had taken advantage of his depressive acquiescence. Also, he clarified his understanding of his medical regimen with his internist. These decisions materially improved Mr. A.'s life and restored his sense of potency and competence. In fact, he reported that in many respects he had never felt so comfortable with himself. He realized that he might again develop HIV-related symptoms like the shingles of 4 years before, and that the transition to acceptance of AIDS would be ongoing. His mood cleared and his depressive symptoms resolved almost entirely.

Case 2 (continued from p. 38)

Ms. B.'s treatment focused on the importance of her resuming her close relationship with her family, particularly a sister who had been her confidante. Ms. B. discussed in therapy her fears of rejection and of burdening others—a shift from her usual caregiving role. Her course was complicated by diabetic complications. When she finally spoke to her sister, after some delay, she steeled herself to the task by abusing diazepam on top of her methadone regimen. Although she felt better for having broken the news to her sister, treatment was interrupted by hospitalization for diazepam detoxification. On this ground we considered her a "treatment failure" but continued to see her after discharge for a total of 16 sessions. When IPT resumed, her footing with her family was restored by her improved communication. She subsequently tolerated the death from AIDS of several friends at her methadone clinic, able to mourn them without resorting to substance abuse. Her glucose was now so well controlled that oral hypoglycemic medication was discontinued. After her final session—admittedly delayed several months past the usual 16 weeks—she was euthymic and hopeful, an almost unrecognizable transformation from her initial presentation.

Ms. B.'s case illustrates the added difficulties in treating a depressed HIV-seropositive patient who is abusing substances (not dual but "treble diagnosis"?), and yet that even so complex a case remains treatable.

The spread of the AIDS epidemic during the last decade carried a message of hopelessness: early death, no cure; doctors could only watch their patients die. There has been progress since then. If HIV still has no cure, hopelessness is surely unwarranted. In the coming years many patients who are depressed and HIV-seropositive will seek psychiatric treatment.

Psychiatrists should not despair when these patients enter their offices. Rather, they can prepare for the challenge and address the patients' medical fears and depressive distortions, effectively treating the depression and facilitating patients' finding optimal medical care for HIV. Psychiatrists may also gain great satisfaction in helping a patient in exigent distress to restore meaning to his or her life. IPT appears to be a valuable modality in treating these patients; other psychotherapeutic approaches may also be effective.

References

American Psychiatric Association: Diagnostic and Statistical Manual of Mental Disorders, 3rd Edition, Revised. Washington, DC, American Psychiatric Press, 1987

Beck AT, Rush AJ, Shaw BF, et al: Cognitive Therapy of Depression. New York, Guilford, 1979

Beckett A: The neurobiology of human immunodeficiency virus infection, in American Psychiatric Press Review of Psychiatry, Vol 9. Edited by Tasman A, Goldfinger SM, Kaufmann CA. Washington, DC, American Psychiatric Press, 1990, pp 593–613

Centers for Disease Control: Human immunodeficiency virus infection in the United States: a review of current knowledge. MMWR 36 (suppl S-6):1–48, 1987a

Centers for Disease Control: Revision of the CDC surveillance case definition for acquired immunodeficiency syndrome. MMWR 36(suppl):1–14, 1987b

Elkin I, Shea MT, Watkins JT, et al: National Institute of Mental Health Treatment of Depression Collaborative Research Program: general effectiveness of treatments. Arch Gen Psychiatry 46:971–982, 1989

Faulstich ME: Psychiatric aspects of AIDS. Am J Psychiatry 144:551–556, 1987

Fernandez F, Levy JK: Psychiatric diagnosis and pharmacotherapy of patients with HIV infection, in American Psychiatric Press Review of Psychiatry, Vol 9. Edited by Tasman A, Goldfinger SM, Kaufmann CA. Washington, DC, American Psychiatric Press, 1990, pp 614–630

Frank E, Kupfer DJ, Perel JM, et al: Three-year outcomes for maintenance therapies in recurrent depression. Arch Gen Psychiatry 47:1093–1099, 1990

Kelly JA, St. Lawrence JS, Hood HV, et al: Behavioral intervention to reduce AIDS risk activities. J Consult Clin Psychol 57:60–67, 1989

Klerman GL, Weissman MM: Interpersonal psychotherapy: efficacy and adaptations, in Handbook of Affective Disorders, 2nd Edition. Edited by Paykel ES. London, Churchill Livingstone, 1992, 501–510

Klerman GL, Weissman MM, Rounsaville BJ, et al: Interpersonal Psychotherapy of Depression. New York, Basic Books, 1984

Manning DW, Frances AJ (eds): Combined Pharmacotherapy and Psychotherapy for Depression. Washington, DC, American Psychiatric Press, 1990

Manning D, Jacobsberg L, Erhart S, et al: The efficacy of imipramine in the treatment of HIV-related depression. Paper presented at the Sixth International Conference on AIDS, San Francisco, CA, June 1990

Markowitz JC, Perry SW: AIDS: a medical overview for psychiatrists, in American Psychiatric Press Review of Psychiatry, Vol 9. Edited by Tasman A, Goldfinger SM, Kaufmann CA. Washington, DC, American Psychiatric Press, 1990, pp 574–592

Markowitz JC, Perry SW: Effects of human immunodeficiency virus on the central nervous system, in American Psychiatric Press Textbook of Neuropsychiatry, 2nd Edition. Edited by Yudofsky SC, Hales RE. Washington, DC, American Psychiatric Press, 1992, pp 499–518

Markowitz JC, Klerman GL, Perry SW: Interpersonal psychotherapy of depressed HIV-seropositive patients. Hosp Community Psychiatry 43:885–890, 1992

Marotta R, Perry S: Early neuropsychological dysfunction caused by human immunodeficiency virus. Journal of Neuropsychiatry and Clinical Neurosciences 1:225–235, 1989

Marzuk PM, Tierney H, Tardiff K, et al: Increased risk of suicide in persons with AIDS. JAMA 259:1333–1337, 1988

Navia BA, Price RW: The acquired immunodeficiency syndrome dementia complex as the presenting or sole manifestation of human immunodeficiency virus infection. Arch Neurol 44:65–69, 1987

Parsons T: Illness and the role of the physician: a sociological perspective. Am J Orthopsychiatry 21:452–460, 1951

Perry SW: Organic mental disorders caused by HIV: update on early diagnosis and treatment. Am J Psychiatry 147:696–710, 1990

Perry SW, Markowitz J: Psychiatric interventions for AIDS-spectrum disorders. Hosp Community Psychiatry 37:1001–1006, 1986

Perry S, Jacobsberg LB, Fishman B, et al: Psychiatric diagnosis before serological testing for the human immunodeficiency virus. Am J Psychiatry 147:89–93, 1990a

Perry S, Jacobsberg L, Fishman B: Suicidal ideation and HIV testing. JAMA 263:679–682, 1990b

Perry S, Fishman B, Jacobsberg L, et al: Effectiveness of psychoeducational interventions in reducing emotional distress after human immunodeficiency virus antibody testing. Arch Gen Psychiatry 48:143–147, 1991

Rabkin JG, Harrison WM: Effect of imipramine on depression and immune status in a sample of men with HIV infection. Am J Psychiatry 147:495–497, 1990

Viederman M: The psychodynamic life narrative: a psychotherapeutic intervention useful in crisis situations. Psychiatry 46:236–246, 1983

Chapter 3

Conceptual Issues in the Psychoanalytic Psychotherapy of Patients With Borderline Personality Disorder

Richard L. Munich, M.D.

T he growing interest in and controversy about the etiology, no-
sology, and psychosocial treatment of personality and/or
character disorders—and more specifically the borderline personality—are intimately connected with psychodynamic theory and
the history of psychoanalysis itself. Several things support this
point of view. Not only do some of Freud's early cases fall into more
recent delineations of borderline personality organization, but his
treatment of these cases showed wide deviations in technique (Lipton 1977). One might also include in the debate on this subject
issues related to the widening scope of psychoanalysis (Stone
1954), and the confusion between the pathogenic role of intrapsychic conflict and that of psychological deficit (London 1973a,

Portions of this chapter were presented at the scientific meeting of the Western
New England Psychoanalytic Society, New Haven, Connecticut, November 10,
1990.
   The author wishes to express his thanks to Ann Appelbaum, M.D., for her considerable help with this manuscript.

61

1973b), as well as the past and recent debate about the seduction theory and the role of real and fantasied early life trauma (Masson 1984).

Another theoretical issue relevant to a discussion of borderline personality is the conflict and interdependence between ego psychology on the one hand and object-relations theory and self psychology on the other (Pine 1985). Much of this conflict was contained within Freud's thinking as his drive theory evolved. A neurobiologist and a romantic philosopher, Freud was concerned both with the force by which drives expressed themselves and with their meaning. The structural model is derived from his considerations of force and is formalized in ego psychology. The representational model is derived from Freud's considerations of meaning and is formalized in object-relations theory and self psychology. Following recent advances in the field of child development, especially those demonstrating the infant's considerable repertoire of interpersonal techniques, *the first premise of this review will be that the development of the ego and that of internalized object relations are parallel rather than prioritized or alternative concepts about mental processes.*

Since the early 1950s, psychoanalytic theory has balanced its interest in the developing infant's internal world with increasing consideration of the infant's external reality. *It is the second premise of this review that internal and external factors are equally relevant in the etiology of psychological difficulty.* Nevertheless, much like the controversy between ego psychologists and object-relations theorists, and more recently between the former two groups and self psychologists, there has emerged a dispute between those who believe borderline pathology derives from an excess of aggression from within and those who believe that it derives from deprivation, trauma, or abandonment from without. This modern-day version of the nature-nurture conflict, like the structural-representational conflict and the deficit-conflict dispute, may have far more theoretical than practical import, particularly in view of the subsequent intermingling of determinants for years before a disturbed patient appears for help. It is along these lines of speculation that this growing field of inquiry is entirely within the realm of psychoanalytic psychology.

In this review I assume a position somewhere between theory

and technique and attempt to integrate approaches to the borderline patient. Compared with more neurotic patients, with whom the primary focus can be on the content of treatment, borderline patients require their psychotherapist to focus at least as much on the framework or conditions of treatment. The conditions of treatment include matters that are dealt with in a treatment contract, but they may involve the management of self-destructive behaviors, extratherapeutic contact, limit setting, and even at times the use of medication and hospitalization. So in addition to the many theoretical questions already raised, this difference of focus in the treatment of neurotic and borderline patients accounts for a great deal of the debate about technique, a debate that mainly centers around the issue of how and when to address, interpret, and manage the negative transference.

Prior to the issue of the negative transference, however, there is the issue of whether various authors are talking about the same population of patients. Is there an important difference between patients who qualify as borderline but who have more affective features, more narcissistic features, or more psychotic features, or in whom identity issues are more prominent? Fulfilling five of eight DSM-III-R criteria (American Psychiatric Association 1987) for borderline personality, for example, can lead to 93 different configurations. Might different technical approaches be more relevant for the patients with these differing features? And finally, might different dynamic theories pertain to different patients?

The Borderline Circle

To help the student, theoretician, and practitioner cope with some of these dichotomies and dilemmas, I am proposing a schematization of the dynamics of the developing mind of an 18-month-old. It is configured with two concentric circles surrounding a central grid made up of two perpendicular axes (see Figure 3–1) and, more realistically, is the graphic representation of the two fundamental premises—structural and object relations, and internal world and external reality.

Ignore for a few moments the outer circle and focus on the elements of the inner circle. On the horizontal axis, the left side emphasizes the structural world of id, ego, and superego. This side represents the view that the ego adds to autonomous functions and is formed from abandoned object cathexes. The other, or right, side emphasizes the world of self and object representations. This side represents the view that it is through object relations that stable self and object representations consolidate. The top of the vertical axis represents influences on the psyche from internal reality—feelings, thoughts, impulses, fantasies, and conflicts. The bottom of the vertical axis represents influences on the psyche

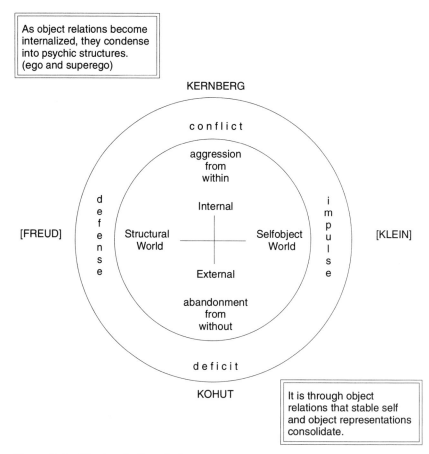

Figure 3–1. The borderline circle.

from the external world, as in the average expectable environment, overinvolvement, abandonment, deprivation, or trauma.
Conflict and deficit are also represented on the vertical axis, but at
a different level of abstraction, just as impulse or drive and defense
represent the corresponding level of abstraction on the horizontal
axis.

As an effort to understand or provide a blueprint for a virtual
Tower of Babel that now encloses the nearly 4,000 articles on borderline personality disorder (BPD), I have tried to arrange some
of the major figures on the subject and their most relevant precursors in the literature around the circumference of the borderline
circle in a way that corresponds to each investigator's primary theoretical position (see Figure 3–2). The net effect of this arrangement is to highlight that what at first seem like widely divergent
points of view are more connected than may appear initially. I have
chosen four key figures to represent the axes, pairings representing stereotypically opposite points of view. On the horizonal axis
are Freud (1923/1961), as the explicator of the structural world,
and Melanie Klein (1946), as the explicator of the object world.
The other pair include Kernberg (1976; Kernberg et al. 1989) and
Kohut (1971), the former starting from the point of view of aggression from within and the latter from that of empathic failure and
abandonment from without. These two axes, each narrowly conceived of as representing divergent points of view, create four
closely interrelated and mutually complementary quadrants that
inform the placement of those investigators who focus on the psychological aspects of the disorder.

Keeping in mind that this schema is for heuristic rather than
explanatory purposes and thus sacrifices depth for breadth, let us
look at the circle. I begin with Otto Kernberg because there is
hardly a paper in the psychological literature on this topic in the
past 20 years that does not agree with, argue with, reject, or take
off from his wide-ranging formulations. Kernberg is located directly between the structural and the representational points of
view and at the top of the axis indicating internal sources for the
disorder. Directly influenced by Helene Deutsch's (1942) writing
about the as-if personality and drawing heavily upon and synthesiz-

ing the work of Edith Jacobson (1964) and Melanie Klein, Kernberg believes the etiology of the borderline personality organization derives from an excess of aggression, most likely on a constitutional basis, which leads to unintegrated good and bad self and object representations. Kernberg does not dismiss environmental factors, nor does he minimize the real disturbances in the patient's primary relationships, but his emphasis and bias shade most clearly toward constitution and internal conflict.

It is perhaps easier to appreciate this emphasis by moving halfway around the circle, to the bottom, where I have located Kohut, and Adler and Buie. On this "external influences" and "deficit"

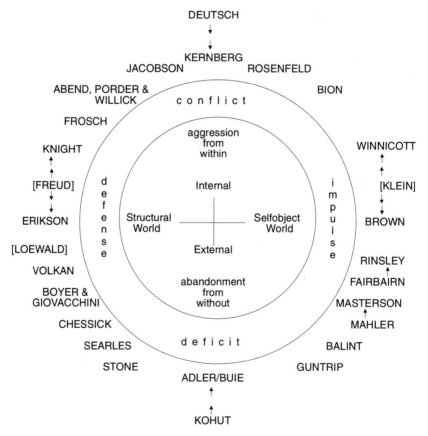

Figure 3–2. The borderline circle: primary theoretical positions of major figures.

side of the circle, there is more emphasis on the empathic failure of selfobjects leading to developmental arrests. This failure and the ensuing arrest lead to what Buie and Adler (1982–1983) see as the incapacity of the child to develop holding and soothing introjects. As noted in reporting Kernberg's position, these theorists are mindful of aggression, but see it as secondary to the disappointments and frustrations children experience in obtaining what they need from the environment.

Michael Stone, among others, has contributed to the emerging awareness of the prevalence of abuse and early trauma in the histories of patients with BPD (see Stone 1988). Therefore, his work places him in the "deficit" area of the diagram. Abuse is an extreme form of empathic failure and of the abandonment of expected caregiving and nurturant roles. Abuse can take many forms, but the psychological common denominator is the abuser's misuse of the child as a means for discharging sexual or aggressive tensions. When this occurs before the child's establishment of mental representations and ego structures, there is a severe inhibition of the establishment of boundaries between self and other, between inside and outside, and between primary and secondary process thinking and impulse and defense, an inhibition that may produce vulnerability to psychosis. Later sexual, physical, and psychological abuse affects the consolidation of these representational and structural aspects of the personality, although other factors such as age at which the abuse is perpetrated may mitigate their impact. These are the factors implicated in the etiology of borderline psychopathology. So much is Stone convinced by the retrospective accounts he has gathered of childhood abuse that he thinks of BPD in much the same way as one might think of posttraumatic stress disorder.

I now return halfway around the circle from Michael Stone to Wilfred Bion (1959). Although he writes about the maternal containing function, an external factor, Bion refers to the role of part objects and the impact of aggression and its destructive consequences for the linkages between thought and affect, and between action and thought—disturbance of these linkages being so much in evidence with borderline patients. By this schema, these consequences are considered internal factors. I include in this quadrant

Herbert Rosenfeld (1987), who, while developing Klein's concept of projective identification to its most useful clinical form, considered it an opportunity for communication between patient and analyst, and discussed the difficulties, by virtue of their destructiveness, of containing the projections of borderline patients. If we follow the circle down from the quadrant represented by the internal and selfobject axis, we pass through Brown (1987), who was influenced by the work of Melanie Klein and Donald Winnicott (1975). In this progression, which encompasses the transitional state between Klein's paranoid-schizoid and depressive positions, we also move down into the next quadrant represented by the selfobject and external axes. Now the 18-month-old infant is postulated as being concerned that his or her aggression will destroy the person upon whom he or she depends as well as the connections with that person. The emphasis has become interpersonal rather than intrapsychic.

This leads us to the work of Fairbairn (1952) and Rinsley (Masterson and Rinsley 1975), and Mahler (1971) and Masterson (1976). Continuing in this overly brief and much too simplified odyssey through major thinkers, it is in these writers that one finds the constellation of ideas around poorly formed and integrated object representations. In this view, the mother's capacity to manage the child's variable need for closeness and autonomy determines the latter's ability to assemble an integrated object representation of the mother. Her incapacity to manage this need leads to abandonment depression or engulfment terror in the child. Or, as Masterson and Rinsley (1975) put it, the mother's unconscious opposition to her child's separation and individuation leads to a fixation during this phase. Beside the emphasis on external factors, the element that puts these formulations on this side of the circle and in this quadrant is that the divergence between withdrawing and rewarding object-relations units is related by these authors to problems in empathic nurturance, thus leading to a defect in the ego's capacity to integrate reality and pleasure.

Reference to the ego, however, propels us to the other side of the circle, back to Edith Jacobson, the ego psychologists, and the quadrant represented by the internal, structural world. Writers located in this quadrant, such as Abend, Porder, and Willick (1983), probably have the most difficulty of any so far mentioned in thinking of the borderline personality as a legitimate diagnosis or a separate and distinct entity. Knight (1953), for example, used the term "borderline states" more to describe alterations from a more neurotic structure than as an independent configuration. That is, as John Frosch (1971) points out in commenting on Knight's work, the variety of presenting symptoms such as phobias, conversion phenomena, compulsive traits, paranoid features, and so forth, are merely defenses—albeit extreme—against basic conflicts. Frosch's "psychotic character"—a term he prefers to "borderline"—has disturbances in its "relationship with reality, the feeling of reality, and the capacity to test reality" (p. 217). These disturbances, which are regressive and lead to a diffusion of ego boundaries, are relatively transient and reversible and are ever present in such patients as a background potential.

Thus, following Knight and Frosch, writers associated with this quadrant see the borderline condition as resulting from the disequilibrium among psychic structures—the intrusion, for example, of drive material into awareness or evidence of archaic superego functioning—and the deneutralization of libidinal and aggressive drives. This disequilibrium and deneutralization are secondary to conflict and, while transitory, are clearly on the way to psychosis. Unlike their colleagues on the opposite side of the circle, the investigators in the internal-structural quadrant assume that the ego, although intimately connected with object relations, comes first and guides the vicissitudes of those object relations. For these classical theoreticians it is the ego's vulnerability to dedifferentiation and regressive processes that is central to the borderline condition rather than object representations that determine the integrity of the ego.

Moving downward from this quadrant to that represented by the axes of structural world and external reality, I have placed Erikson (1950), Volkan (1987), Boyer and Giovacchini (1967/1980), Chessick (1977), and Searles (1986) in roughly that order. Many of these figures treat these patients on the couch and refer to their approach as "classical psychoanalysis," but of greater relevance for this section of our review is their similar orientation toward etiology. Although coming directly from a traditional ego psychological background, Erikson is the first to fall below the internal-external axis because of his central interest, captured by the title *Childhood and Society* (1950), in the role of the external world on personality development and his epigenetic schemata. Even his speculations about identity—a central aspect of the borderline personality—include not only what the individual thinks of himself or herself, but also and equally what those in the environment think. Giovacchini (1979) writes about poorly structuralized self representations leading to the fixation of the individual in a transitional space where there are blurred boundaries between internal and external worlds. Just as previously described when I was locating abandonment in the same quadrant as abuse, Giovacchini believes that this fixation results from an early caretaking in which there was either very little sensory input from mother to child beyond the basic care of bodily needs, or a situation in which the mother used the child as an object for sexual or aggressive gratification.

For Searles (1986), the borderline personality represents a stage of ego development prior to any clear differentiation between inner and outer world, and prior to the child's coming to function as a whole person with others being experienced as whole persons. Clearly citing environmental factors as etiological, Searles believes the parents of these patients with "dual or multiple identity processes" are not predominately whole, well-integrated individuals themselves. Rather, they are a collection of poorly integrated, seemingly innumerable introjects. To complete this circular odyssey and taking off from Searles' innumerable, unintegrated introjects, I refer you again halfway around the circle to Bion, who is interested in the role of internalized part objects in addition to the aggressive destruction of linkages in the etiology of the disorder.

Finally, for the sake of completeness, I have added Grinker's (1977) four subtypes of borderline individuals to the circle and have attempted to locate the importance of the role of constitutional factors. The theoretical points of view espoused by the major writers and practitioners connected with this subject are repre-

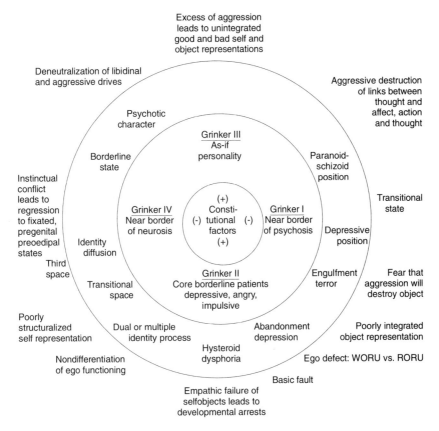

Figure 3–3. The borderline circle: theoretical points of view, including Grinker's subtypes.

sented in Figure 3–3. We will now consider clinical features and, finally, psychotherapeutic technique.

Consonance and Dissonance in the Psychotherapy of Patients With Borderline Personality Disorder

According to Waldinger and Gunderson (1987; see also Waldinger 1987) in their overview of psychodynamic therapy with borderline patients, most writers agree that there are eight basic "tenets" of "safe and effective intensive treatment" (p. 8):

1. Ensuring stability of the framework of treatment
2. Increasing the therapist's activity
3. Tolerating the patient's hostility
4. Making self-destructive behaviors ungratifying
5. Establishing a connection between the patient's actions and feelings in the present
6. Blocking acting-out behaviors
7. Focusing early clarification and interpretations on the here and now
8. Paying careful attention to countertransference feelings

It is after this general agreement that widespread conflict and divergence appear. Waldinger and Gunderson go on to identify the areas of disagreement:

◆ Interpretation and the usefulness of content versus creation of a holding environment and the importance of process
◆ The origins and the primacy of positive versus negative transference
◆ The timing of interpretations of the transference and the provision of corrective experiences in therapy

I would add to these areas of disagreement whether one should focus on the identification and interpretation of impulses or on the systematic analysis of defenses. With the possible exception of the therapist's response to the patient's behavior, it is worth noting that these guidelines and controversies might well be applied to all psychotherapies.

By returning to our circle, it is not hard—at least from a theoretical point of view—to place the various actors with respect to these issues. If you believe, with Buie and Adler, for example, that a patient's borderline disturbance results from a failure to internalize soothing and nurturant introjects, then you will provide as an invariable aspect of your psychotherapy a holding tolerant atmosphere in the face of hostility and distorted perceptions from your patient. If, on the other hand, you believe that the patient's hostility and distorted perceptions emerge directly from an excess of aggression that results in unintegrated good and bad self and object representations, then you will, as Kernberg does, respond more rapidly with confrontation and interpretation of these negative transference distortions.

Similarly, if you are a therapist who believes in the inevitable depressive consequences of abandonment, as do Masterson and Rinsley, then you will look for, point out, and interpret this connection at every opportunity. Moving back across our circle, if you believe that conflict between drive and defense leads to borderline pathology, then you will, very much like a classical psychoanalyst, interpret along inter- and intrasystemic lines. If, as Stone does, you think there is trauma, you will want to uncover and work it through; or if you believe the trauma is nonspecific, you might want to provide corrective emotional experiences. And finally, if you believe that splitting and projection are prominent, then, as with Rosenfeld, the identification and interpretation of part objects and the reconnection of severed linkages will inform your technique.

Patients, however, defy categorization; therefore, while we may categorize etiological theories, we cannot translate them into prescriptions. Etiological theories can alert the therapist to moment-to-moment developments in the treatment, but they cannot determine a course. The continuing and vexed history of Axis II—discrete clusters notwithstanding—is graphic testament to this. As suggested earlier, it is probably true that different technical approaches might be relevant for differing symptom configurations.

Based on areas that overlap the quadrants of the borderline circle previously outlined, for example, I would divide the eight borderline anchor points into four constellations, represented on the circle along with the corresponding therapeutic technique, in Figure 3–4.

The first constellation would include inappropriate, intense anger or lack of control of anger and impulsiveness in self-damaging activity, including such antisocial and sadistic behaviors as promiscuity, reckless driving, and manipulation and splitting of the therapeutic frame. The latter includes lying, attempting to control the therapy and therapist, and conscious withholding of data, as well as manipulative self-mutilation. As you might suspect, I believe Kernberg's approach has much to offer for the psychotherapy of borderline patients presenting in this way. A clear spelling out of the framework of the treatment, confrontation, and early interpretation of destructive behaviors and of transference distortions in the here and now are the hallmarks of this approach.

The second constellation includes those symptoms associated with unstable and intense interpersonal relationships, micropsychotic episodes, schizoid phenomena, and nonpsychotic paranoia. This constellation is the one in which projection and projective identification are most visibly operative as the individual desperately tries to locate himself or herself in others. The psychotherapy associated with this approach would also benefit most from responding to here-and-now issues—that is, how the behavior is

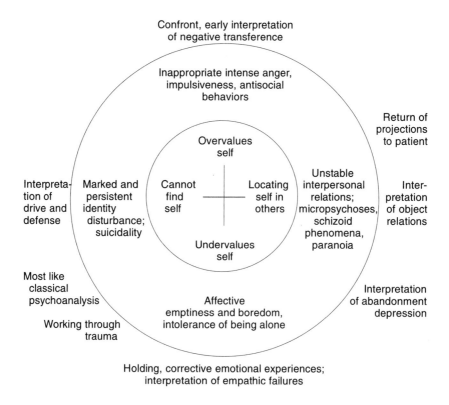

Figure 3–4. The borderline circle: patient clusters and therapeutic technique.

being enacted in the transference—but with the added link with genetic material primarily around disturbed object relationships and the patient's fear of his or her own intensity, neediness, and aggression, and the alternate fear of being overwhelmed and engulfed by the other. This approach, associated most closely with the British object-relations theorists, is different from that which I will advocate for the fourth constellation in that I would focus more on the impulses and longings rather than on the defenses against them. As I understand the literature, English psychoanalysts, unlike their more classical American counterparts, have always considered borderline patients as being in their domain.

The third constellation of symptoms that may require a unique psychotherapeutic stance includes those associated with affective instability, marked shifts from baseline mood to depression, chronic feelings of emptiness and boredom, intolerance of being alone, and the clinging, dependent, and masochistic behaviors so often seen in patients with this disorder. While it is beyond the domain of this review, this constellation, of course, is the one most closely connected with Axis I affective disorders, so a careful diagnostic differentiation must always be made. Once you have established that this constellation is characterological, then the psychotherapeutic approach would be that which is identified with a patient, tolerant holding environment, with efforts to identify and locate areas of empathic failure and to gradually interpret them in those terms or in terms of working through early trauma. In this context and borrowing from the identity disorders of the next constellation, I would also include the notion of a damaged identity. The psychotherapeutic stance in this constellation, as well as that in the first, is more forthcoming and, under special circumstances, may include elements of supportive psychotherapy and corrective emotional experiences. It is when the clinging has controlling elements that trouble often emerges in the therapeutic relationship, controversy about management begins, and the risks of countertransferential acting out are greatest.

Marked and persistent identity disturbance characterizes the fourth, and final, constellation of symptoms. In DSM-III-R, this disturbance is in part characterized by uncertainty about at least two of the following: self-image, sexual orientation, long-term goals or career choice, type of friends desired, and preferred values. While I am in essential agreement with these, I tend to add *identity diffusion, multiple and negative identity* to this constellation from the analytic literature. Insofar as I believe perverse sexuality is connected with defects in self representation and often represents an effort to find oneself, I include it here as well as self-mutilation in the original sense of the word. The psychotherapeutic approach most appropriate to this constellation is closest to classical psychoanalysis as practiced in modified form by Chessick, Boyer, Giovacchini, Volkan, and Searles with borderline patients. In this approach the analyst acts as a neutral screen onto which instinctual conflicts and defenses against those conflicts are projected and through which interpretation is made. My language in this work would often center around psychosexual stages, including oral, anal, and phallic fixations and the dysfunctional condensations of genital and pre-genital trends. At the same time, I would be linking these to actual defective parenting. Finally, my focus would be on the defenses against this material rather than the material itself, and my stance would be somewhat less forthcoming.

Clinical Material

Let me conclude these abstractions with an example illustrating some of these dilemmas. Ms. B., a lawyer in her mid-50s and never married, was referred for psychotherapy by a consulting analyst. She presented with a chief complaint of being increasingly depressed that she had never been able to form an attachment to a man—sexual or otherwise—and was beginning to despair of a life of unfulfillment and loneliness. Ms. B. reported in detail in this first session her fear of being considered homosexual and a social outcast in the community, her two previous failed treatments with respected psychoanalysts, and her considerable professional status and responsibilities.

Ms. B. was the second born of identical twins and the fifth child of middle-class parents. Because her mother was apparently overwhelmed with having twins and already somewhat ill, there were many caretakers. Her father was busy with two and sometimes three jobs. When Ms. B. was 8 years old, her mother died of Bright's disease, a circumstance the child was informed of upon returning home from school on the afternoon of her mother's death. She remembered virtually nothing about her first 8 years, her mother, or her reaction to her mother's death.

What the patient did remember in much more detail was that after the death, she received care but no comfort. In particular, she was bitterly resentful of her father's appearance to the world as a nice guy, his quick remarriage after 6 months, his apparent lack of concern for the fate of the twins, his threats to break up the family when she complained, lack of time spent with her, and her own uneasy adjustment to the new stepmother. No physical or sexual abuse was described; rather the theme of deprivation of contact with parents was echoed in her failed relations with her older siblings and with a succession of significant others for the rest of her life.

The first year of our work together was characterized by an idealized transference, a flood of details from her daily life and legal practice, and many phone calls to obtain more contact with me. Selecting the seat farthest away, she established dominion over my office, researched my credentials, and constructed a narrative that placed men in the position of enemy or, like her father, as being unresponsive, self-centered, and thoughtless. She never missed or was late to a session, and she promptly paid her bill, occasionally with the smug comment that she made more than I did, certain of my obvious envy. The next 2 years were characterized by the emergence, with the same energy and intensity of the first year's idealization, of an angry, contentious, devaluing, and difficult negative phase and transference. I could do no right: if I talked, I was missing the point; if I did not talk, I was not being empathic and responsive. The patient also complained bitterly that our work was proceeding too slowly. Because time was running out for her, she wanted "breakthroughs" similar to those she had read about in books. She protested vigorously when I had to be away, demanding to know where I was going and staying. Often distorting a comment or interpretation, she added to her growing list of indictments. She sought consultation from eminent psycho-analysts, the recommendation from which was for me to assume a less analytic and more supportive approach.

I cannot locate or remember the precise shift in the valence of Ms. B.'s attitude toward me; but early during the fourth year of treatment she began saying that, even though I had several prob-lems, I might be a "good enough" psychotherapist. There was evi-dence that she was benefiting from treatment in that her life was more settled and her interpersonal relations less chaotic; but, more important from my point of view, she was beginning to un-derstand her difficulty with close relationships as emanating at least as much from her own ambivalence about them as from the unfortunate circumstances of her early life or the distance from her father. There was a hint that her depression and despair about her situation were tempered with regret and sadness about her role in bringing it about; however, for various reasons, these gains were fleeting. In the 4 years of treatment, however, this sadness was never translated into tears.

Combining supportive, interpretive, holding, and (occasion-ally) confrontive techniques, I would characterize my style with her as analytically eclectic. More recent material in therapy centered around Ms. B.'s difficulties feeling closer to me, while her resis-tances included a growing pressure for me to advise her about sit-uations in her practice and office and financial matters. Much of the above, and, in addition, her multiple previous careers and gen-der identity dysphoria, conform to a diagnosis of BPD with narcis-sistic, paranoid, and depressive traits as well as the more or less expectable treatment course.

Because of hospital construction, I was temporarily relocated to an office in the front of the building. What is important here is that in the new setting there was no way the patient could sit as far away from me as usual. In fact, compared with our usual 10 to 12 feet apart, Ms. B. and I were at the time of the material I will pres-ent 5 to 6 feet apart, with only a coffee table separating us. Another item of importance is that I could see the front parking area of the hospital.

In the week preceding the following vignette, Ms. B. felt saddened to discover that an acquaintance who had recently lost his wife was enamored of another woman. She had hoped to connect with him, fantasizing a permanent relationship; but in this week she spent most of one session unhappily outlining the man's self-centered, passive, and clinging features. She compared him unfavorably to me and sadly wondered if she would ever find someone. She was especially worried because she was able to notice me more closely now and was made anxious by our closeness in the room. If she leaned forward, she explained, it would not be difficult to touch me. She could not go further with these thoughts and defended herself by raising concern about the expense of her summer house and our previous discussions and requests for advice about where all of her money was going. She ended the week by mentioning a couple whom she was helping with their separation and divorce, all complicated by the wife's being pregnant with twins.

Session No. 364

When I came in to work I noticed Ms. B.'s car parked as usual, so I was surprised she wasn't waiting at the office. After waiting 5 minutes, I looked out the front window and noticed her opening and closing her car door. She continued to fuss with it and finally engaged someone to help her. Finally, they solved whatever the problem was, and she arrived at the appointed hour almost 15 minutes late. With a brief word about her car door and being late, she announced that she really had to talk about the couple she mentioned the previous week. Acknowledging that she was avoiding therapy issues, she began by asking me a complicated question about how to bill for the previously mentioned couple's legal work. I did not understand the question. She explained that in spite of their having a combined income of over $200,000, they were already complaining about her fee. She explained that in a divorce action, couples usually do not come to the same lawyer. Should she charge them double? She said each obviously needed psychiatric treatment, but she feared they would use money as an excuse not to undertake consultation. Again she pressured me to tell her what to do. I said that I did not understand these financial issues, and that it seemed more important that she felt under so much pressure about the case.

"Yes," she replied, "I am under enormous pressure. Still," she continued, "I really need advice." I listened as she outlined in detail the situation of the couple, the news of impending twins, the mother's concern about her career, and how little time the mother spent with their 3-year-old daughter. My patient then went through all the steps she was taking to help this couple get help, including everything from intensive psychotherapy and couples therapy, to household help and a nanny for the children for a minimum of 5 years. What was making the situation so tense, she explained, was that the couple seemed on the verge of accepting none of the recommendations, terminating their contact with Ms. B., and finding a lawyer who would get them divorced.

Again, I commented on how much pressure Ms. B. seemed under, and wondered if she were pushing her clients somewhat further than what I understood to be the usual legal intervention. She replied that she was only doing what was right and that, in fact, she had commented to the couple that a few thousand dollars now would save tens of thousands of dollars in therapy bills later. I wondered what there was about this couple that was generating so much involvement and intensity. She responded that it was her sensitivity to the situation of the twins, but mainly how very cold the expectant mother seemed.

It was the end of the abbreviated hour. I said I would see her Wednesday and opened the first door, and she said I could open the second door for her. I had a vaguely uneasy, out-of-touch feeling about the session, but had seen this kind of near-panicky pressure before and mainly attributed it to the session's uncharacteristic brevity.

Session No. 365

Ms. B. was waiting for me as usual, and the session began at its usual time. Even before reaching her seat, she began by commenting on how angry she was with me when leaving the previous session. That's why, she reported, she asked me to open the door. She was angry, she continued, because I had totally missed the point in the previous session. She was abruptly reminded of how insensitive and unempathic I could be. I was making light of her concern about the family; she claimed to notice a sneer on my face as I let her out, something disrespectful.

It was true, she continued, that I commented on the pressure she was under, but if I had really understood that the twins were in danger, just as she and her sister had been in danger, then I would not have been so concerned about all the arrangements she was making. A really good psychotherapist would have been more responsive to his patient's pressure and more supportive and empathic, and would have called the patient in the evening, scheduled an extra session for the next day, and even come in 45 minutes early if necessary.

I commented that she seemed angry but that all of this was quite complicated, particularly since she was so clear at the beginning of the hour that she wanted my advice about the couple. She sat back in her chair, shook her head, and spoke of how tired she was. She said she had met once again with the couple, who had begun by saying they did not want to hassle over the money. Nevertheless, they both decided to see another lawyer, but somehow the patient felt relieved about it. She didn't think she had the energy to deal with the wife's coldness. In a way, the husband, for all his self-centeredness, seemed more concerned and spent more time with the daughter and on the house than did his wife. There was a silence.

I asked what she was thinking. She reached over for some tissues, got up, blew her nose, and walked over to the desk and threw the tissues in the wastebasket. She looked at the desk and came back and sat down. Then she began complaining again about me, how I had missed the point. She repeated again that I had noticed her pressure on Monday and commented on it, but did not go far enough. She seemed almost confused. Again I said that this seemed quite complicated, but this time I wondered if she were on the verge of remembering something.

She said she had been thinking of an image or a memory of a time in the old house—it must have been before her mother died. She had awakened early and come downstairs to the kitchen. It was morning but there was no one there yet. The room seemed very large and very empty. That's all she remembered. There was a pause. I asked if anything else came to mind. Nothing did. Again she spoke of feeling tired. Work was piling up on her desk. The birds and deer in her backyard were coming up to the house looking for food. She had not put any out. We were both quiet.

After another pause, she remarked again how cold this wife she evaluated seemed. I now commented that all of this, as well as her feelings about my coldness, might be a way of remembering her mother. For the first time in our work together, tears welled up in her eyes, and she shook her head back and forth, looked at her watch, and then gazed out the window. She asked when I would be moving back to the regular office. I told her the plan was in less than 2 weeks.

In the last part of the session, Ms. B. returned to the idea that a truly empathic person would have called after the hour on Monday, and how she felt I had let her down. She fingered a plant on the coffee table and commented that I was letting it die. She remembered another thing that bothered her about me on Monday, and that was how relaxed I was listening to her—another sign that I did not care. Looking at her watch again and seeing the time was almost up, she left—something she often did as a means of reestablishing control over the situation.

The next session began with Ms. B. raising questions about terminating. She did not; but it took several months for this memory to recur or be elaborated. More to the point, I think this brief vignette demonstrates many of the technical issues and controversies alluded to earlier. Following the second session, I reexamined my feeling of uneasiness at the end of the first one. It seemed to me that a perfectly reasonable approach for me to have taken during the abbreviated hour in this fourth year of treatment that was supposedly going well would go something like this: "I can see you are under a lot of pressure about this couple and very much want my advice, but I couldn't help notice that even though you were here on time today, you were 15 minutes late coming in, and I'm having trouble putting those two things together. What do you think?"

*   *   *

Unlike my more traditional approach, this more confrontive intervention, very much in the style of Kernberg, might have short-circuited Ms. B.'s attack, limited her sadistic and controlling behavior, and redirected attention to her defensive and provocative efforts to obfuscate her concerns about our closeness of the previous week. Waldinger and Gunderson (1987) have detailed the successful psychotherapy of five cases of patients with BPD, and in none of them is historical material or genetic reconstruction a significant focus. Kernberg would agree that historical material is less important than the patient's efforts to control the therapeutic interaction. His question about this intervention would be that 4 years is much too late in the game and that irreparable damage to the hopes for success with such a patient was done by not addressing her controlling, distorting behaviors early on.

Or one might have formulated an intervention from the second quadrant of the circle: "This cold mother in your office puts you in mind of how little you feel you get from me in this one—better you should keep a distance from such withholding influences." This intervention would have identified Ms. B.'s schizoid maneuvers, her paranoid fear of intrusion, and her difficulty integrating split object representations. As in Rosenfeld, this interpretation tries to return the projected indifference back to the patient.

Finally, one could take the patient at her literal word, acknowledge that an important empathic failure had occurred in the previous hour, and join with the patient in exploring its vicissitudes. In this quadrant, historical material, especially in the case of abuse, may be very important. This Kohutian-like intervention would hopefully provide a holding, soothing experience for the patient by acknowledging her pain, detoxifying the noxious stimulus, and making comprehensible her anger as secondary to not being heard.

The different kinds of approaches not only vary in terms of

therapeutic activity and material interpreted, they also involve changing from a focus on the *here and now* to one on the *there and then* as well as shifting from the internal world to external reality. With this patient who presents with mixed characterological features, I believe a good case can be made for all four. I have made a similar argument for technical flexibility in the psychotherapy of patients with narcissistic character pathology (Munich 1986). However, as suggested by this review, much of the controversy about theory and technique with borderline patients results from discussions about different patient types, and specific theories and techniques are differentially relevant depending on the kind of borderline patient you are treating. At different times in the treatment of a single patient, furthermore, different approaches might be more relevant. It is, however, the therapeutic dyad's harmony and disharmony—consonance and dissonance, if you will—that signals the need for shifts in technique and the evidence for genuine change in the patient. Too much harmony or too much dissonance can be either stultifying in a way that leads to overlooking important material or overstimulating in a way that disrupts useful exchange—and vice versa. One might contrast the point of view I have presented about the therapist's changing stances according to the patient's presentation with Waldinger and Gunderson's first recommendation that the therapeutic frame be as stable as possible. This is not an inconsiderable problem. If, however, the therapist can be reliable in the sense of consistency in the conditions of treatment, then adapting to the symptom picture with which the patient presents offers the patient the opportunity of integrating disparate elements in his or her psychic structure and representational life.

The tenuous relationship between theory and practice is no more evident than in the psychotherapeutic treatment of patients with BPD, an area fraught with ambiguity and unclarity. This is because the structural world, the representational world, and the world of the therapeutic interaction are constantly shifting in harmonious and disharmonious ways that challenge the further development of psychological theory and its coordination with technique.

References

Abend SM, Porder MS, Willick MS: Borderline Patients: Psychoanalytic Perspectives. New York, International Universities Press, 1983

American Psychiatric Association: Diagnostic and Statistical Manual of Mental Disorders, 3rd Edition, Revised. Washington, DC, American Psychiatric Association, 1987

Balint M: The Basic Fault. New York, Brunner/Mazel, 1979

Bion WR: Attacks on linking. Int J Psychoanal 40:308–315, 1959

Boyer LB, Giovacchini PL: Psychoanalytic Treatment of Schizophrenic, Borderline and Characterological Disorders. New York, Jason Aronson, 1967 [See also 2nd Edition, Revised and Expanded, 1980]

Brown LJ: Borderline personality organization and the transition to the depressive position, in The Borderline Patient. Edited by Grotstein JS, Solomon MF, Lang JA. NJ, Analytic Press, 1987, pp 147–180

Buie DH, Adler G: Definitive treatment of the borderline personality. International Journal of Psychoanalytic Psychotherapy 9:51–87, 1982–1983

Chessick RD: Intensive Psychotherapy of the Borderline Patient. New York, Jason Aronson, 1977

Deutsch H: Some forms of emotional disturbance and their relationship to schizophrenia. Psychoanal Q 11:301–321, 1942

Erikson E: Childhood and Society. New York, WW Norton, 1950

Fairbairn WRD: Psychoanalytic Studies of the Personality. London, Tavistock, 1952

Freud S: The ego and the id (1923), in The Standard Edition of the Complete Psychological Works of Sigmund Freud, Vol 19. Translated and edited by Strachey J. London, Hogarth Press, 1961, pp 11–66

Frosch J: Technique in regard to some specific ego defects in the treatment of borderline patients. Psychiatr Q 45:216–220, 1971

Giovacchini PL: Treatment of Primitive Mental States. New York, Jason Aronson, 1979

Grinker RR: The borderline syndrome: a phenomenological view, in Borderline Personality Disorders. Edited by Hartocallis P. New York, International Universities Press, 1977, pp 159–172

Guntrip H: Schizoid Phenomena, Object Relations and the Self. New York, International Universities Press, 1969

Jacobson E: The child's discovery of his identity and his advance to object relations and selective identifications, in The Self and the Object World. New York, International Universities Press, 1964, pp 49–69

Kernberg OF: Object-Relations Theory and Clinical Psychoanalysis. New York, Jason Aronson, 1976

Kernberg OF, Selzer MA, Koenigsberg HW, et al: Psychodynamic Psychotherapy of Borderline Patients. New York, Basic Books, 1989

Klein M: Notes on some schizoid mechanisms. Int J Psychoanal 27:145–174, 1946

Knight RP: Borderline states. Bull Menninger Clin 17:1–12, 1953

Kohut H: The Analysis of the Self. New York, International Universities Press, 1971

Lipton SD: The advantages of Freud's technique as shown in his analysis of the rat man. Int J Psychoanal 58:255–273, 1977

Loewald HW: Psychoanalytic theory and the psychoanalytic process, in Papers on Psychoanalysis. New Haven, CT, Yale University Press, 1980, pp 277–301

London NJ: An essay on psychoanalytic theory: two theories of schizophrenia, Part I: review and critical assessment of the two theories. Int J Psychoanal 54:169–178, 1973a

London NJ: An essay on psychoanalytic theory: two theories of schizophrenia, Part II: discussion and restatement of the specific theory of schizophrenia. Int J Psychoanal 54:179–193, 1973b

Mahler MS: A study of the separation-individuation process and its possible application to borderline phenomena in the psychoanalytic situation. Psychoanal Study Child 26:403–424, 1971

Masson JM: The Assault on Truth: Freud's Suppression of the Seduction Theory. New York, Farrar, Strauss & Giroux, 1984

Masterson JF: Psychotherapy of the Borderline Adult: A Developmental Approach. New York, Brunner/Mazel, 1976

Masterson JF, Rinsley DB: The borderline syndrome: the role of the mother in the genesis and psychic structure of the borderline personality. Int J Psychoanal 56:163–177, 1975

Munich RL: Some forms of narcissism in adolescents and young adults, in Adolescent Psychiatry: Developmental and Clinical Studies, Vol 13. Edited by Feinstein SC, et al. Chicago, IL, University of Chicago Press, 1986, pp 85–99

Pine F: Developmental Theory and Clinical Process. New Haven, CT, Yale University Press, 1985

Rosenfeld H: Projective identification and the problem of containment in a borderline psychotic patient, in Impasse and Interpretation: Therapeutic and Anti-Therapeutic Factors in the Psychoanalytic Treatment of Psychotic, Borderline, and Neurotic Patients. London, Tavistock, 1987, pp 191–208

Searles HF: My Work With Borderline Patients. Northvale, NJ, Jason Aronson, 1986 [See, especially, Chapter 3: Non-differentiation of ego functioning in the borderline individual and its effect on this sense of personal identity (pp 57–78).]

Stone L: The widening scope of indications for psychoanalysis. J Am Psychoanal Assoc 2:567–594, 1954

Stone M: Toward a psychobiological theory of borderline personality disorder: is irritability the red thread that runs through borderline conditions? Dissociation 1:1–15, 1988

Volkan V: Six Steps in the Treatment of Borderline Personality Organization. Northvale, NJ, Jason Aronson, 1987

Waldinger RJ: Intensive psychodynamic therapy with borderline patients: an overview. Am J Psychiatry 144:267–274, 1987

Waldinger RJ, Gunderson JG: Effective Psychotherapy With Borderline Patients: Case Studies. New York, American Psychiatric Press, 1987

Winnicott DW: Through Paediatrics to Psycho-Analysis. New York, Basic Books, 1975

Chapter 4

Assessment and Management of the Suicidal Patient

Howard C. Blue, M.D.
Claudia Bemis, M.D.
William H. Sledge, M.D.

S uicide is the eighth leading re- ported cause of death in the United States, with a rate of 12.5 per 100,000. Among young adults, the suicide rate has tripled over the past 30 years (Vaillant and Blumenthal 1990).

It is difficult to obtain an accurate rate of suicide because it is underreported on death certificates. Furthermore, some accidents and other violent deaths are suicidal acts. It is estimated that approximately 1,000 suicides occur each day worldwide (Centers for Disease Control 1985). Compared with death from other causes such as cardiovascular disease and cancer, suicide is a low-frequency event representing less than 1.5% of deaths from all causes in the United States. However, the tremendous impact that suicide has on a family, on a community, and on society as a whole underscores the urgent need for improved recognition of risk factors and the implementation of preventative interventions. Among the more tragic aspects of suicide as a cause of death is that it is mostly preventable. Whatever the multiple determinants of suicide, the individual uniqueness of the act of suicide and its low frequency make the assessment of the suicidal person a complex process (Motto 1989).

In this chapter our purpose is to provide an overview of suicide, with an emphasis on clinical risk factors. Case vignettes are used to demonstrate common and uncommon presentations of suicidal patients to guide the clinician's awareness toward careful assessment and management practices. We also present a pragmatic approach to clinical evaluation and intervention, in addition to discussing some medicolegal aspects of evaluating suicidal patients. Finally, the impact of suicide on survivors (family, friends, and clinicians) is identified, and the different aspects of bereavement for those deaths versus deaths from other causes are discussed.

Conceptual Bases

Sociological Studies

Throughout history suicide has been viewed both as a rational, honorable act in the face of injustice and defeat and as a form of madness or depravity. The first large sociological study of suicide was undertaken by Durkheim (1897/1951), who attempted to compare suicide rates in several European countries and the United States with social variables. Durkheim proposed that social, political, and economic forces acted on the individual and his or her capacity to be integrated and regulated by the society. Durkheim proposed four types of suicide based upon society's degree of integration and regulation of the individual: egoistic, altruistic, anomic, and fatalistic. Sociologists after Durkheim have emphasized the role of dynamic forces, such as the loss of social status and downward mobility and its relation to suicide. Limitations in sociological studies because of large population samples and the multiplicity of variables have been addressed by more detailed ecological studies of the social environment, to which we now turn.

Ecological Studies

Ecological studies of suicide have attempted to explore the social environment of the individual and its relation to suicide rates.

Sainbury (1955) compared the social characteristics of completed suicides in 28 boroughs in London, England, with epidemiological factors of 409 suicides in North London during the same periods. Higher rates of suicide were found among urban areas with high numbers of boardinghouses and hotels with transient populations. Suicide victims from North London, when compared with the general population, were often found to have been living alone, elderly, unemployed, and widowed, divorced, or separated from a spouse. Social isolation, social mobility, and social disorganization were concluded to be significantly correlated with suicide.

Maris (1969), in a study of Chicago communities, found that substandard housing correlated with high suicide rates. Findings of the direct impact of unemployment on suicidal behavior have been mixed. Platt (1984) found evidence indicating that attempted suicides occur more frequently among the unemployed than the employed. The duration of unemployment may be a significant risk factor for suicide because lengthy unemployment may contribute to a sense of hopelessness and other cumulative risk factors for suicide, such as poor self-esteem, poverty, family tension, alcoholism, and psychiatric illness.

Psychoanalytic Perspective

The classic psychoanalytic theory of suicide is derived from Freud's paper "Mourning and Melancholia" (1917[1915]/1957), in which he proposed that under conditions of ambivalent feelings toward a lost object, individuals introjected the object, including the negative and positive feelings. Under the circumstances of loss, rage of murderous proportions was stimulated and directed toward the introjected lost object now integrated within the self. The result could be self-murder. This idea of ambivalently held introjected object loss and subsequent rage and murderous intention has been the basis for the psychoanalytic theory of suicide. However, others have emphasized other perspectives. Menninger (1933) emphasized the primary role of the death instinct and conceptualized that the wish to kill was a superego or conscience function in response to a need for punishment. Menninger elaborated on the wish to kill, the wish to be killed, and the wish to die as being possible motivations for suicide.

The modern-day psychodynamic conception of suicide emphasizes the multidetermined and variable nature of the unconscious motivation for suicide. It is probably not the case that there is a single motivational structure for suicide. However, the psychodynamic understanding of the role of suicidal ideation in a particular individual is critical for effective evaluation, treatment, and management.

One of the motivations that has been emphasized by a variety of authors (see, e.g., Gabbard 1990) has been the element of *hostility*. Indeed, many suicidal patients have been noted to wish to harm the survivors of their act by killing themselves. In addition to the role of sadistic tormentor, suicidal victims think of themselves as victims tormented by others. Other motivational complexes have emphasized fantasies of reunion, merger, and, at times, hostile dependency (Dorpat 1973).

Biological Studies

Biologically mediated factors in suicide have received growing attention in the past 15 years. Much of this attention has been focused on the serotonergic system. Åsberg et al. (1976), in their landmark study, reported that persons with depression who attempted and completed suicides had low levels of the serotonin metabolite 5-hydroxyindoleacetic acid (5-HIAA) in their cerebrospinal fluid (CSF). Subsequent studies demonstrated lower CSF 5-HIAA levels in suicidal depressed individuals when compared with nonsuicidal depressed individuals (Agren 1980; Montgomery and Montgomery 1982; Palaniappan et al. 1983; van Praag 1982). Similar findings have also been reported for suicidal persons with schizophrenia, alcohol dependency, borderline personality disorder, and antisocial personality disorder when compared with nonsuicidal patients (Banki et al. 1986; Brown et al. 1979, 1982; Ninan et al. 1984; van Praag 1983). Decreased ^{3}H-labeled imipramine binding in tissue from the frontal cortex has also been found during postmortem examination of persons who completed suicide

(Stanley and Mann 1988). [³H]Imipramine binding is associated with pre- and postsynaptic 5-hydroxytryptophan (5-HT) neurons; reduced [³H]imipramine is suggestive of decreased functioning of the serotonergic terminals. Abnormal results on the dexamethasone suppression test and elevated levels of urinary metabolites of cortisol have also been found in suicide completers. Moreover, these findings have been associated with clinical depression. It is not clear whether any of these biological findings will define useful clinical markers for suicide potential, nor is it clear whether there are significant interactions between biological factors and psychosocial factors in increasing one's risk for suicide.

Suicide and Parasuicide

A large body of evidence exists that indicates that individuals who attempt suicide (i.e., parasuicide) are different as a group from those who complete suicide (Table 4–1).

Farberow and Shneidman (1961) estimate that there are at least eight suicide attempts for every completed suicide. Follow-up studies of persons who have attempted suicide indicate that 1% to 2% actually kill themselves within a year following their initial at-

Table 4–1.   Comparison of patients who either completed or attempted suicide

	Completed suicides	**Suicide attempts**
Gender	Predominantly male	Predominantly female
Age	Elderly	Majority under 35
Psychiatric disorders	Majority with affective disorder and/or alcoholism	No disorder or presence of personality disorder only
Means	Firearms—more lethal and rapid	Ingestions, wrist slashings—ineffective and requiring time to culminate in death
Communication of intent	Usually no	Yes
Setting	Isolated	Public, high potential for exposure to others

tempt. Approximately 10% of the total number of persons attempting suicide will complete suicide at a later time (Kreitman 1977).

Risk Factors for Suicide

Recognition of risk factors for suicide is key for the prevention of suicide and the targeting of programs for education and intervention. It is important to consider that risk factors change across the life cycle and will depend upon the population being studied. For example, risk factors for hospitalized psychiatric patients are different from those for ambulatory psychiatric patients. Some of the factors associated with higher and lower risk for suicide are compared in Table 4–2.

Table 4–2.   Risk factors for suicide

Characteristic	Higher-risk group	Lower-risk group
Age	Adolescents, young adults, elderly	Middle adult years
Gender	Male	Female
Race	Whites, American Indians, Alaskan natives	Blacks, Hispanics
Marital status	Single, divorced, living alone	Married
Religion	Protestantism	Catholicism, Judaism
Geographic region (United States)	Mountain states	Middle Atlantic states
Psychiatric disorder	Affective disorders, panic disorder, alcohol and substance abuse	Somatization, OCD
Genetics	Monozygotic twin of suicide victim, family history of suicide	Dizygotic twin of suicide victim
Biological	Possible low levels of 5-HIAA in CSF	Normal levels of 5-HIAA in CSF

Note.   OCD = obsessive-compulsive disorder; 5-HIAA = 5-hydroxyindoleacetic acid; CSF = cerebrospinal fluid.

Psychiatric Disorder

The most frequently associated risk factor for suicide is the presence of a psychiatric disorder. It has been estimated that over 90% of persons who commit suicide suffer from a psychiatric disorder (Barraclough et al. 1974; Buda and Tsuang 1990; Dorpat and Ripley 1960; Robins 1981). Major affective disorders comprise the largest single diagnostic group among completed suicides. Guze and Robins (1970) estimated that approximately 15% of patients with affective disorders, including unipolar and bipolar disorders, will eventually kill themselves. Studies have been mixed as to whether suicide risk is greater or less in patients with bipolar disorder when compared with patients with unipolar disorder (Angst et al. 1979; Black et al. 1987; Dunner et al. 1976; McGlashan 1984; Morrison 1982). Compared with rates in other diagnostic groups, the suicide rate in depressed patients ranges from 3.5 to 4.5 times higher and is from 22 to 36 times higher than in the general population (Pokorny 1964; Temoche et al. 1964).

It has been estimated that nearly 10% of patients with schizophrenia will commit suicide (Miles 1977; Tsuang 1978). Likewise, some investigators have estimated that 10% of chronic alcoholic individuals will kill themselves (Miles 1977). Intoxication at the time of death, as measured by blood alcohol levels, may be associated with suicide in 90% of alcoholic persons compared with 40% of nonalcoholic individuals (Dorpat and Ripley 1960). Other drugs of abuse frequently accompany suicide and suicide attempts.

Recent studies indicate that panic disorder is associated with higher rates of suicide attempts than are found in the general population (Johnson et al. 1990; Weissman et al. 1989). On the other hand, somatization and obsessive-compulsive disorders have not been associated with increased suicide risk (Coryell 1981); however, a coexisting Axis I disorder such as major depression may increase the risk of suicide.

Personality disorders have not been studied sufficiently by themselves to establish their contribution to suicide rates. Difficulties lie in the high frequency of comorbid Axis I disorders and substance-use disorders in patients with personality disorders. Persons with borderline personality disorder and antisocial personality disorder have suicide rates of 4%–10% and 5%, respectively (Akiskal et al. 1985; Maddocks 1970; Miles 1977; Paris et al. 1987; Pope et al. 1983). The risk of suicide is broken down by particular diagnosis and presented in Table 4–3.

The characteristics of suicide in affective disorders, schizophrenia, and alcohol dependency are given in Tables 4–4, 4–5, and 4–6, respectively.

Age

The overall rate of suicide for all ages has not changed in the past 20 years in the United States; however, significant shifts have occurred among specific age groups. Suicide rates are highest in the over-65 age group, which comprises 11% of the population but contributes to 17% of all suicides (McIntosh 1985). Compared with younger populations, the elderly communicate their suicidal intent less openly to others and use more violent and lethal means; they infrequently use suicide attempts as a cry for help and may be more concerned about health problems (Copeland 1987; Osgood and Thielman 1990).

The suicide rate among adolescents has risen from 2.6 to 8.5 per 100,000 over the past 30 years and represents the second leading cause of adolescent deaths (Blumenthal 1988; Centers for Disease Control 1985; Shaffer and Fisher 1981). Klerman and Weissman (1989) suggest that changing environmental factors interacting with genetic liability have played a role in shifting both depression and suicide to younger age groups. In cases where psychological autopsy was used to render diagnoses, affective disorders and substance-use disorders were frequently found (Brent et al. 1988; Shafii et al. 1985).

Gender

Males commit suicide at greater rates than females among all age groups. When gender and age are viewed together over time, the ratio of male to female suicide has increased dramatically in the 15-

Table 4–3. Number of suicides (broken down by psychiatric diagnosis)

	Men		
Diagnosis	Observed deaths	Expected deaths	SMR[a]
Organic mental disorders	1	0.34	2.94
Schizophrenia	9	0.29	31.00[*]
Acute schizophrenia	3	0.12	25.00[**]
Affective disorder	9	0.57	15.79[*]
Neuroses	4	0.11	36.36[**]
Depressive neuroses	1	0.11	9.09
Personality disorder	5	0.42	11.91[**]
Alcohol and other drug abuse	3	0.27	11.11[***]
Adjustment disorder	2	0.16	17.50
Psychophysiological disorders and special symptoms	0	0.07	0
Total	37	2.46	14.98

	Women		
Diagnosis	Observed deaths	Expected deaths	SMR[a]
Organic mental disorders	0	0.08	0
Schizophrenia	5	0.08	62.51[*]
Acute schizophrenia	2	0.03	66.67[***]
Affective disorder	13	0.21	61.91[*]
Neuroses	1	0.06	16.67
Depressive neuroses	4	0.05	80.06[**]
Personality disorder	2	0.12	16.67
Alcohol and other drug abuse	3	0.05	60.00[**]
Adjustment disorder	1	0.05	20.00
Psychophysiological disorders and special symptoms	0	0.02	0
Total	31	0.75	41.33[*]

[a]Indicates *standardized mortality ratio,* which is the ratio of observed to expected deaths. These data suggest that a male with a diagnosis of schizophrenia is 31 times more likely to commit suicide than someone from the general population.

[*]Observed mortality significantly different from that expected ($P < .001$).

[**]Observed mortality significantly different from that expected ($P < .01$).

[***]Observed mortality significantly different from that expected ($P < .05$).

Source. Reprinted from Black DW, Warrack G, Winokur G: "The Iowa Record Linkage Study, I: Suicide and Accidental Deaths Among Psychiatric Patients." *Archives of General Psychiatry* 42:71–75, 1985. Copyright 1985, American Medical Association. Used with permission.

to 19-year-old age group: from 0.7 to 1 in 1911 to 4.7 to 1 in 1980 (Buda and Tsuang 1990).

Race

White persons commit suicide at two times the rate of nonwhite persons. The ratio of suicides by white persons to those by non-

Table 4–4. Risk factors in affective disorders

Risk factor(s)	Study	Comments
Single, living alone, prior history of attempt	Roy (1983)	21 depressed suicide and 21 depressed control subjects matched for gender and age
Living alone	Murphy and Robins (1967)	Review of 134 consecutive suicides
Hopelessness	Beck et al. (1985)	5- to 10-year follow-up of 207 patients hospitalized for suicidal ideation
Psychosis	Roose et al. (1983)	Study of hospitalized psychotically depressed patients
	Black et al. (1988) Wolfersdorf et al. (1987) Coryell and Tsuang (1982)	Longer-term follow-up showing no predisposition with psychosis

Table 4–5. Characteristics of suicide in persons with schizophrenia

Characteristic	Studies
Early in course of illness	Lindelius and Kay (1973)
Higher educational level	Drake et al. (1984)
Nonpsychotic phase of illness	Breier and Astrachan (1984); Roy (1982a)
No communication of intent	Allebeck et al. (1987); Breier and Astrachan (1984)
Less than 30 years old	Breier and Astrachan (1984); Roy (1982b)
Unemployment	Roy (1982b)
Chronic relapsing course	Farberow et al. (1966); Roy (1982b)
Prior depression	Cohen et al. (1964); Roy (1982b)

Table 4–6. Characteristics of suicide in persons with alcohol dependency

Characteristic	Study
Long duration of alcoholism	Robins et al. (1959)
Comorbidity with other psychiatric disorders, especially depression	Barraclough et al. (1974)
Recent interpersonal loss	Murphy and Robins (1967)
Poor physical health	Motto (1980)
Poor work history in previous years	Motto (1980)
History of previous attempts	Motto (1980)

white persons changes across age categories, with the smallest ratio across the 15- to 24-year-old and the 25- to 34-year-old age groups; the largest ratio occurs for those over age 75 (Buda and Tsuang 1990).

Marital Status

Suicide is more prevalent in single, separated, divorced, and widowed individuals. People in intact marriages with children have the lowest rates of suicide (Buda and Tsuang 1990; Durkheim 1951; Maris 1969).

Religion

Religion as a variable demonstrates that suicide rates among Protestants are greater than those among Catholics and Jews (Durkheim 1951).

Geography

The mountain states in the United States have the highest suicide rates in the country; the middle Atlantic states have the lowest rates. Worldwide, the Eastern European nations, Switzerland, Scandinavia, and Japan have the highest rates of suicide. Italy and Spain are the nations with the lowest suicide rates (Buda and Tsuang 1990).

Family History

A family history of suicide has been shown to be a significant risk factor. Twin studies have demonstrated a higher concordance rate of suicide in monozygotic twin pairs when compared with dizygotic twin pairs (Haberlandt 1967). Adoption studies have shown there is a significantly higher incidence of suicide in the biological relatives of adoptees who committed suicide when compared with adoptive relatives (Wender et al. 1986). Family stress and psychiatric disorders as shared risk factors are confounding variables that were not controlled in these genetic studies. Tsuang et al. (1980) demonstrated an increased incidence of schizophrenia and affective disorders among the biological relatives of persons with schizophrenia and manic-depressive illness. Tsuang (1983) and Roy (1983) both demonstrated a significantly greater incidence of suicidal behavior in the families of patients who committed suicide. The findings of these studies have contributed to the debate over whether suicides in families are a result of a genetic predisposition to psychiatric disorders or of psychological processes related to the suicidal death of a relative.

Life Events

Studies have shown that individuals with suicidal behavior also have more extensive histories of negative life events, such as occupational problems, change in residence, and object loss, particularly in the weeks and months prior to the suicidal event (Cochrane and Robertson 1975; Hagnell and Rorsman 1980; Isherwood et al. 1982; Paykel et al. 1975). Many studies have also demonstrated a high degree of recent interpersonal conflict prior to attempted and completed suicides (Adam 1985; Goldney and Burvill 1980; Stengel 1964; Weissman 1974). The latter factor has been particularly demonstrated in alcoholic persons (Murphy and Robins 1967).

The impact of early parental loss has been examined as a contributor to increased suicide risk. Many of these studies have been methodologically flawed because of their failure to define early parental loss and to control for confounding variables. Comparison of studies demonstrates considerable variability in the definition of early parental loss and failure to discriminate between loss due to death, separation, or divorce. There has been little attention to the duration of the loss (i.e., permanent vs. time-limited) or the impact of the gender of the "lost parent" and the quality of relationship with that parent prior to the separation. Few studies have utilized structured interviews. Most have relied on self-reports, which are frequently unreliable for detailed accounts of early childhood experiences.

Physical Illness

Chronic debilitating diseases, such as cancer, Huntington's chorea, epilepsy, rheumatoid arthritis, multiple sclerosis, and acquired immunodeficiency syndrome (AIDS), have been associated with higher suicide risk (Chandler et al. 1960; Dorpat et al. 1968; Farberow et al. 1963; Kahana et al. 1971; Louhivuori and Hakama 1979; Marshall et al. 1983; Marzuk et al. 1988; Matthews and Barabas 1981; Muller 1949; Pokorny 1960; Whitlock 1978). Physical illness can initiate or exacerbate a psychiatric illness. Suicide and suicide attempts in physically ill persons rarely occur in the absence of psychiatric disorders (usually depression or alcoholism) (Dorpat et al. 1968; MacKenzie and Popkin 1987; Robins 1981; Robins et al. 1959). The so-called rational suicides in the context of terminal illness appear to be infrequent (Robins et al. 1959; Sainbury 1956; Seager and Flood 1965).

Assessment and Management

In this section we focus on the evaluation and management of the suicidal patient and address some of the consequences of completed suicides for survivors—both the clinician and the patient's family. This section is oriented for work within emergency rooms and other crisis-oriented centers; however, the general principles apply to any clinical setting.

The suicidal patient presents the psychiatric clinician with one of the true emergencies of psychiatric medicine. The risk that a patient may elect to die and is the agent of his or her own destruction will raise anxiety and perhaps anger in the evaluator. A careful and respectful evaluation of the patient provides the best chance for the patient to be understood and for the most appropriate treatment intervention to be made. It is also important for the clinician to recognize that the management of the suicidal patient is influenced by clinical findings as well as legal considerations.

The clinician's effectiveness in assessing suicidal patients will be enhanced if patients are approached with empathy and circumspection. It is crucial that the clinician maintain what some have described as "compassionate detachment" when working with suicidal patients, such that the clinician is able to empathize with the person's level of distress but not become overwhelmed by the affects that may be generated by this often difficult clinical situation.

Clinical Issues of Assessment

In order to arrive at the most appropriate interventions for suicidal patients, the clinician must be able to form an effective rapport with patients and to perform a comprehensive assessment of the circumstances that may contribute to the patient's level of distress.

There are five key areas that the clinician must address in his or her evaluation of the patient:

1. The clinician must establish rapport with the patient so that the patient feels free to disclose his or her personal feelings.
2. The clinician should elicit the patient's thoughts, feelings, and motives for the suicidal thinking or the suicide attempt. If the patient has performed a suicidal act, then the clinician must determine the circumstances of that act. For example, was the patient secreted away to perform the act or did he or she do it in a manner so as to be discovered quickly? What method was used? What was the anticipated outcome? Was the act impul-

sive or well planned? Was the individual sober or under the influence of intoxicants? and so forth.

3. The clinician should determine if the patient feels hopeless and, if so, to what degree.

4. The clinician must determine if there are signs and symptoms of psychopathology by performing a thorough mental status examination that assesses mood, thought processes, perceptual experiences, cognitive style, degree of insight and judgment, and the presence or absence of internal controls that may help the patient refrain from acting on suicidal thoughts. It is critically important to determine the patient's reaction to surviving a suicide attempt—for example, does he or she feel remorseful or relieved about surviving?

5. The clinician must assess the patient's social environment, paying particular attention to the quality and reliability of the patient's emotional supports.

The aforementioned key areas of evaluation are applicable to any clinical setting, regardless of whether the patient is well known to the clinician or meeting the clinician for the first time.

Assessment Scales

Scales to assess suicide risk have been criticized because of the relatively small samples involved in their development, the nongeneralizability of critical factors in suicide, the individual uniqueness of the act of suicide, and problems demonstrating reliability and validity of instruments in general. Scales are not useful in helping clinicians predict who will kill themselves. The most appropriate use of scales is as a supplement to clinical judgment to help guide the clinician in ascertaining those factors associated with increased suicide risk.

Patterson et al. (1983) developed the SAD PERSONS Scale to aid clinicians in assessing the relative risk of suicide for patients presenting with defined characteristics. The scale includes the following items: sex, age, depression, previous history, ethanol use, rational thinking loss, lack of social support, lack of spouse, organized suicide plan, and sickness. A total score is derived from the presence or absence of one of these 10 items, and the score is used to guide decisions about disposition.

Beck et al. (1974) have developed a Suicide Intent Scale (SIS) for suicide attempters. The SIS is used to examine defined aspects of the suicide attempt, including precautions against discovery, level of planning, communication of attempt, perceived level of lethality of method, and relationship between substance use and the attempt.

Both the SAD PERSONS Scale and the SIS provide guides in the decision-making process regarding suicidal patients; however, the ultimate clinical interventions will be based on a synthesis of multiple clinical and psychosocial findings.

Interventions

The management of the suicidal patient will be determined by the clinician's findings during the assessment, the circumstances under which the patient presents, and the characteristics of the expression of suicidal behavior (i.e., ideation only, ideation with a plan, or postsuicide attempt). If the patient has made a suicide attempt, the medical condition of the patient is paramount and must be attended to before an appropriate psychiatric disposition can be instituted. Emergency rooms have established protocols for the evaluation and management of patients who present after overdoses, and the medical attention that other patients who have attempted suicide receive will depend on the method used in the attempt. The clinician must always be aware of the secretive "self-poisoner" and monitor the suicidal person for signs of overdose.

There are two options when developing treatment plans for the suicidal patient; 1) the patient is hospitalized or 2) the patient is referred for outpatient treatment.

Inpatient treatment.   The decision to hospitalize a patient is a serious matter and represents the most restrictive of available interventions. In general, decisions to hospitalize a patient will be based upon a combination of clinical and psychosocial factors.

Guggenheim (1984) has suggested absolute and relative indications for hospitalization. Among those findings that he indicates strongly support hospitalization after a suicide attempt are psychosis, age 40 or older (unless there has been a history of multiple manipulative gestures without any increase in the degree of risk taken or an increase in attempts to avoid rescue), and a premeditated near-lethal attempt. Although diagnosis and symptoms may influence decisions to hospitalize patients, they should not dictate the decision. Inpatient treatment is obligatory only when there is a need for 24-hour medical supervision of the patient, if it is necessary to remove the patient from a social environment that is noxious and likely to exacerbate suicidal intention, or if adequate social and clinical supports cannot be mobilized to maintain the patient in outpatient treatment safely.

After a patient is hospitalized, care must be taken to remain aware that suicidal behavior and attempts to act on the suicidal impulses and thoughts can continue during the hospitalization. Suicide precautions must be employed, including continuous monitoring of the patient and restriction of the patient's access to objects that could be used as suicide weapons (belts, sharp instruments, etc.). It is also important to remain attentive to the possibility that staff will assume inappropriately that simply being in the hospital reduces the risk for the patient. Staff may also assume, erroneously, that the rapid diminution of suicidal ideation upon admission suggests that the patient may be ready for an early discharge. The hospital provides patients with a level of support that cannot be replicated outside the hospital, and in some cases the patient's suicidal impulses may decrease while hospitalized but reemerge upon discharge because adequate and reliable supports are absent. It is important to be aware that patients have eloped from hospitals and killed themselves and have even killed themselves while in the hospital.

Outpatient treatment. Outpatient treatment of the suicidal patient may include day hospital; outpatient crisis intervention, involving frequent and intensive contact; or mobile outreach. The choice of outpatient treatment will be made if the clinician determines that the relative risk of suicide is low and that adequate supports are in place. The particular outpatient treatment intervention will depend on the intensity of follow-up required. If the patient is symptomatic enough to require daily contact but has fairly good social supports, then day-hospital treatment may be the optimal treatment choice. If the patient requires frequent contact but does not require daily supervision, then an outpatient crisis intervention model that ensures therapist availability and flexibility may be reasonable and appropriate. Regardless of the treatment modality chosen, the clinician must develop a plan of action that underscores therapist availability and the availability of other treatment and social supports. No patient who presents with suicidal ideation or who has made a suicide attempt should be discharged from any setting until follow-up care is clearly defined and arranged.

The following cases will be used to illustrate applications of the evaluation and management principles that should be involved in assessing the suicidal individual:

Case 1

Ms. A., a 37-year-old divorced mother of two, has been in various types of psychiatric treatment since age 13. She has had approximately 16 hospitalizations since age 14 for the treatment of anorexia, depression, and suicidal ideation or intent. Her two sons (ages 15 and 12) live with their father in accordance with a custody agreement; however, Ms. A. has liberal visitation rights. Although trained as a legal secretary, she is unable to "tolerate the pressure of a law office" and chooses to work for a temporary employment agency. Because of her considerable knowledge and skill, she has no difficulty in finding work.

As noted above, Ms. A. has had multiple hospitalizations because of suicidal ideation or actual suicide attempts. She has made three nearly lethal attempts over the past 5 years and has presented on multiple occasions to her therapists with intense suicidal ideations. She states that she is never "not suicidal" because "life has no real meaning." She experiences mild to moderate depressions but has only had two major depressive episodes. She sees herself as a failure in all her endeavors and is particularly sensitive to actual or perceived criticisms. She is certain that anyone she "gets close to" will abandon her. She feels unable to trust others and fails to see that she "makes any difference to anyone's life." Two of her most severe suicide attempts occurred when her therapists were on vacations. She has shifted therapists on many occasions, usually citing their lack of understanding of her as the reason for leaving the therapy. In actuality, the disruptions in treatment often followed periods of intense work and much self-revelation and self-examination.

She has been with her current therapist for the past 19 months, her longest period of treatment with one person. During this time she has made nearly a dozen suicide attempts. Typically, she attempts suicide by ingesting sublethal doses of medications or by cutting her wrists in ways that require minimal surgical intervention. More substantial attempts are made in a context where rescue is guaranteed. At times, issues raised in therapy initiate an increase in suicidal thinking; however, at other times, no identifiable precipitant is present. During the past 19 months she has had one brief hospitalization after becoming intensely anxious and acutely suicidal during her therapist's vacation. Prior to the therapist's vacation, Ms. A. had become increasingly angry and was demanding to end therapy. She took an overdose of barbiturates that she obtained from her internist. Recent increases in suicidal thinking began when she recalled a period of sexual abuse by her father. She believed her mother knew about the sexual abuse but "looked the other way."

The chronically suicidal patient in a clinical practice presents many challenges to the therapist. These patients may not present with any precipitating crisis and are more likely to engender anger in clinicians than patients presenting with precipitating crises (Dressler et al. 1975). The therapist is constantly presented with the need to assess shifts in the patient to determine the seriousness of the patient's suicidal intent within the ongoing therapeutic relationship. Contracts with the patient not to harm himself or herself are frequently not reliable and may serve to provide false reassurance to the therapist. In an attempt to ensure safety the therapist may also err by not prescribing medication that may be indicated, because of fears that a patient may use it to overdose.

In therapy with the suicidal patient, the therapist must be ever attentive to his or her own activity level, availability, degree of tolerance of the suicidal thoughts and behaviors, and the particular feelings engendered by the patient. The therapist must do all that can be done to ensure that he or she will respond to the patient appropriately and empathically. Understanding, whenever possible, the dynamics of the suicidal actions is extraordinarily helpful in developing one's responses. The therapist must have some appreciation of the meaning of the patient's actions and of any underlying clinical or environmental factors that may contribute to the patient's self-destructiveness.

Self-destructive action may not be a wish to die. It may be the patient's attempt to deal with intolerable affects such as rage, despair, emptiness, and deprivation (Buie and Adler 1972). In many instances patients acknowledge a sense of relief after a self-destructive or self-mutilating action. Suicidal action may be an attempt to mitigate intense feelings of loneliness and isolation. It may feel like the only conceivable option for someone who feels helpless and hopeless. Some suicides may be psychotically based and may represent an opportunity to achieve a reunion with someone who has already died, or they may represent delusional responses to feeling controlled by alien forces living within the person. Other suicides may be symbolic and represent an intent to hurt or injure someone else. A myriad of possible motives may exist and may be unique for each individual suicidal action.

In the preceding case, the patient's panic over the therapist's absence during vacation and her angry reactions to it led to a suicidal crisis. The patient's limited sense of object constancy and the fragile sense of herself as a cohesive and autonomous being crumbled under the intense feelings of perceived abandonment by the therapist, and primitive defenses were evoked to cope with the pain of her perceived loss. Some of her suicidal actions were probably precipitated by hostility and a desire to punish the therapist for abandoning her. Frosch (1990) comments that

> in reaction to loss, there may be a feeling of hatred and anger to the loss, and a feeling of guilt at one's culpability in contributing to this loss. The hatred and aggression may have been primary

and played a role in creating this loss. The guilt feeling may be due either to having done something to contribute to the loss, or not doing something to prevent it. (p. 381)

Under such circumstances, the patient's self-esteem may suffer further and may eventuate in a suicide attempt. In the case of Ms. A., the patient's capacity for trust is compromised by her experiences with sexual molestation by her father and her belief that her mother tacitly concurred with his actions; hence, the relationship with the therapist is bound to be fraught with ambivalence. Her frequent therapy terminations suggest that close and caring relationships are difficult for her to manage. The struggles that she has exhibited with other therapists are possibly derived from her sense that these individuals could not or would not respond to her needs even if she reached out to them. In much the same way her own mother could not or would not reach out to her and protect her. Her acting out may be a result of the hostile dependency that she tends to form. She desires to be taken care of but resents having such needs. In many patients the hostile dependency of their relationships and the devalued sense of self may be causative agents in their self-destructiveness. The therapist must attend to issues of self-worth and self-esteem in patients who have failed to develop a sense of autonomy, whose self-worth is in question, and who feel that they do not matter. The therapist must reach out to them and respond consistently and honestly.

Jacobs (1989) comments that in treating suicidal patients the "challenge is to be where the patient is—a place where, under ordinary circumstances, we would not choose to go" (p. 341). He further notes that "the issue of responsibility should not be confused with overprotectiveness nor omnipotence—it is merely being sensitive to and facing the gravity of the patient's situation" (p. 341). Within these comments are the framework for working with suicidal patients. That is, the therapist must 1) develop the ability to empathize with the patient's pain, 2) be attentive to the meaning of a suicidal action and why death is desirable for some people, and 3) be aware that suicide occurs across a spectrum of illnesses and circumstances. Understanding these dimensions of a suicidal patient enhances one's capacity to respond appropriately. For a chronically suicidal patient the therapist has to emphasize that the decision to live or die is ultimately under the control of the patient and is the patient's responsibility. The therapist's role may be that of protector whenever it is possible; however, the therapist's primary function must be aimed toward reinforcing more adaptive responses and actions.

Case 2

Mr. B., a 79-year-old twice-widowed white male, was brought to the emergency room by ambulance after his live-in girlfriend summoned 911 for assistance after finding Mr. B. covered with blood. Mr. B. claimed that he had accidentally cut himself when the knife he was using to slice bread slipped. Mr. B. was evaluated by a surgical resident in the ER who noted that in addition to a 3"-by-1" gaping wrist laceration, there were also a number of fresh smaller cuts. The surgical resident requested a psychiatric consultation to assess Mr. B.'s suicide risk. Mr. B. appeared mildly intoxicated at the time of admission to the ER, and his blood alcohol level was indeed 130 mg %.

Mr. B. vehemently denied that he was suicidal to the consulting psychiatrist and insisted that he was simply the victim of a careless accident. He denied that he had any problems at all. However, his girlfriend and family gave a differing account. Mr. B.'s girlfriend and two of his daughters stated that Mr. B. had become more depressed recently and had started drinking excessively. He had been arrested twice in the past 6 months for driving while intoxicated and had had his driver's license suspended. He had also begun to complain about some visual problems and was afraid that he would go blind. Additionally, his golden retriever had to be "put to sleep" because of advancing age and illness. His girlfriend stated that Mr. B. spoke of wanting to be "put to sleep too" because he no longer felt useful. These comments were mostly in the context of intoxication. Mr. B.'s girlfriend was convinced that he had tried to kill himself and that he may have succeeded if she had not returned home earlier than she had intended. Mr. B.'s girlfriend had asked him to talk to a counselor; however, he rejected her suggestions, stating, "Ain't no shrink gonna dig around in my head. I ain't never needed one before and I don't need one now."

Mr. B. appeared mildly to moderately depressed. Initially, he was pleasant and accommodating, but became more irascible as the interview went on. He became tearful when talking about his dog. He denied suicidal ideation, insisting that the wrist injury was an accident. When asked about the other cuts, he denied having any.

The emergency room is likely to be the site where most suicidal individuals will be encountered. The evaluation and management of suicidal patients in this setting may be a considerably complicated matter. Often, the clinician is confronted with making decisions about the likelihood of suicide in someone whom they are seeing for the first time. The decision making is complicated by the wide spectrum of emotional disorders of which suicidal ideation or action is a manifestation and by the clinician's lack of accuracy in predicting suicidal behavior.

Emergency-room settings often require rapid decision making in a context of high patient volume and limited resources. In evaluating suicidal intent, the clinician is faced with the knowledge that not every self-destructive act is indicative of a desire to die. Deciding which act is a cry for help and which act is a desire to die fuels the affect associated with evaluating and treating suicidal patients. The clinician may be pressed by feelings of anxiety, fear, anger, pity, or hopelessness in confronting such an individually unique phenomenon as suicide. Such feelings may jeopardize the establishment of a relationship that permits the patient to feel understood and validated. Management of these feelings is necessary so that the patient does not experience the clinician as rejecting or indifferent to his or her distress. The patient must be able to sense that the evaluating clinician will attempt to understand the patient's pain and respond with tolerance, patience, and flexibility. Inexperienced clinicians often feel compelled to find immediate solutions to the patient's dilemma; however, it is unlikely that these solutions will be found in a transient relationship. Nevertheless, the emergency-room clinician may be able to set the tone for future therapeutic relationships by providing a benign, permissive environment for the patient to examine his or her feelings.

Although Mr. B. has multiple risk factors for suicide (i.e., advanced age, alcohol abuse, depressive symptoms, evidence of a recent suicide attempt, medical problems, and recent losses), he denies suicidal intent and is reluctant to contemplate treatment. In such instances, the evaluating clinician must make every effort to elicit information from the patient's close associates and family to develop a better profile of the patient. It would be a mistake to discharge this man from the emergency room without a comprehensive treatment plan that seemed reasonable and acceptable to the patient as well as to the patient's associates and family. In this case, the patient's denial that anything is wrong or that there is any need for treatment forces the clinician to be more conservative in his plans. The most reasonable response to this circumstance is hospitalization of the patient for further evaluation so that better, more detailed assessment can be made of his depression, alcohol abuse, and physical problems.

Once the immediate plan has been implemented, the course of action will depend upon a clinician's ability to engage Mr. B. in a trusting, caring relationship. One should not expect this immediately; however, it is possible that the level of concern shown by those evaluating him in the ER may lead to more self-disclosure and comfort in talking about difficult and painful emotions. If he can get past his presumptions about therapists and find some value in psychotherapy, it may be possible to explore his concerns and feelings about his declining function and independence.

Case 3

Mr. C., a 57-year-old married white male, presented to an emergency walk-in clinic on a Friday afternoon with his wife of 10 years. Mr. C.'s wife was the identified patient at the time of their presentation, although both Mr. and Ms. C. had extensive psychiatric histories. The couple had presented to the clinic requesting assistance in getting Ms. C.'s family to give them a place to live. The couple had arrived in the area several weeks prior to their presentation and had been assisted by Ms. C.'s daughter in locating a temporary place to live and in being connected to ongoing outpatient treatment. Because of their history of mismanaging money, Ms. C.'s daughter requested that the couple allow her to become payee for their social security disability checks to ensure that rent and utilities were paid and that the couple had spending money. Ms. C. objected to this arrangement, stating that the family should pay for the couple's housing. When the family refused to do this, the couple moved into a local shelter. Their experiences in the shelter led to their presentation to the clinic. Ms. C.'s daughter confessed to one of the clinicians that she might consider housing her mother alone but did not feel any desire or obligation to house Mr. C.

Although Mr. C. had an extensive psychiatric history, he did not exhibit any evidence of thought disorder, psychosis, or mood disturbance. In fact, he appeared euthymic and pleasant throughout his interviews with the clinic staff. There was some evidence of borderline intellectual functioning. He denied any suicidal ideation but readily described a remote suicide attempt via overdose after an argument with his wife over "cigarettes." He did admit to past auditory hallucinations that instructed him to "dress in women's clothes." His only current complaint was about epigastric pain, which had been persistent for 2 to 3 days.

A comprehensive treatment plan was developed for the couple and included the provision of temporary housing by the daughter, the setting up of appointments with the homeless health care clinic for the following morning to evaluate Mr. C.'s epigastric pain, and a return to the clinic on the following Monday for further clarification of the couple's treatment and housing options. The couple and the daughter were informed of the clinic's availability throughout the weekend if problems emerged. All parties seemed pleased with these plans.

Approximately 48 hours after leaving the clinic, Mr. C. hung himself. He did not leave a suicide note. He was discovered by his wife when she and her daughter returned from morning church services. While preparing for a review of the suicide, the clinic that had most recently treated Mr. C. revealed that his last suicide attempt occurred after he was excluded from a family party that his wife attended.

This case is a tragic reminder that patients may kill themselves even if you have done the most comprehensive assessment. It also reminds us that demographic characteristics are only useful when combined with the clinical state of an individual. Because psychological functioning is a dynamic process, one may expect that a person's social environment can lead to changes in this functioning. The circumstances related to Mr. C.'s suicide will never be fully understood. One may speculate that something transpired in his environment that made him believe that he had no option except death. His previous attempt occurred within the context of feeling excluded and peripheral. Amid this current crisis and his step-daughter's reluctance to assist him, he may have felt peripheral again and burdensome to others. Additionally, he may have felt inadequate because of his own mental illness and his inability to provide for his wife. This narcissistic injury, with its resultant diminution of self-esteem, may have stimulated significant anger and rage that led to self-destruction. Also, the patient's limited intellectual functioning may have interfered with his ability to create a more adaptive response. Although he exhibited neither psychotic symptoms nor disorganized behavior at the time of his initial evaluation, it is certainly possible that under stress he became more psychotic and that this contributed to the actions that eventually led to his death. Although death was the result, we cannot be certain that the actual intent of this man's action was death.

Legal Issues

All states allow persons to be committed to a hospital if they are judged likely to kill themselves. State legislatures have adopted procedures and rules that regulate mandated psychiatric hospitalization. These regulations vary from state to state in regard to a number of parameters, including definitions of mental disorder, length of time a patient can be committed to a hospital involuntarily, and the threshold for involuntary commitment. All states have procedures for patient appeal of involuntary commitment to a hospital as well as procedures for voluntary patients to seek release if the hospital does not concur with the patient's request to be discharged. Every state requires that a patient be mentally disordered upon commitment. The statutory definitions of mental disorder may be explicit or they may be relatively vague. For example, some states have excluded personality disorders specifically, while others have excluded mental retardation from categorization as a mental disorder.

States have granted themselves the power to act in the presumed best interest of their citizens. For the psychiatrically ill, these *parens patriae* powers are invoked to provide treatment when it is deemed that the patient is unable to obtain these services on his or her own and is in need of treatment because of danger to self or others. These powers may act in concert with a state's police powers to ensure the safety of the individual and the community. Thresholds for involuntary commitment on the basis of danger to self are usually contained within the regulating statutes; however, these may be ambiguous and difficult to implement, because these statutes may give arbitrary time frames (e.g., within 72 hours or within 30 days) or use vague expressions (e.g., "in the near future" or "in imminent danger"). These statutes place considerable burden on the clinician to predict if and when suicide is likely to occur despite empirical analysis that demonstrates the inability of psychiatrists to predict suicide accurately (Pokorny 1983). The statutory language defining the various aspects of involuntary commitment differs from jurisdiction to jurisdiction; hence, the clinician must be aware of the mental health codes that regulate his or her particular setting. The clinician's responsibilities are 1) to determine the clinical rationale for involuntary commitment, 2) to document that reasoning based upon the patient characteristics and the determined level of risk, and 3) to provide a safe environment for intervention.

The legal consequences of a completed suicide vary according to the circumstances and may have profound effects on the individual clinician, the family and friends of the victim, the community, and the institution. It is possible that the clinician and his or her institution may face allegations of malpractice when someone under their care commits suicide; they also may face civil proceedings aimed toward demonstrating that the clinician or institution did not deliver the proper care to prevent the suicide. The leading reasons for malpractice litigations against mental health care providers are suicide and attempted suicide (Besharov 1985; Slawson 1984 [cited in Amchin et al. 1990]). Although the payment of malpractice claims is unusual, in suicides and attempted suicides the likelihood that a tort will be successful is increased if the clinician has not properly documented the assessment of the individual and the rationale for the kinds of interventions he or she used. Amchin et al. (1990) point out that "professional liability for the suicidal behavior of patients is frequently decided by determining whether there was a breach of duty, as defined by failing to meet the standard of ordinary and reasonable care" (p. 650). Typically, breach of duty may result from failure to assess for suicide potential or from failure to provide treatment for someone already diagnosed as suicidal.

Special Considerations

Therapist Countertransference

Suicidal patients often arouse strong feelings in the evaluating clinician. The feelings aroused in the clinician will be determined by the clinical circumstances, but may include anxiety and anger. It is critical to be aware of these feelings and the ways in which they may interfere with the objective assessment of the patient. Maltsberger and Buie (1974) have described countertransference hate in the treatment of the suicidal patient. They have described malicious and aversive aspects of countertransference and suggest that the aversive aspect may be especially influential in precipitating suicidal action. The aversive aspect of countertransference leads the therapist to withdraw from the patient or act in ways that precipitate patient flight from the therapist. This withdrawal of support at a time when the patient may need the therapist the most may lay the foundation for a patient suicide. Suicidal patients may also evoke a sense of hopelessness in the clinician. These feelings may be intolerable, and the clinician's capacity to tolerate being with the patient may be compromised. Such feelings in the therapist may be manifested by indifference toward the patient, and, therefore, the risk of suicidal behavior will be increased.

Sacks (1989) states that "ambivalence toward patients is a major aspect of any therapist's confrontation with the reality of a patient killing himself" (p. 575). He notes that one must remain cognizant that the wish to help or save the patient may also be accompanied by wishes to reject, hurt, or even murder the patient. Suicidal patients often present significant challenges to the clinician's societally sanctioned role as a help-giver, particularly because the object of the patient's actions is in contrast to the clinician's efforts. The clinician may feel impotent to effect change and may react with hostility and rage toward the patient if the clinician is not attentive to these feelings. It is advisable for any clinician treating a complicated suicidal patient to seek advice, assistance, or supervision in an effort to avoid the pitfalls that negative countertransference reactions may present.

Another problematic countertransference reaction that is frequently seen in caring for suicidal patients is the fantasy of the therapist as savior. Chronically suicidal patients have a tendency to assign others the responsibility for keeping them alive (Hendin 1982). To the extent that the therapist unwittingly accepts this unrealistic bargain, the patient will have the capacity to torture the therapist and wreak havoc on the treatment. The idea of saving the patient at all costs allows the patient to experience only one side of the ambivalence, that is, the wish to die. Under some such circumstances, it is important for the therapist to adopt a balanced position, assisting the patient to live in the fullest manner possible, but not taking on the ultimate responsibility for the patient's life.

Consequences of Completed Suicides

Completed suicide may have profound effects on the victim's family as well as the clinician. The therapist, because of the expectation to diagnose and prevent suicide, may feel particularly vulnerable after the death of a patient by suicide. Feelings may follow the course of normal bereavement or normal responses to traumatic events and may include experiences of guilt, anger, denial, and repression, or there may be experiences of shock and disbelief, self-blame, and feelings of personal inadequacy. Kahne

(1968) found that after the suicide of a patient, psychiatrists were prone to feelings of guilt, decreased confidence, and feelings of blame. Ruben (1990) warns that clinicians must expect an unavoidable negative impact on their professional functioning and be careful to ensure that any negative effects do not cause harm to other patients in their care. Sacks (1989) points out that there has been little attention paid to the process of the therapist's grief in the context of patients killing themselves; he suggests that it is the responsibility of a clinician's peers to evaluate the clinician's work yet provide needed support during a period of increased personal and professional stress.

Reviews of patient suicides should attempt to evaluate the circumstances that preceded the deaths. This should not be a mission in search of blame and fault, but one in search of the factors that may have been related to the suicide. Many institutions review all suicides and serious suicide attempts routinely as a matter of quality assurance, risk management, and peer review. In the ideal situation, these reviews will also serve to provide support to the clinician and others involved in the patient's treatment. In a solo practice, the experience may be particularly lonely, and hence it becomes imperative that the clinician find ways to process his or her feelings with colleagues. In addition to dealing with his or her personal reactions to losing a patient, the clinician, when feasible, should reach out to the patient's family to offer support and counseling. This may be done either directly by the clinician or by a colleague.

Resnik (1969) suggests that it is critical to visit or talk to the patient's family within 24 hours of the death to begin discussions of what the suicide signifies, what motivated it, and what the consequences might be. This begins a process of helping the family work through their mourning and provides a conduit for referral of the family to appropriate sources of support. It is always a mistake to avoid the family if the family seeks the clinician out. Such avoidance may complicate the family's ability to cope and mobilize negative reactions toward the clinician.

There is not much systematic data on the sequelae of bereavement resulting from suicide; however, there is considerable anecdotal evidence that the bereavement resulting from suicide may follow a more difficult course (Cain and Fast 1972; Dunne et al. 1987; Shneidman 1969). Emotional reactions to a death in a family due to suicide are often more intense than reaction to death from other causes and may be more difficult for family survivors to comprehend and work through. One must be aware that the family may also possess ambivalent feelings toward the deceased and may feel both sadness and relief with the patient's death. Ness and Pfeffer (1990) reviewed bereavement over suicide and bereavement resulting from other kinds of death and found that the former was characterized by greater preoccupations of the bereaved with finding meaning in the tragedy. Additionally, societal attitudes were more blaming of bereaved individuals when death resulted from a suicide. Postsuicide counseling can help bereaved families better understand the complexity of suicidal actions and to attenuate feelings of self-blame.

Conclusions

Despite the accumulated knowledge on the subject of suicide and the proliferation of suicide prevention centers, suicide hotlines, and community mental health centers with available psychiatric care, the overall rate of suicide in America has not changed significantly in the past 20 years. Because suicide is such a heterogeneous phenomenon and such an individualized act, the precise prediction of the outcome of suicidal thinking is virtually impossible. However, the clinical and demographic profile of a particular patient can aid in detecting someone who is at greater risk for suicide. It is critical for both primary care physicians and specialty physicians to develop the ability to recognize risk factors of suicide, because nearly 50% to 80% of patients who commit suicide will have seen their primary care physician within the weeks to months preceding the act (Blumenthal 1988). The ability to recognize risk factors for suicide and develop appropriate interventions is key to suicide prevention.

References

Adam KS: Attempted suicide. Psychiatr Clin North Am 8:183–201, 1985

Agren H: Symptom patterns in unipolar and bipolar depression correlating with monoamine metabolites in the cerebrospinal fluid, II: suicide. Psychiatry Res 3:225–236, 1980

Akiskal HS, Chen SE, Davis GC: Borderline: an adjective in search of a noun. J Clin Psychiatry 46:41–48, 1985

Allebeck P, Varla A, Kristjansson E, et al: Risk factors for suicide among patients with schizophrenia. Acta Psychiatr Scand 76:414–419, 1987

Amchin J, Wettstein RM, Roth LH: Suicide, ethics, and the law, in Suicide Over the Life Cycle: Risk factors, Assessment, and Treatment of Suicidal Patients. Edited by Blumenthal SJ, Kupfer DJ. Washington, DC, American Psychiatric Press, 1990, pp 637–663

Angst J, Felder W, Frey R: The course of unipolar and bipolar affective disorders, in Origin, Prevention, and Treatment of Affective Disorder. Edited by Schou M, Stromgren E. London, Academic, 1979, pp 215–226

Åsberg M, Thorén P, Träskman L, et al: Serotonin depression: a biochemical subgroup within the affective disorders? Science 191:478–480, 1976

Banki CM, Arató M, Kilts CD: Aminergic studies and cerebrospinal fluid cautions in suicide, in Psychobiology of Suicidal Behavior. Edited by Mann JJ, Stanley M. New York, New York Academy of Sciences, 1986, pp 221–230

Barraclough B, Bunch J, Nelson B, et al: A hundred cases of suicide: clinical aspects. Br J Psychiatry 125:355–373, 1974

Beck AT, Steer RS, Kovacs M, et al: Hopelessness and eventual suicide: a 10-year prospective study of patients hospitalized with suicidal ideation. Am J Psychiatry 142:559–563, 1985

Beck RW, Morris JB, Peck AT: Cross-validation of the Suicide Intent Scale. Psychol Rep 34:445–446, 1974

Besharov DJ: The Vulnerable Social Worker: Liability for Serving Children and Families. Silver Spring, MD, National Association of Social Workers, 1985

Black DW, Warrack G, Winokur G: The Iowa Record Linkage Study, I: suicide and accidental deaths among psychiatric patients. Arch Gen Psychiatry 42:71–75, 1985

Black DW, Winokur G, Nasrallah A: Effect of psychosis on suicide risk in 1,593 patients with unipolar and bipolar affective disorders. Am J Psychiatry 145:849–852, 1988

Black DW, Winokur G, Nasrallah A: Suicide in subtypes of major affective disorder: a comparison with general population suicide mortality. Arch Gen Psychiatry 44:878–880, 1987

Blumenthal SJ: Suicide: a guide to risk factors, assessment, and treatment of suicidal patients. Med Clin North Am 72:937–971, 1988

Breier A, Astrachan BM: Characterization of schizophrenic patients who commit suicide. Am J Psychiatry 141:206–209, 1984

Brent DA, Perper JA, Goldstein CE, et al: Risk factors for adolescent suicide: a comparison of adolescent suicide victims with suicidal inpatients. Arch Gen Psychiatry 45:581–588, 1988

Brown GL, Goodwin FK, Ballenger JC, et al: Aggression in humans correlates with cerebrospinal fluid amine metabolites. Psychiatry Res 1:131–139, 1979

Brown GL, Ebert MH, Goyer PF, et al: Aggression, suicide, and serotonin: relationships to CSF amine metabolites. Am J Psychiatry 139:741–746, 1982

Buda M, Tsuang MT: The epidemiology of suicide: implications for clinical practice, in Suicide Over the Life Cycle, Risk Factors, Assessment, and Treatment of Suicidal Patients. Edited by Blumenthal SJ, Kupfer DJ. Washington, DC, American Psychiatric Press, 1990, pp 17–37

Buie DH Jr, Adler G: The uses of confrontation with borderline patients. International Journal of Psychoanalytic Psychotherapy 1:90–108, 1972

Cain AC, Fast I: The legacy of suicide: observation of the pathogenic impact of suicide upon marital partners, in Survivors of Suicide. Edited by Cain AC. Springfield, IL, Charles C Thomas, 1972, pp 145–154

Centers for Disease Control: Suicide Surveillance 1970–1980. Atlanta, GA, Violent Epidemiology Branch, Center for Health Promotion and Education, 1985

Chandler JH, Reed TE, DeJong RN: Huntington's chorea in Michigan. Neurology 10:148–153, 1960

Cochrane R, Robertson A: Stress in the lives of parasuicides. Social Psychiatry 10:161–171, 1975

Cohen S, Leonard CV, Farberow NL, et al: Tranquilizers and suicide in the schizophrenic patient. Arch Gen Psychiatry 11:312–321, 1964

Copeland AR: Suicide among the elderly: the Metro-Dade County experience, 1981–1983. Med Sci Law 27:32–36, 1987

Coryell W: Diagnosis-specific mortality: primary unipolar depression and Briquet's syndrome (somatization disorder). Arch Gen Psychiatry 38:939–942, 1981

Coryell W, Tsuang MT: Primary unipolar depression and the prognostic importance of delusions. Arch Gen Psychiatry 39:1181–1184, 1982

Dorpat TL: Suicide, loss and mourning. Suicide Life Threat Behav 3:213–224, 1973

Dorpat TL, Ripley HS: A study of suicide in the Seattle area. Compr Psychiatry 1:349–359, 1960

Dorpat TL, Anderson WE, Ripley HS: The relationship of physical illness to suicide, in Suicidal Behaviors: Diagnosis and Management. Edited by Resnik HLP. Boston, MA, Little, Brown, 1968, pp 209–219

Drake RE, Gates C, Cotton PG, et al: Suicide among schizophrenics: who is at risk? J Nerv Ment Dis 172:613–617, 1984

Dressler DM, Prusoff B, Mark H, et al: Clinician attitudes toward the suicide attempter. J Nerv Ment Dis 160:146–155, 1975

Dunne EJ, McIntosh JL, Dunne-Maxim K (eds): Suicide and Its Aftermath: Understanding and Counseling the Survivors. New York, WW Norton, 1987

Dunner DL, Gershon ES, Goodwin FK: Heritable factors in the severity of affective illness. Biol Psychiatry 11:31–42, 1976

Durkheim E: Suicide: A Study in Sociology (1897). Translated by Spalding JA, Simpson G. New York, Free Press, 1951

Farberow NL, Shneidman ES: The Cry for Help. New York, McGraw-Hill, 1961

Farberow NL, Shneidman ES, Leonard CV: Medical Bulletin 9: Suicide among general medical and surgical hospital patients with malignant neoplasms. Washington, DC, Department of Medicine and Surgery, Veterans Administration, February 1963, pp 1–I1

Farberow NL, Shneidman ES, Neuringer C: Case history and hospitalization factors in suicides of neuropsychiatric hospital patients. J Nerv Ment Dis 142:32–44, 1966

Freud S: Mourning and melancholia (1917[1915]), in The Standard Edition of the Complete Psychological Works of Sigmund Freud, Vol 14. Translated and edited by Strachey J. London, Hogarth Press, 1957, pp 237–260

Frosch J: Psychodynamic Psychiatry: Theory and Practice, Vol II. Madison, CT, International Universities Press, 1990

Gabbard GO: Psychodynamic Psychiatry in Clinical Practice. Washington, DC, American Psychiatric Press, 1990

Goldney RD, Burvill PW: Trends in suicidal behaviour and its management. Aust N Z J Psychiatry 14:1–15, 1980

Guggenheim FG: Management of suicide risk in the psychiatric emergency room, in Manual of Psychiatric Consultation and Emergency Care. Edited by Guggenheim FG, Weiner MF. New York, Jason Aronson, 1984, pp 23–32

Guze SB, Robins E: Suicide and primary affective disorders. Br J Psychiatry 117:437–438, 1970

Haberlandt W: Aportacion a Ia genetica del suicido. Folio Clinica Internationale 17:319–322, 1967

Hagnell O, Rorsman B: Suicide in the Lundby study: a controlled prospective investigation of stressful life events. Neuropsychobiology 6:316–332, 1980

Hendin H: Psychotherapy and suicide, in Suicide in America. Edited by Hendin H. New York, WW Norton, 1982, pp 160–174

Isherwood J, Adams KS, Hornblow A: Life events stress, psychosocial factors, suicide attempts, and auto-accident proclivity. J Psychosom Res 26:371–383, 1982

Jacobs D: Psychotherapy with suicidal patients: the empathic method, in Suicide: Understanding and Responding. Edited by Jacobs D, Brown HN. Madison, CT, International Universities Press, 1989, pp 329–342

Johnson J, Weissman MM, Klerman GL: Panic disorder, comorbidity, and suicide attempts. Arch Gen Psychiatry 47:805–808, 1990

Kahana E, Leibowitz U, Alter M: Cerebral multiple sclerosis. Neurology 21:1179–1185, 1971

Kahne MJ: Suicide among patients in mental hospitals: a study of the psychiatrists who conducted their psychotherapy. Psychiatry 31:32–43, 1968

Klerman GL, Weissman NM: Increasing rates of depression. JAMA 261:2229–2235, 1989

Kreitman N (ed): Parasuicide. New York, Wiley, 1977

Lindelius R, Kay DWK: Some changes in the pattern of mortality in schizophrenia in Sweden. Acta Med Scand 49:315–323, 1973

Louhivuori HA, Hakama M: Risk of suicide among cancer patients. Am J Epidemiol 109:59–65, 1979

MacKenzie TB, Popkin MD: Suicide in the medical patient. International Journal of Psychiatry 17:3–22, 1987

Maddocks PD: A five year follow-up of untreated psychopaths. Br J Psychiatry 116:511–515, 1970

Maltsberger JT, Buie DH: Countertransference hate in the treatment of suicidal patients. Arch Gen Psychiatry 30:625–633, 1974

Maris R: Social Forces in Urban Suicide. Homewood, IL, Dorsey Press, 1969

Marshall JR, Burnett W, Brasure J: On precipitating factors: cancer as a cause of suicide. Suicide Life Threat Behav 13:15–27, 1983

Marzuk PM, Tierney H, Tardiff K, et al: Increased risk of suicides in persons with AIDS. JAMA 259:1333–1337, 1988

Matthews WS, Barabas G: Suicide and epilepsy: a review of the literature. Psychosomatics 22:515–524, 1981

McGlashan TH: The Chestnut Lodge follow-up study, II: long-term outcome of schizophrenia and the affective disorders. Arch Gen Psychiatry 41:586–601, 1984

McIntosh JL: Survivors of suicide: a comprehensive bibliography. Omega 16:355–370, 1985

Menninger KA: Psychoanalytic aspects of suicide. Int J Psychoanal 14:376–390, 1933

Miles CP: Conditions predisposing to suicide: a review. J Nerv Ment Dis 164:231–246, 1977

Montgomery SA, Montgomery D: Pharmacological prevention of suicidal behavior. J Affective Disord 4:291–298, 1982

Morrison JR: Suicide in a psychiatric practice population. J Clin Psychiatry 43:348–352, 1982

Motto JA: Suicide risk factors in alcohol abuse. Suicide Life Threat Behav 10:230–238, 1980

Motto JA: Problems in suicide risk assessment, in Suicide: Understanding and Responding. Edited by Jacobs D, Brown HN. Madison, CT, International Universities Press, 1989, pp 129–142

Muller R: Studies on disseminated sclerosis with special reference to symptomatology, course, and prognosis. Acta Med Scand (Suppl) 222:1–214, 1949

Murphy GE, Robins E: Social factors in suicide. JAMA 199:303–308, 1967

Ness DE, Pfeffer CR: Sequelae of bereavement resulting from suicide. Am J Psychiatry 147:279–285, 1990

Ninan PT, van Kammen DP, Scheinin M, et al: CSF 5-hydroxyindoleacetic acid levels in suicidal schizophrenic patients. Am J Psychiatry 141:566–569, 1984

Osgood NJ, Thielman S: Geriatric suicidal behavior: assessment and treatment, in Suicide Over the Life Cycle: Risk Factors, Assessment, and Treatment of Suicidal Patients. Edited by Blumenthal SJ, Kupfer DJ. Washington, DC, American Psychiatric Press, 1990, pp 341–379

Palaniappan V, Ramachandran VI, Somasundaram O: Suicidal ideation and biogenic amines in depression. Indian Journal of Psychiatry 25:286–292, 1983

Paris J, Brown R, Nowlis D: Long-term follow-up of borderline patients in a general hospital. Compr Psychiatry 28:530–535, 1987

Patterson WM, Dohn HH, Bird J, et al: Evaluation of suicidal patients: the SAD PERSONS scale. Psychosomatics 24:343–349, 1983

Paykel ES, Prusoff BA, Myers JK: Suicide attempts and recent life events: a controlled comparison. Arch Gen Psychiatry 32:327–333, 1975

Platt S: Unemployment and suicidal behavior: a review of the literature. Soc Sci Med 19:93–115, 1984

Pokorny AD: Characteristics of forty-four patients who subsequently committed suicide. Arch Gen Psychiatry 2:314–323, 1960

Pokorny AD: Suicide rates in various psychiatric disorders. J Nerv Ment Dis 139:499–506, 1964

Pokorny AD: Prediction of suicide in psychiatric patients: report of a prospective study. Arch Gen Psychiatry 40:249–257, 1983

Pope HG Jr, Jonas JM, Hudson JI, et al: The validity of DSM-III borderline personality disorder: a phenomenologic, family history, treatment response, and long-term follow-up study. Arch Gen Psychiatry 40:23–30, 1983

Resnik HLP: Psychological resynthesis: a clinical approach to the survivors of death by suicide, in Aspects of Depression. Edited by Schneidman ES, Ortega NJ. San Francisco, CA, Jossey-Bass, 1969, pp 213–224

Robins E, Murphy GE, Wilkinson RH Jr, et al: Some clinical considerations in the prevention of suicide based on a study of 134 successful suicides. Am J Public Health 49:888–899, 1959

Robins E: The Final Months: A Study of the Lives of 134 Persons Who Committed Suicide. New York, Oxford University Press, 1981

Roose SP, Glassman AH, Walsh BT, et al: Depression, delusions, and suicide. Am J Psychiatry 140:1159–1162, 1983

Roy A: Risk factors for suicide in psychiatric patients. Arch Gen Psychiatry 39:1089–1095, 1982a

Roy A: Suicide in chronic schizophrenia. Br J Psychiatry 141:171–177, 1982b

Roy A: Family history of suicide. Arch Gen Psychiatry 40:971–974, 1983

Ruben HL: Surviving a suicide in your practice, in Suicide Over the Life Cycle: Risk Factors, Assessment, and Treatment of Suicidal Patients. Edited by Blumenthal SJ, Kupfer DJ. Washington, DC, American Psychiatric Press, 1990, pp 619–636

Sacks MH: When patients kill themselves, in American Psychiatric Press Review of Psychiatry, Vol 8. Edited by Tasman A, Hales RE, Frances AJ. Washington, DC, American Psychiatric Press, 1989, pp 563–579

Sainbury P: Suicide in London: An Ecological Study (Maudsley Monographs No 1) London, Chapman & Hall, 1955

Sainbury P (ed): Suicide in London. New York, Basic Books, 1956

Seager CP, Flood RA: Suicide in Bristol. Br J Psychiatry 111:919–932, 1965

Shaffer D, Fisher P: The epidemiology of suicide in children and young adolescents. Journal of the American Academy of Child Psychiatry 20:545–565, 1981

Shafii M, Carrigan S, Whittinghill JR, et al: Psychological autopsy of completed suicide in children and adolescents. Am J Psychiatry 142:1061–1064, 1985

Shneidman ES: Prologue: fifty-eight years, in On the Nature of Suicide. Edited by Shneidman ES. San Francisco, CA, Jossey-Bass, 1969, pp 1–30

Slawson PF: The clinical dimension of psychiatric malpractice. Psychiatric Annals 14:358–364, 1984

Stanley M, Mann JJ: Biological factors associated with suicide, in American Psychiatric Press Review of Psychiatry, Vol 7. Edited by Frances AJ, Hales RE. Washington, DC, American Psychiatric Press, 1988, pp 334–352

Stengel E: Suicide and Attempted Suicide. Harmondsworth, Middlesex, UK, Penguin, 1964

Temoche A, Pugh TF, MacMahon B: Suicide rates among current and former mental institution patients. J Nerv Ment Dis 138:124–130, 1964

Tsuang MT: Suicide in schizophrenics, manics, depressives, and surgical controls: a comparison with general population suicide mortality. Arch Gen Psychiatry 35:153–155, 1978

Tsuang MT: Risk of suicide in the relatives of schizophrenics, manics, depressives, and controls. J Clin Psychiatry 44:396–400, 1983

Tsuang MT, Winokur G, Crowe RR: Morbidity risks of schizophrenia and affective disorders among first degree relatives of patients with schizophrenia, mania, depression, and surgical conditions. Br J Psychiatry 137:497–504, 1980

Vaillant GE, Blumenthal SJ: Introduction: suicide over the life cycle—risk factors and life-span development, in Suicide Over the Life Cycle: Risk Factors, Assessment, and Treatment of Suicidal Patients. Edited by Blumenthal SJ, Kupfer DJ. Washington, DC, American Psychiatric Press, 1990, pp 1–14

Van Praag HM: Depression, suicide, and the metabolism of serotonin in the brain. J Affective Disord 4:275–290, 1982

Van Praag HM: CSF 5-HIAA and suicide in non-depressed schizophrenics. Lancet 2:977–978, 1983

Weissman MM: The epidemiology of suicide attempts, 1960 to 1971. Arch Gen Psychiatry 30:737–746, 1974

Weissman MM, Klerman GL, Markowitz JS, et al: Suicidal ideation and suicide attempts in panic disorder and attacks. N Engl J Med 321:1209–1214, 1989

Wender PH, Kety SS, Rosenthal D, et al: Psychiatric disorders in the biological and adoptive families of adopted individuals with affective disorders. Arch Gen Psychiatry 43:923–929, 1986

Whitlock FA: Suicide, cancer, and depression. Br J Psychiatry 132:269–274, 1978

Wolfersdorf M, Keller F, Steiner B, et al: Delusional depression and suicide. Acta Psychiatr Scand 76:359–363, 1987

Chapter 5

Psychotherapy With the Self-Destructive Borderline Patient

Eric M. Plakun, M.D.

By Christmas the gently rolling Berkshire hills of western Massachusetts, just south of the Vermont border, were covered by a beautiful but forbidding and impenetrable blanket of snow and ice, a description that also suited Ms. A., a 35-year-old married woman with a borderline personality organization. When Ms. A. failed to appear at her Christmas Eve therapy session, the therapist was puzzled but not especially alarmed, even though she had been referred because of a near-lethal suicide attempt 6 months earlier. Ms. A., like the Berkshires, seemed blanketed under a frozen, inscrutable, often impenetrable surface. It had not been the therapist's inclination to push too hard at what lay buried beneath. An hour later, though, when Ms. A.'s husband called asking if his wife had kept her appointment, because she was now an hour late for a lunch engagement with him, it was clear something had in fact happened. Three hours later Ms. A. was found by the police in her car in a parking lot, comatose from ingestion of 2 grams of amitriptyline.

The therapist felt a mixture of intense emotions: betrayal (Those were my pills! I thought we had an agreement?), anger (How could she do this—on Christmas Eve yet? I'll be dealing with this all holiday.), guilt (Did I miss something? Have I blown this case? Will she die because of me? How could I try to work with someone so suicidal in psychotherapy?), a wish for revenge (I'll kill her if she lives, or at least I'll end the therapy), and calm expectation (Aha! The game is begun. Now maybe we'll see what the ice and snow have been hiding).

There will be more to say about Ms. A. later. For now it is enough to note that this kind of experience is a familiar one for psychotherapists who work with borderline patients.

This chapter is concerned with principles of psychotherapeutic work with such patients. Treatment of the borderline patient has long been recognized as a formidable therapeutic challenge because of the primitive defenses, self-destructive acting out, and intense countertransference responses frequently encountered. The introduction of DSM-III in 1980 (American Psychiatric Association 1980) was a watershed event in the empirical study of borderline patients, for the first time delineating specific, discrete criteria for borderline personality disorder (BPD). It should be noted that patients with DSM-III or DSM-III-R (American Psychiatric Association 1987) BPD probably represent a subset of a wider group of borderline patients, best categorized by Kernberg's (1975, 1984) description of *borderline personality organization,* which includes most of the DSM-III and DSM-III-R personality disorders.

Retrospective follow-up studies by McGlashan (1983a, 1983b), Stone et al. (1987), Paris et al. (1987), and Plakun (1989; Plakun et al. 1985) in the past decade have contributed to the establishment of the validity of BPD as a discrete diagnostic entity. These studies have demonstrated considerable outcome heterogeneity in BPD patients. Perhaps as many as 75% of these patients achieve relatively good outcomes at long-term follow-up, but the risk of suicide in once-hospitalized BPD patients approaches 10% (Paris et al. 1987; Stone et al. 1987). Several of these researchers have also studied predictors of outcome in BPD (McGlashan 1985; Plakun 1991). It was reported by Plakun (1991), and replicated by McGlashan (1990), that the presence of self-destructive behavior during, but not preceding, the index hospitalization correlated with better long-term outcome. Although the amount of outcome variance accounted for by this variable is less than 5%, it is worth noting that it is the only treatment-related, rather than historical or clinical, variable that appeared predictive of outcome. Half of Plakun's BPD patients engaged in preadmission self-destructive or suicidal acts, but fewer than 10% did during the mean 14-year follow-up interval. This finding further suggests that treatment might have an impact on self-destructive behavior. Indeed, scrutiny of the case records of these patients, coupled with thousands of hours working with self-destructive borderline patients and 15 years observing the work of colleagues at the Austen Riggs Center in Stockbridge, Massachusetts, has led the present author to hypothesize a number of principles that facilitate successful psychotherapy with self-destructive patients, especially self-destructive borderline patients.

A cautionary note is appropriate at this point. A single chapter is certainly not adequate to do justice to the range of technical and conceptual considerations required to cover a topic as complex as the psychotherapy of borderline patients. Numerous authors (Adler 1981; Kernberg 1975, 1984; Kernberg et al. 1989; Masterson 1983; Rinsley 1982, among others) have written extensively on the subject. In Chapter 3 of the present volume, Dr. Munich summarizes some of these issues. Psychotherapy is more art than science and thus is not easily amenable to empirical study. The model offered here has not been subject to empirical investigation, but this type of investigation is planned and will be reported in the future. Finally, it is worth noting that any effort to distill essential principles from a complex interpersonal process like psychotherapy leads to the dangers of reductionism and oversimplification. The hope is that these principles will provide a framework allowing a therapist to examine meaningfully with a patient a pattern of dangerous behavior, while at the same time holding the patient responsible for the behavior and emphasizing the vulnerability of the therapeutic collaboration.

A few orienting remarks and definitions are in order. These principles have been derived from the study of inpatients at the Austen Riggs Center, where patients are seen weekly in 4 hours of intensive psychoanalytic psychotherapy in a fully open hospital setting, with no use of seclusion, restraints, or a privilege system. Patients participate in a community program that includes group meetings designed to hold patients responsible for their own behavior and for setting standards for the behaviors tolerated in the patient community. Although 24-hour nursing care is provided, there is minimal emphasis on one-to-one interactions, with nurses functioning primarily as model community members. For example, patients receiving medication are expected to appear at the medication dispensing area at scheduled hours to request medication, rather than have nursing staff pursue patients. Although these principles are derived from scrutiny of patients in such an inpatient setting, the openness, the antiregressive demands of the milieu, and the position of the hospital staff that they cannot and will not attempt to control patients allow for translation of this approach to work with outpatients, as well as to work with patients in nonhospital residential settings or partial hospital programs. The model is appropriate for insight-oriented psychodynamic psychotherapy (expressive psychotherapy) conducted from a position of technical neutrality, with a focus on interpreting transference and resistance. Although derived from a treatment setting offering 4 hours of psychotherapy weekly, the model has been used successfully with patients seen less often but at least once weekly. The approach described here is not appropriate for treatments with a primarily supportive focus or for those that focus on management of behavior rather than its interpretation.

The concept of *countertransference* is central in psychotherapy with borderline patients. The term will be used in its broadest sense here, including both the therapist's "transference" to the patient (i.e., neurotic projections from the therapist onto the patient) and the complete range of feelings the therapist has in response to the patient. Self-destructive behavior as conceptualized in this chapter refers to a wide range of suicidal and parasuicidal behaviors, including suicide attempts, suicide gestures, and suicide threats. Nonsuicidal overdoses, self-starvation, and cutting, burning, and other self-mutilating behaviors may also be appropriately dealt with using this model if the behaviors pose a threat to life or to the continuation of treatment. In all these instances it is the potential of the behavior to terminate the treatment that is the foundation upon which these principles are based. Two brief clinical vignettes illustrate this point:

Case 1

Ms. B., a 22-year-old anorexic and borderline patient with a history of cutting and pseudoseizures, was referred to a long-term hospital by a case management organization that was concerned because the patient had required nearly 100 hospitalizations in the preceding several years. The patient's weight and metabolic status were frequently marginal; she often induced vomiting, abused laxatives, and failed to comply with prescribed medications. In a previous outpatient therapy Ms. B. had severely cut herself during a session. Her alarmed outpatient therapist had called an ambulance, then cradled her in his arms until it arrived, while the patient had a series of pseudoseizures. First, in an extended consultation with the patient about the possibility of admission for long-term hospital treatment, then after admission in the initial stages of establishing a therapeutic contract, the admissions officer, then the therapist and the nursing staff, clearly and unambivalently but nonpunitively stated the reality that neither the hospital nor the therapist had the ability to control the patient's weight or to preserve her treatment. The patient responded with genuine interest and relief to this recognition that the behavior was under her control; she then went on to form a good working alliance with her therapist and the hospital.

There were numerous early close calls in which the patient required confrontation about the way she was threatening her treatment. In her first week of long-term hospital treatment, Ms. B. produced a knife in a therapy session, threatening to kill herself. The therapist responded by calmly asking the patient why she was trying to destroy her treatment so soon after deciding to begin it. Ms. B. handed the knife to the therapist. Three months later Ms. B. had lost 20 pounds, leading the hospital internist to declare an unwillingness to continue caring for Ms. B. unless she gained at least 5 pounds in the next 6 weeks. Although Ms. B. protested about the impossibility of meeting such a goal and claimed she would continue to lose weight, the therapist insisted it was the patient's responsibility to maintain a weight that allowed the internist to feel comfortable with her metabolic status.

By the specified date, Ms. B. had gained 8 pounds and preserved her treatment. Eighteen months after admission Ms. B. had managed not to interrupt the treatment relationship and was virtually pseudoseizure free, productively grappling with the determinants of her disorder in therapy, maintaining her weight, and resuming age-appropriate behaviors. A year into the patient's treatment her case manager sent a letter thanking the hospital and its staff for their work, noting that not only was the patient improving but several thousand dollars had been saved over the cost of treatment in the year preceding long-term hospitalization, during which the patient had required multiple short-term hospitalizations.

Case 2

Ms. C., a 19-year-old woman with a dysthymic disorder and mixed personality disorder with borderline, schizotypal, narcissistic, and avoidant traits, had a several-year history of superficial cutting of her arms, abdomen, and thighs. The cuts had never required sutures. The patient was referred for long-term treatment because of failure to benefit adequately from outpatient psychotherapy, medication trials, or two short-term hospitalizations in a 6-month period, and an exacerbation of her chronic suicide risk. Ms. C. had a suicide plan of hanging herself from a specific tree in her hometown. The patient's cutting was ego-syntonic and experienced as both providing relief from episodes of intense dysphoria and giving her an alternative to carrying out her suicide plan.

Ms. C., upon admission to a long-term hospital at a time of administrative turmoil and anxiety, was assigned a new and inexperienced therapist. The patient quickly engaged in cutting, which she exhibitionistically brought to the attention of patients and staff. Nurses and the therapist focused their interventions on the need for the patient to cease her cutting behavior, expressing their countertransference discomfort with the behavior and failing to first establish a therapeutic contract that clarified the patient's responsibility for modulating anxiety about her cutting. The patient responded to the focus on cutting by threatening to leave the hospital. The therapist, who retreated to a position of advising the patient not to leave so that her problems could be worked on, was on the defensive and unable to establish an effective alliance. Soon after, the patient left the hospital.

In the first vignette the hospital and therapist successfully engaged Ms. B. in treatment through a meaningful dialogue, clarifying the limitations of the hospital and therapist and Ms. B.'s responsibility for preserving the treatment. Although the patient tested the limits of the hospital and therapist with a threat to kill herself, loss of weight, and other behaviors, limits were consistently made clear and the patient responded well.

In the second vignette a combination of factors, including the therapist's inexperience and staff anxiety about administrative matters, undermined the establishment of a clear treatment contract with Ms. C. The therapist and nursing staff focused excessively and prematurely on Ms. C.'s superficial cutting, although this behavior did not really threaten the continuity of the treatment. While it was known that the patient became anxious with scrutiny and that the cutting was unlikely to be serious, often representing an alternative to more serious suicidal behavior, the staff overlooked these data in an overly anxious and premature countertransference response to her cutting. Unlike Ms. B.'s threat to kill herself with a knife, Ms. C.'s cutting did not pose a threat to continuation of the treatment, yet it was incorrectly treated as if it did. It is not known if Ms. C. was prepared to engage in the kind of treatment offered; however, it is clear that there was an over-response to her superficial cutting at the expense of a focus on the establishment of a therapeutic alliance.

The model offered here pertains to psychotherapy with those patients whose behaviors threaten the continuity of the psychotherapy—a reality that must be made an explicit part of the therapeutic contract.

The Initial Evaluation

Prior to establishing a therapeutic contract, most experienced therapists first meet with patients in a period of evaluation. Clarifying what the patient would like to change about himself or herself, potential treatability, and diagnosis are foci of an evaluation period, but not of this chapter. However, a few words about diagnosis and medication are in order because they have such a profound impact on the treatment.

The self-destructive borderline patient may present with a borderline disorder alone, or with a borderline state comorbid with a complicating Axis I disorder, such as a superimposed affective disorder or substance dependence. Untreated substance dependence mitigates against treatability and should be dealt with appropriately before therapy for BPD can begin. A careful diagnostic evaluation for comorbidity is particularly important in determining the role of medication in the treatment of a borderline patient.

Akiskal (1981) conceptualizes the borderline syndrome as a variant of affective disorder, viewing medication as essential. Gardner and Cowdry (1985) report benefit from carbamazepine, while Soloff et al. (1986) have described response to low-dose neuroleptics in borderline patients. In fact, virtually every class of psychoactive medication has been advocated for borderline patients.

In my experience many BPD patients have been psychopharmacological nonresponders despite adequate doses for adequate duration. These patients and their doctors have often lost hope that medication will make much difference for them and recognize the way these patients may have previously abused medication through overdose or intoxication. My own preference is to avoid medication with noncomorbid self-destructive borderline patients. The presence of clear comorbidity, particularly with a unipolar or bipolar affective disorder, generally requires medication. Suicidality or self-destructiveness, though, can and does exist in borderline patients without comorbid affective disorders, and this behavior should not be construed as being an indication for an antidepressant per se. Although some therapists (Kernberg et al. 1989) prefer to avoid prescribing medication for their own patients, I have often found it workable. When it is clear from past history or from experience with a patient that talking about the medication becomes a resistance to the psychotherapeutic work, or when one is confounded by the clash of treatment paradigms, there should be no qualms about enlisting a colleague to prescribe a patient's psychopharmacological regimen. The task of being a psychotherapist to these patients can be more than enough of a challenge.

The Therapeutic Contract

After adequate evaluation, a therapeutic contract must be established. It is a sine qua non of intensive psychotherapy that the therapeutic contract negotiated at the outset of the work must define the responsibilities of each participant. When the therapist is working with the self-destructive patient, in addition to the usual arrangements about fee, scheduling of sessions, the patient's obligation to speak freely about what is on his or her mind, and the therapist's responsibility to listen, understand, and provide therapeutic interventions, the contract should be modified to include clarification of the patient's responsibilities and the therapist's limits with respect to self-destructive behavior.

Many borderline patients come to psychotherapy with an implicit request that the therapist or hospital assume the task of keeping them alive, leaving the patients the job of making themselves dead. Although short-term acute-care hospitals sometimes have no choice but to engage with patients in this way, in outpatient psychotherapy or voluntary settings it should be made clear from the inception of the therapeutic contract that this is not possible. Therapist and patient reach mutual agreement to work toward a set of achievable goals over time. This cannot be accomplished unless the two meet. Any behavior that the patient or an important third party has demonstrated in the past that undermines and threatens the continuity of the therapy should be addressed in the therapeutic contract. This is true whether the issue is nonpayment of bills from a previous therapist, a history of premature termination, a history of behavior likely to lead to arrest and incarceration, or a history of suicidal or other self-destructive behavior serious enough to interfere with the continuity of the treatment.

The therapist should clarify the patient's responsibility for managing self-destructive feelings and outline a sensible sequence of steps for the patient to take if the patient finds himself or herself dealing with serious self-destructive impulses. Such a sequence may vary with the patient, the doctor, the treatment setting, or the locale, but generally includes a clearly communicated obligation of the patient to contain the impulses or, failing that, to communicate promptly his or her need for help and make an effort to bring himself or herself to an appropriate place for evaluation and assistance. One works toward the goal of the patient's developing a capacity for tolerating these feelings without action and, instead, bringing them to the next scheduled session. Until that is achieved the patient may need to get himself or herself to an emergency room for evaluation (or to nursing staff in other settings) if the patient has already ingested pills or otherwise initiated a suicide attempt or feels unable to refrain from doing so. The interposition of a relationship with another person during self-destructive crises is the goal, but it is preferable for the therapist not to make himself or herself available in such crises. Such availability usually creates an incentive for the patient to be in crisis because of the extra attention made available. All too often therapists working with self-destructive borderline patients fail to establish and maintain a clear, mutually honored contract, allowing the therapy to become a kind of ongoing crisis intervention in which therapist and patient are always recovering from the last self-destructive crisis or fending off the next one. Searles' (1979) helpful paper on the dangers of therapeutic zeal, especially for "dedicated physicians," is well worth recalling.

Certainly a suicide attempt is a complex, multidetermined act in a troubled individual. The primary method of psychoanalytic psychotherapy is to analyze the meaning in the transference of such behavior, but first it must be possible for therapy to continue. It is important to clarify with patients that a failed suicide attempt will not be met simply with relief that the patient did not die, but rather with the inference that the patient has made a decision to end the therapy. Such a decision must be examined and reversed before resumption of the work can be considered. The model delineated below cannot be implemented without the prior clarification of these issues in the therapeutic contract, so addition of this parameter to the contract from the outset is essential. Should awareness of such risk emerge only after treatment has begun, it is essential to modify the therapeutic contract.

It is, of course, one thing to note what a therapeutic contract should include, but quite another to negotiate such a contract with a patient using a firm but collaborative, empathic approach, without sadism or harsh judgment. Both parties must recognize the commonsense reality that the patient's participation in the therapy requires him or her to be alive and to come to sessions, which only the patient can assure. If a patient is to find the courage to take the considerable risk involved in entering such an agreement with a stranger, the therapist will have to be able to communicate understanding, empathy, and warmth, as well as firmness, so that the terms of the agreement do not scare off the patient through their potential to be perceived as rejecting.

The Five Principles

In many instances clarification of the therapeutic contract in the manner described above is a new experience for a patient whose previous therapists may have been less clear about responsibility and limits. For some minimally self-destructive borderline patients, clarification of the patient's responsibility for managing self-destructive behavior may allow treatment to unfold without such behavior; it is hard, however, to imagine how such a treatment could be useful if the patient were not struggling with self-destructive impulses within the therapeutic work. A failure of these issues to emerge suggests that they are dissociated or dangerously encapsulated, a situation that demands exploration in the therapy. In most instances, the patient does threaten to engage in, or actually engages in, self-destructive behavior. Once appropriate interventions have been made to protect the patient's life, the therapist's response should be consistent with the therapeutic contract without being rigid, punitive, or inflexible. The five principles described below are an approach to working with the patient once self-destructive acting out has occurred. They are based on the therapist's inference that the patient has made a decision to end the treatment. This notion should be reintroduced in a balanced and flexible way, avoiding two extreme positions. One of these is the rage-related refusal to work further with a patient, although sometimes the end of treatment will result from following these principles. The other extreme is a guilty response to the patient's suicide attempt, as if the behavior was in some way the fault of the therapist. This type of response, as illustrated in the following example, may lead the therapist to feel responsible for trying harder, renouncing any possibility of ever abandoning the therapeutic work:

Case 3

Mr. D., a 42-year-old married engineer and father of three young children, manifested a dysthymic disorder and BPD with prominent schizoid and narcissistic features. He had for many years struggled with depression, a profound sense of alienation, and a tendency toward isolation. Mr. D. resided in an isolated home in a harsh northern New England climate, commuting long distances to work and to his twice-weekly psychotherapy sessions with a senior resident at a teaching hospital. The resident also prescribed numerous medication trials without significant benefit. Shortly after learning his resident therapist would complete his training and leave the area in another year, the patient announced suicidal intent in a telephone call to his therapist. Mr. D. refused to disclose his whereabouts, other than to say that he was leaving in his pickup truck with a loaded rifle. Only after an extensive search were police able to locate the patient with his loaded gun on an isolated mountain road.

Once hospitalized, Mr. D. said he wished to end treatment with the resident, but the latter and the hospital treatment team decided the work should continue, coercing the patient into signing a written contract to continue the outpatient therapy. Over the next year the resident was led on a merry chase by the patient, who repeatedly voiced his objections to continuing therapy. These objections were regularly countered by the therapist invoking the signed contract to require the patient to continue therapy. Numerous suicide threats were made, leading to additional hospitalizations. The resident was determined not to terminate the therapy because of his own zeal and the advice of his supervisors that it was too dangerous to allow this patient not to be in treatment. The end of the therapist's residency was discussed in the therapy, but with an emphasis on how transfer of Mr. D. to a new resident when the current therapist left would minimize the problem. Eventually the patient was referred for evaluation for long-term hospitalization.

Because the patient's family life and job performance were adequate, long-term hospitalization did not appear necessary to the admissions officer. The patient expressed relief at the admission officer's recognition that outpatient therapy would be long-term and thus Mr. D. needed a therapist who could see it through to completion, if the patient could. The admissions officer recommended that the patient terminate treatment with the resident and begin psychotherapy with a more experienced therapist who would not be leaving the area and who would hold the patient responsible for the continuity of the therapy relationship, rather than proceed as if it were the therapist's job to keep the patient in therapy and to keep him alive.

As illustrated in the opening remarks of this chapter concerning Ms. A., therapists commonly respond with a mixture of countertransference feelings in response to self-destructive behavior. Mr. D.'s therapist responded with a zealous dedication to the treatment and failed to recognize that the patient's self-destructiveness was in part a communication of distress that he would lose his therapist in less than a year while his need for therapy would continue.

It is important to keep in mind that the five principles presented below are not a substitute for the primary work of the therapy, which includes analyzing the transference and making conscious the unconscious meanings of self-destructive behavior and other issues the patient brings to the therapy.

Engagement of Affect

The first principle emphasizes engaging with the patient around the self-destructive behavior in a way that makes a meaningful, genuine affective connection. Although in some respects this sounds obvious, frequently the behavior has occurred in the context of mutual withdrawal by both therapist and patient. For example, a failure of affective engagement was illustrated by Ms. C's therapist's retreat from the psychotherapeutic position into advice giving (see Case 2).

It should be clear here that this principle is one that emphasizes the need for direct, genuine relating, and should not be misconstrued as implying that therapist and patient need to engage with a lot of affect, for example, in an angry or tearful confrontation. Therapist and patient need to speak personally and honestly, not necessarily loudly. Affect must be engaged in a way that generates more light than heat. Dissociation is a common phenomenon in borderline patients. In fact, dissociation and self-destructive behavior are often linked, with dissociation frequently preceding and/or following self-destructive behavior. The therapist must not only engage with the patient in a way that bridges the patient's dissociative withdrawal, but must also be wary of his or her own potential affective withdrawal from the patient in the aftermath of self-destructive behavior. The therapist may retreat because of countertransference rage, become overly solicitous because of countertransference guilt, or withdraw from meaningful affective connection with a subtle shift from the psychotherapeutic to the medical model, viewing the self-destructive behavior as a manifestation of the patient's "illness" that must be "managed" better. Many psychiatrists with a serious commitment to psychotherapy but a training emphasis on the medical model at the expense of adequate training in psychotherapeutic technique become "fair weather psychotherapists," who are comfortable enough with psychotherapy until acting out begins. At this point they may shift to a view of the behavior as something caused by the patient's illness rather than as having meaning in the therapeutic dyad.

Nonpunitive Interpretation of the Patient's Aggression

Once the therapist has reviewed his or her countertransference responses, met with the patient to discuss the status of their relationship, and found a way to satisfactorily engage affects, it is time to remind the patient of the therapist's inference that the self-destructive behavior represents a decision to end the treatment, although the reasons for such a decision are probably unknown at this point. The patient has made a unilateral decision to revise the terms of the treatment contract in a way that aggressively attacks the relationship between therapist and patient. This is best articulated to the patient in a nonpunitive, nonaccusatory, non–guilt-inducing way. I view this principle as a necessary but not sufficient step in the process of understanding with the patient the unconscious meaning in the transference of the self-destructive behavior, in the service of bringing the self-destructive behavior under conscious control.

In many inpatient and outpatient settings, self-destructive behavior is dealt with as an indication for limits to be set. The patient is heard to be asking for hospitalization or, if already an inpatient, for seclusion, restraint, or restriction. All too often this becomes a justification for punitive retaliation against the patient. Such acting out of the therapist's or hospital staff's countertransference anger becomes an instance of joining the patient in making the therapy a power operation rather than a collaboration. In fact, the psychotherapy should only continue if the underpinnings of the patient's decision to change the therapeutic collaboration into a unilateral power operation can be understood and the collaborative process restored.

Assignment of Responsibility for Preservation of the Treatment to the Patient

Self-destructive behavior is viewed as the patient's assault on the therapy and as invariably raising the question of whether the patient has changed his or her mind about wishing to be in the treatment. Having noted the patient's aggression and apparent decision to end the treatment, the therapist may open up the possibility of the preservation of the therapy, but from a position that holds the patient responsible for such an outcome. It is often a new experience for a borderline patient to be confronted with the view that his or her behavior has meaning in the therapeutic dyad and that he or she has the power essential to preserve or end the relationship and the behavior. In most instances, if the therapy has become an important attachment and a useful collaboration, the patient will be eager to preserve it. If affects are genuinely engaged, the patient can internalize the essential recognition that he or she must modulate self-destructive behavior to preserve the therapy.

A Search for the Perceived Empathic Failure by the Therapist That May Have Precipitated the Self-Destructive Behavior

The therapist, as well as the patient, is held responsible for self-destructive behavior, but in markedly different ways. In most instances, the emergence of self-destructive behavior in a borderline patient follows the patient's perception of a significant narcissistic injury or empathic failure that has led to a dramatic shift in the patient's experience of the therapy. In what Cooperman (1989) has called "the defeating process," the patient suddenly makes a retaliatory attack against the therapist and the treatment. Shifting the treatment into a vengeful power operation has become more important than preserving the therapeutic collaboration. When such behavior occurs in the course of the therapy, it is important to join the patient in searching for, and then acknowledging, the perceived empathic failure or other injury to the patient. Often the failure or injury is something as inevitable as a vacation or weekend, but it may also be a substantial error on the part of the therapist, such as an important misunderstanding of communication from a patient, failure to listen in a therapeutic attitude, or a sadistic or condescending remark or tone on the part of the therapist. If there has been an error by the therapist, generally a genuine apology is in order. Frequently a patient's self-destructive behavior follows a perceived abandonment because of the therapist's vacation or necessary weekend separation. In this case an apology would be an obvious error, but a dismissive statement of the patient's perception of abandonment as unjustified because of the inevitability of such separations in life would be little better. Indicating that the patient's perception is heard, understood, and appreciated (but unlikely to lead to a change in the therapist's future behavior) would be far more appropriate.

Paradoxically, some borderline patients, particularly those engaged in a negative therapeutic reaction, may respond to an empathic "success" by engaging in self-destructive behavior. The principle of searching for perceived empathic failure still holds in such instances, but the focus will be on clarifying how the therapist's successful understanding of the patient is unacceptable to the patient.

Provision of an Opportunity for Reparation

Ultimately, the successful resolution of the crisis in the therapy precipitated by self-destructive behavior depends on the provision of an opportunity for repair. Unless a patient can be given space to repair the damage done to the therapeutic relationship, continuation is foolish. Repair here means something more than simply an apology by the patient, although this may be part of the process. In most instances how the damage can be repaired becomes apparent as a result of what has been learned in the implementation of the other four principles.

In some respects the most important reparation is the patient's genuinely communicated realization of the therapist's limits, the patient's internalization of the reality of his or her responsibility for preserving the treatment, and the patient's intention to manage self-destructive feelings differently in the future. If, in addition, part of the process of reparation includes an advancement of mutual understanding of the meaning of the patient's behavior in the transference, so much the better. Then a phoenix can truly be said to have arisen from the ashes of an aggressive assault on the treatment relationship.

These principles are illustrated in the following case example, which returns to the outpatient psychotherapy of Ms. A., whose case was discussed at the beginning of this chapter.

Case Example: Ms. A.

About a year before Ms. A.'s Christmas Eve suicide attempt, she and her children had followed her husband to the Berkshires. Not long after this move, the patient's eldest teenage son had become uncontrollable, refusing to accept parental limits and acting out with drugs and the law, leading to arrests and a referral for family therapy. The family therapist focused on assisting the parents in filing a court petition that would lead to foster placement of the son. Meanwhile, Ms. A. began to feel guilty and depressed, feeling that everyone would be better off if she were dead. She carefully planned and executed a suicide attempt by carbon monoxide poisoning, but it was interrupted when one of her children returned home unexpectedly.

Ms. A. refused further family therapy, leading to referral to a new psychiatrist, who became the therapist in the aftermath of this interrupted but potentially lethal suicide attempt. Ms. A. gave a history of being the eldest and least favored child of her cold, punitive fundamentalist Christian parents, who were opposed to too much education, especially for girls. She reported a poorly recalled psychiatric hospitalization at age 14. Ms. A.'s marriage at age 18 had been a way of escaping her parents.

Ms. A. appeared depressed, but when the possibility of the use of antidepressants was raised, the patient stated a striking but unexplained refusal to take medication. Ms. A. and the therapist agreed to meet twice weekly for evaluation of her situation. Although hospitalization was considered, Ms. A. declined and was able to assure the therapist that she felt safe now that her suicide attempt had been aborted. In the first several evaluation sessions Ms. A. provided more history, particularly reporting her upset about her husband's series of past affairs. Within 2 weeks suicidal ideation returned and she felt more alone and hopeless, leading the therapist to recommend again a trial of amitriptyline up to 200 mg qhs, to which the patient reluctantly agreed, but without much response.

During the evaluation period various options were developed for the patient, including a medication approach, a family therapy focus, individual psychotherapy, or inpatient treatment. After 10 sessions the patient stated her preference for individual psychotherapy. The therapist agreed to provide this, negotiating a verbal therapeutic contract with the patient for twice-weekly outpatient psychoanalytic psychotherapy that held the patient responsible for keeping herself alive and made explicit the therapist's limitations in protecting the patient. Steps to take if the patient became suicidal were explored. Ms. A. was agreeable to the contract but suspicious that the therapist was primarily interested in money. A family meeting was held with the patient's husband to inform him of the terms of the therapeutic contract and its risks and benefits. Mr. A. was in agreement with the plan. At this point the therapist's diagnostic impression was of a probable major depressive episode in a woman with an adjustment disorder of adult life, but there were troubling hints of an underlying personality disorder.

Ms. A. was frequently silent and suspicious of the therapist in the hours. When she did speak there was an empty, ahistorical quality to her verbalizations, most of which were reports of details of the vicissitudes of her interactions with her children and husband. She seemed devoid of an inner mental life. Ms. A. struggled with suicidal ideation, but the therapist never had any sense of linkage between suicidal feelings, life events, and the history, and struggled with a countertransference feeling that Ms. A. might be unsuitable for psychotherapy. Ms. A. complained of feeling taken for granted by her husband and of fears that her eldest son was becoming psychopathic because of his remorseless struggles with the law.

In an early December session Ms. A. revealed she was increasingly concerned by an issue she had not mentioned and that had not been taken seriously by her husband: an accusation that her eldest son had sexually molested his younger female cousin. Ms. A. felt a time bomb was ticking inside her but was unable to put the details of this feeling into words. In the last session before Christmas Eve, Ms. A. reported she had not taken in a stray dog because of her husband's objections, but overnight the dog had nearly died in the cold. Ms. A. was furious at herself for following her husband's feelings instead of her own, but had difficulty voicing her anger. She felt that the therapist agreed with her husband's view that she was just "crazy" and not to be taken seriously. In that same hour the therapist told her of his week's vacation early in the New Year.

Ms. A. did not come to her next appointment on Christmas Eve. As described earlier, she overdosed on 2 grams of amitriptyline and was discovered comatose in her car, at which time she was hospitalized in an intensive care unit. One day after Christmas the therapist spoke to Ms. A. briefly by phone. He would not consider discussing the possibility of resuming the work unless she now agreed to a psychiatric hospitalization. Ms. A. voiced anger at the therapist, feeling that he, like her husband, was cold and cared only about money and his track record. The therapist also learned that Ms. A. had had a Christmas gift to bring to the Christmas Eve session and had been in a struggle about whether or not to come to the session and bring it.

After a week in an inpatient psychiatric unit Ms. A. met with her therapist. She spoke of herself as a dead person, wondering whether she wanted to come back to life and resume her therapy. She was aware that her attachment to the therapist was important but felt abandoned by the inference that she had terminated her treatment and by being held responsible for her actions. She realized there was much she did not remember from her early life, questioning whether she wanted to remember a painful past and if she wanted to be in an uncovering psychotherapy. Ms. A. feared that she would die without the therapy but might go crazy with it. The patient acknowledged that her struggle over the Christmas gift and the announcement of the therapist's vacation had had a frightening effect on her that she had been unable to understand.

At this point the therapist felt he and Ms. A. were having some success engaging affects genuinely. The therapist did not feel burdened any longer by his initial anger and guilt toward Ms. A. for her suicide attempt. The patient's aggression toward the therapy had been interpreted, and there was some preliminary understanding of the therapist's announcement of his vacation having been experienced by Ms. A. as an empathic failure, especially in the context of her intensely ambivalent dependent attachment to the therapist, with wishes both to flee the therapy and to give the therapist a gift. In the therapist's mind, an opportunity for repair was available to the patient, but it was not clear she would choose to make reparation or exercise the option to preserve the treatment. Ms. A.'s view of herself as dead, her uncertainty about whether she wished to come back to life, and her fear of what psychotherapy might uncover were clear. There was some suggestion that her son's possible molestation of his cousin and her husband's refusal to take this seriously were important issues. Ms. A. felt that husband, son, and therapist all viewed her as crazy and not to be taken seriously. Feeling it essential to take the patient seriously, to acknowledge her doubts about proceeding, and to hold her responsible for the preservation of the therapy and for repairing damage to it, the therapist suggested they suspend further meetings unless and until Ms. A. decided she wished to resume this kind of therapy.

Ms. A. remained hospitalized on a short-term unit for 3 weeks while consulting with two other psychiatrists about outpatient work. Finding those consultations unsatisfactory, Ms. A. asked to meet with her original therapist again. Ms. A. reported that in the hospital she had been among people who expected doctors to change them. This had brought home a realization that what the therapist had been saying was correct: she was the only one who could keep herself alive. Ms. A. asked if the therapist would resume outpatient therapy with her under the previous terms. Although much about the overdose remained unknown and unexplored, the therapist agreed to resume their twice-weekly work. Ms. A. was discharged from the hospital still on amitriptyline, but with the agreement of the inpatient treatment team that it seemed to be of little benefit.

After the sessions resumed, Ms. A. revealed she had begun to experience frightening tactile hallucinations of sexual penetration that made her fear she was losing her mind. She became tearful for the first time in the therapy as she reported recovery of the memory of a gang rape when she was 13 years old. Ms. A., who had never spoken about dreams or sexual material before, now revealed long-standing repetitive dreams of being raped, dreams that had troubled her but whose origin now for the first time she understood. Ms. A. asked for help in recalling what had happened in her past, but she was terrified of psychosis and of the therapist's presumed power over her. With great dread, Ms. A. explained that as a preteen she had felt so stifled by her parents' controlling, bigoted values that she would sneak out her bedroom window at night while her parents slept. By age 13 some of this time was spent visiting with a group of manifestly friendly older boys in a neighborhood clubhouse. On one occasion she had been given a drink laced with chloral hydrate. She had a hazy, terrifying memory of struggling to resist the power of the drug while attempting to fight off the boys who took turns raping and beating her. She also felt considerable guilt for having found the experience sexually arousing. Ms. A. had concealed the rape from her parents, claiming she was sick in order to avoid school. She recalled believing she had been damaged internally because of vaginal bleeding and numerous bruises, fearing she would probably die, but preferring death to letting her parents know what had happened. She was already familiar with her parents' intolerance of sexual experimentation and their tendency to blame a woman for whatever happened to her. The best way to deal with the rape had been to pretend it had never happened. Ms. A. felt she now had an explanation for a previously inexplicable finding on a routine chest X-ray, which showed several old rib fractures. It became clear that Ms. A.'s initial reluctance to take medication from the therapist was related to this repressed memory. Her suspicion and mistrust of the therapist were also related to the experience of the rape, but there was more.

A year after the rape, at age 14, Ms. A. had been hospitalized. Gradually Ms. A. pieced together that this "breakdown" had followed a boy's sexual interest in her. Ms. A. had been hospitalized and was treated by a psychiatrist who also was giving ECT to the elderly woman in the next bed. The teenage Ms. A. had believed ECT was used by that psychiatrist as a punishment and that if she did not comply she would be given the same treatment and then locked away forever. She had become a good patient to gain discharge, including agreeing to outpatient meetings with the psychiatrist. Shortly after beginning this teenage outpatient work, Ms. A. had begun to speak boastfully about her sexual knowledge, possibly as a prelude to revealing the rape to the doctor. Ms. A. recalled pleasure that the psychiatrist of her teenage years had seemed to find her attractive. When he suggested that she demonstrate her sexual prowess, she complied, feeling flattered, but also terrified of saying no to the "ECT doctor." Over the next 2 months Ms. A. had been forced to perform oral sex on the doctor in sessions, with the explicit threat that otherwise he would do to her what he had learned she feared most—that is, have her committed and given ECT. Terrorized but also aroused, Ms. A. had begun engaging in compulsive promiscuous sex with older boys. Knowing she would not otherwise be believed by her parents, Ms. A. had fantasized slashing the doctor's genitals during oral sex, twice having gone to sessions with a razor to implement this plan, but she was too frightened to try and feared her parents would blame her anyway. When the fall school term began, Ms. A. was able to convince her parents she no longer needed therapy. Her life became focused on forgetting the sexual traumata.

A number of important things seemed to fall into place in the therapy. The onset of Ms. A.'s son's sociopathic behavior, particularly the alleged sexual molestation of his cousin and Ms. A.'s husband's indifference to this, touched on long repressed material that stimulated the emergence of suicidal behavior without a conscious context. Also, Ms. A.'s husband had matter-of-factly assumed she was having a sexual relationship with the current therapist at around the time of the Christmas Eve suicide attempt. She liked the therapist and had been struggling with whether or not to bring him a gift, but her affectionate, dependent, and sexual longings, coupled with her husband's calm expectation of an affair, had been a source of intense turmoil immediately before the suicide attempt. Ms. A.'s sexual relationship with a previous therapist greatly complicated her ability to trust this therapist or to take seriously his commitment to the terms of the therapeutic contract, including refraining from a sexual relationship. Ms. A. had understandably come to view men as able to talk about principles and ethics only until they had an erection, at which point they would insist on sex. One of her solutions to this problem had been to become good at pleasing them sexually. In a sense, she repetitively prevented repetition of the rape by willingly providing sex to her husband whenever and however he wished. Men were feared and viewed with contempt, but in some way also seen as preferable to women, toward whom the patient felt disdain, and for which reason she preferred a male therapist, despite the fear (and wish) that never left her that the therapist was biding his time for the right moment to force her into a sexual relationship.

The recovery of the memory of the rape had a powerful consolidating effect on the therapeutic alliance. Antidepressants were soon tapered and discontinued without ill effects, but suicide did not disappear as an issue. Ms. A. frequently brought suicidal feelings to the therapy, struggling to keep herself from acting on these impulses more because she wanted the therapy to continue if she were going to stay alive than because she felt her life was worth living. Indeed, she made it clear she would have preferred dying in one of her suicide attempts.

Around the 200th psychotherapy hour there was a second suicide attempt that occurred in the context of Ms. A.'s terrifying awareness of intense dependency on the therapist while she was seriously considering separation from her husband. Ms. A. had taken the therapist's admonition that one should be cautious about deciding to separate during intensive psychotherapy as siding with the husband's view of her. The five principles described above were again operationalized, but space does not permit a detailed recounting of this process. It emerged in the aftermath of this attempt, though, that the patient wanted a marital separation not for the reasons she had offered, which had led the therapist to offer his admonition, but because of her husband's previously undisclosed pattern of awakening her from sleep by biting, pinching and hitting her, and then forcing her to submit to sex. The patient had felt the therapist's caution about separation during therapy was an abandonment of her to her husband's abuse, an empathic failure that the therapist could not possibly have anticipated because the behavior had been concealed.

More than 500 hours of psychotherapy have occurred in the 6 years since Ms. A. was first referred. Suicide dropped out as an active issue after the 200th hour. Ms. A. has divorced her husband, is completing a bachelor's degree at a competitive college, and plans to go on to graduate school. She is engaged in a rewarding relationship with a man. Shortly before termination, Ms. A. spoke of herself as having experienced a mental death after the rape, living her life only on the surface, but as having recovered her mental life and her ability to use her intellect through the therapy.

Conclusions

The case of Ms. A. is complex. The material presented is not meant to be a complete description of the therapy or of all the dynamic issues, but rather an illustration of how establishing a clear therapeutic contract and using the principles described in this chapter can provide a schema for psychotherapeutic work with self-destructive patients. Such a schema not only allows such work to proceed but facilitates it. Winnicott (1965) has noted that the emergence of self-destructive acting out that can be contained within the holding environment of the therapy may be a hopeful sign of useful therapeutic engagement. The use of these principles can provide a framework through which this observation can be operationalized.

It is not my experience or contention that these five principles need be applied in any particular sequence or that in any one instance of self-destructive behavior their utilization will lead a self-destructive patient to change. Rather, dealing with self-destructive behavior with the above schema in mind leads to clarification of the reality of the responsibilities and limitations of the therapeutic relationship. The principles may require repetition on more than one occasion, but they provide an opportunity eventually to work through and internalize a new object relationship. Such an outcome will not always be the case, though, and some therapies will fail. When the self-destructive behavior is more valuable to the patient than the therapeutic relationship, the treatment will end, with referral to a new therapist or to a new form of treatment. Nor is such an ending necessarily a failure. More than one borderline patient has learned something important by losing a therapist who was pushed beyond his or her limits, rather than being inseparably linked in a sadomasochistic dyad.

There is also the reality that following this schema will not always prevent suicide. For example, Ms. A.'s survival of her suicide attempts was largely a matter of luck. Of course, there is no treatment that can guarantee that self-destructive borderline patients will not attempt or commit suicide. No therapist who works with such patients can be useful if excessively burdened by the reality that some of his or her patients will commit suicide. This is not intended to absolve therapists of careful scrutiny of the quality of their work with patients or of their countertransference responses. In fact, these principles are offered in the hope that they will allow therapists to do their work better and to scrutinize their approach more effectively.

References

Adler G: The borderline-narcissistic personality disorder continuum. Am J Psychiatry 138:46–50, 1981

Akiskal HS: Subaffective disorders: dysthymic, cyclothymic and bipolar II disorders in the "borderline" realm. Psychiatr Clin North Am 4:25–46, 1981

American Psychiatric Association: Diagnostic and Statistical Manual of Mental Disorders, 3rd Edition. Washington, DC, American Psychiatric Association, 1980

American Psychiatric Association: Diagnostic and Statistical Manual of Mental Disorders, 3rd Edition, Revised. Washington, DC, American Psychiatric Association, 1987

Cooperman MC: Defeating processes in psychotherapy, in Psychoanalysis and Psychosis. Edited by Silver AS. Madison, CT, International Universities Press, 1989, pp 339–357

Gardner DL, Cowdry RW: Suicidal and parasuicidal behavior in borderline personality disorder. Psychiatr Clin North Am 8:389–403, 1985

Kernberg OF: Borderline Conditions and Pathological Narcissism. New York, Jason Aronson, 1975

Kernberg OF: Severe Personality Disorders. New Haven, CT, Yale University Press, 1984

Kernberg OF, Selzer MA, Koenigsberger HW, et al: Psychodynamic Psychotherapy of Borderline Patients. New York, Basic Books, 1989

Masterson JF: Countertransference and Psychotherapeutic Technique: Teaching Seminars on Psychotherapy of the Borderline Adult. New York, Brunner/Mazel, 1983

McGlashan TH: The borderline syndrome, I: testing three diagnostic systems. Arch Gen Psychiatry 40:1311–1318, 1983a

McGlashan TH: The borderline syndrome, II: is it a variant of schizophrenia or affective disorder? Arch Gen Psychiatry 40:1319–1323, 1983b

McGlashan TH: The prediction of outcome in borderline personality disorder: part V of the Chestnut Lodge follow-up study, in The Borderline: Current Empirical Research. Edited by McGlashan TH. Washington, DC, American Psychiatric Press, 1985, pp 61–98

McGlashan TH: Impulsivity in borderline personality disorder: longitudinal perspectives. Paper presented at the 143rd annual meeting of the American Psychiatric Association, New York, May 1990

Paris J, Brown R, Nowlis D: Long-term follow-up of borderline patients in a general hospital. Compr Psychiatry 28:530–535, 1987

Plakun EM: Narcissistic personality disorder: a validity study and comparison to borderline personality disorder. Psychiatr Clin North Am 12:603–620, 1989

Plakun EM: Prediction of outcome in borderline personality disorders. Journal of Personality Disorders 5:93–101, 1991

Plakun EM, Burkhardt PE, Muller JP: 14-year follow-up of borderline and schizotypal personality disorders. Compr Psychiatry 26:448–455, 1985

Rinsley DB: Borderline and Other Self Disorders. New York, Jason Aronson, 1982

Searles HF: The "dedicated physician" in the field of psychotherapy and psychoanalysis, in Countertransference and Related Subjects: Selected Papers. New York, International Universities Press, 1979, pp 71–88

Soloff PH, George A, Nathan RS, et al: Progress in pharmacotherapy of borderline disorders: a double-blind study of amitriptyline, haloperidol, and placebo. Arch Gen Psychiatry 43:691–697, 1986

Stone MH, Hurt SW, Stone DK: The PI 500: long-term follow-up of borderline inpatients meeting DSM-III criteria, I: global outcome. Journal of Personality Disorders 1:291–298, 1987

Winnicott DW: Psychotherapy of character disorders (1963), in The Maturational Process and the Facilitating Environment. New York, International Universities Press, 1965, pp 203–216

Chapter 6

Psychotherapeutic Approaches to Masochism

Arnold M. Cooper, M.D.

Patients whose lives are characterized by behaviors that result in seemingly needless disappointment, defeat, and suffering form a significant portion of psychotherapeutic practice. These patterns of self-inflicted, self-defeating behaviors have been of interest to psychiatrists at least since the work of Kraft-Ebbing in 1895 (Kraft-Ebbing 1895). He coined the term *masochism,* giving credit to Leopold von Sacher-Masoch, who in his novel *Venus in Furs* (Sacher-Masoch 1870/1971) described a man who ruined his life through his enthrallment to a woman. The 1931 movie *The Blue Angel* (*Der blaue Engel* [1930]), directed by Josef von Sternberg, with Marlene Dietrich and Emil Jannings, adapted from the book of Heinrich Mann, similarly described the total enslavement and humiliation of a self-respecting schoolteacher who is infatuated with a nightclub singer.

Freud adopted Kraft-Ebbing's term masochism to describe two related, but different, psychic situations. In his early writings Freud was primarily concerned with perversion masochism (Freud 1905/1953), in which there is a clear, conscious sexual pleasure that accompanies painful experience, whether the pain is self-inflicted or not. He later took up the problem of moral or psychic masochism (Freud 1924/1961), in which the individual relentlessly pursues psychologically painful, humiliating, or self-defeating outcomes and seems to avoid opportunities for pleasure and success. In these instances, sexual satisfaction is usually not a component of the overt behavior patterns. Freud puzzled over these curious reversals of the pleasure principle and suggested in the course of his work a variety of possible explanations. Although Kraft-Ebbing and Sacher-Masoch before him had described this behavior in male patients, Freud and some of his followers, noting the passivity that seemed so much a part of the character structure of masochistic individuals, assumed that this passivity represented a feminine characteristic, and through this logic regarded masochism as a feminine trait. Helene Deutsch (1944), in particular, emphasized masochism as being innate to femininity and related it to the sexual act of being penetrated and the painful circumstances of giving birth. The error of equating passivity with femininity was pointed out quite early (Rado 1956) in the psychoanalytic literature, but it persisted until the feminist critique of the past several decades put to rest that unfortunate culturally determined misunderstanding.

More recently, residues of this heritage linking masochism and femininity led to fierce debate over the inclusion of the category of "masochistic personality disorder" in DSM-III-R (American Psychiatric Association 1987). Feminist clinicians feared that such a category would be used prejudicially against women, would make women to blame when they were the objects of abuse by men, and would lead the judicial system toward exoneration of men guilty of violence against women. In an attempt to reach a compromise over these concerns, the framers of DSM-III-R agreed to drop the term "masochism" because of its earlier psychological linkage with femininity, and they substituted the phrase "self-defeating personality disorder" (SDPD). Furthermore, the category was placed among the "proposed diagnostic categories needing further study" (American Psychiatric Association 1987, pp. 371–374).[1]

---

[1] In this chapter the terms "self-defeating" and "masochistic" will be used interchangeably.

Description of the Syndrome of Self-Defeating Personality Disorder

The DSM-III-R criteria (American Psychiatric Association 1987, pp. 371–374) for SDPD are given in Table 6–1.

Table 6–1. DSM-III-R criteria for self-defeating personality disorder

A. A pervasive pattern of self-defeating behavior, beginning by early adulthood and present in a variety of contexts. The person may often avoid or undermine pleasurable experiences, be drawn to situations or relationships in which he or she will suffer, and prevent others from helping him or her, as indicated by at least five of the following:

1. Chooses people and situations that lead to disappointment, failure, or mistreatment even when better options are clearly available.

2. Rejects or renders ineffective the attempts of others to help him or her.

3. Following positive personal events (e.g., new achievement), responds with depression, guilt, or a behavior that produces pain (e.g., an accident).

4. Incites angry or rejecting responses from others and then feels hurt, defeated, or humiliated (e.g., makes fun of spouse in public, provoking an angry retort, then feels devastated).

5. Rejects opportunities for pleasure, or is reluctant to acknowledge enjoying himself or herself (despite having adequate social skills and the capacity for pleasure).

6. Fails to accomplish tasks crucial to his or her personal objectives despite demonstrated ability to do so, e.g., helps fellow students write papers, but is unable to write his or her own.

7. Is uninterested in or rejects people who consistently treat him or her well, e.g., is unattracted to caring sexual partners.

8. Engages in excessive self-sacrifice that is unsolicited by the intended recipients of the sacrifice.

B. The behaviors in A do not occur exclusively in response to, or in anticipation of, being physically, sexually, or psychologically abused.

C. The behaviors in A do not occur only when the person is depressed.

Source. Reprinted from American Psychiatric Association *Diagnostic and Statistical Manual of Mental Disorders,* 3rd Edition, Revised. Washington, DC, American Psychiatric Association, 1987, pp. 373–374. Copyright 1987, American Psychiatric Association. Used with permission.

There has been an increasing number of empirical studies of SDPD during the past several years. These studies are the subject of an exhaustive review by Fiester (1991), who concludes:

> Data from existing studies show a relatively high prevalence, slightly higher female:male sex ratio, good internal consistency, significant overlap with several other personality disorders (particularly borderline, dependent, and avoidant personality disorders), some possible inherent sex bias in the criteria, an apparent lack of sex bias in the application of the criteria by clinicians, and lack of differentiation of patients with SDPD from patients with other disorders in terms of demographic factors other than gender. (p. 207)

Fiester also concludes that the research is not yet adequate to decide upon the inclusion of this category in DSM-IV.

Theories of Masochism

The psychodynamic and psychophysiological understanding of the ways in which people can derive pleasure or satisfaction from painful circumstance—or are at least more comfortable with defeat than with success—has been a topic of major significance since the very beginnings of psychoanalysis. I have elsewhere (Cooper 1988) reviewed our clinical knowledge of and theoretical constructions for an understanding of masochistic behavior, so I will not detail them here. In general, these explanations fall under several headings:

1. Attitudes of passivity, harmlessness, and nonaggression are unconsciously adopted as a defense against dangerous competitive impulses and fear of retaliation.
2. Suffering, helplessness, and defeat represent a cry for love and are unconsciously intended to ensure loving care, which is otherwise perceived not to be available.
3. Early, severe, inescapable painful traumas lead to defensive efforts to cope with the trauma by learning to enjoy it, adopting it as one's own.

4. Early injuries to the infantile sense of omnipotent control are adapted to defensively by the fantasy of control over disappointing, powerful parents and by defensively claiming the disappointment as directed by oneself.
5. Experiences of pain result in endorphin release in the attempt to ease the pain, and one becomes self-addicted to endorphin release, pursuing painful events for this end (van der Kolk 1987).
6. Children reared under abusive conditions nonetheless attach to their abusing caretakers. For these persons with damaged self-esteem and fears of abandonment, maintaining the safety of familiarity takes precedence over potential pleasure that entails the anxiety of the new.
7. The Lesch-Nyhan syndrome, in which, among other things, children are born with what seems to be a defective capacity for experiencing protective pain responses and they engage in severe self-mutilating behaviors, has been suggested as a biologic model for psychological self-inflicted pain (Dizmang and Cheatham 1970). There is, however, no evidence that would connect these two quite different conditions.

These explanations are not mutually exclusive, and it is likely that in every masochistic individual there is an amalgam of several of these attempts at adaptation, with one or another group of defense mechanisms predominating in a particular patient. However, except for the Lesch-Nyhan syndrome, all of these explanations share the view that individuals who develop SDPD were, at least in their own perception, the victims of unempathic or abusive childhood settings, and clinical experience would seem to confirm that abused children are prone to developing sadistic and masochistic relationships in later life. Again with the exception of the Lesch-Nyhan syndrome, the explanations all posit early failure to support the child's budding self-esteem and to provide the atmosphere of safety required for adequate development of healthy narcissism and assertion. As I shall attempt to demonstrate in this chapter, the understanding of masochism is enhanced by understanding the narcissistic roots of the masochistic defenses that lead to self-defeating behavior.

The Narcissistic-Masochistic Personality Disorder

Although the DSM-III-R description of SDPD is generally in accord with clinical experience, it can be enhanced by providing a richer clinical texture and an attempt to understand the psychodynamics that are part of the behaviors. My description will be colored by my conviction that masochistic patients are a variant of narcissistic personality disorder, and that in every masochistic patient one finds prominent narcissistic traits. I have in a series of papers suggested that self-defeating (or masochistic) personality disorder is best understood as a constellation involving narcissistic and masochistic conflicts (Cooper 1984, 1988, 1989) and is more accurately classified as the *narcissistic-masochistic personality disorder.*

Very briefly, masochistic patients are those who as children were especially intolerant of the hurts to their self-esteem that regularly accompany frustration, or who experienced an actual excess of such hurts. Rather than admit to the defeat, or to the state of relative childhood helplessness, or to the need for the benign intervention of others to provide their satisfactions, they resort to a special defense. In effect, they deny their childhood helplessness by claiming control over their frustrators, especially the mother of the preoedipal period, inwardly asserting that the frustrations were delivered because the child forced the parent to do so. Moreover, the child claims to be so powerful that the parent cannot really hurt him or her because the child enjoys the injury that has been suffered. If the child does feel hurt, it proves the extraordinary power and malice of the parents who are mistreating him or her. All this goes on out of awareness and arouses its own guilty responses, requiring conscious denial of pleasure in pain by exaggerating one's feelings of hurt, thereby proving one's innocence of self-defeating intentions.

Phenomenologically, behind a thin facade, these patients behave as if motivated by a need for defeat and victimization, and they pursue humiliation and defeat. Success seems to make them uncomfortable, whereas they experience a sense of act completion—that is, the sense of an ending—when finally they feel hurt. With the feeling of victimization, the drama has come to what feels to the masochistic person like an appropriate and expected end-ing—like the child who comes to the end of a favorite fairy tale whose ending he or she knows very well—and there is a sense of familiarity and relief and closure. One can now go on to other things.

It is implicit in the definition of all personality disorders or neuroses that they handicap adaptation. What is specific to the masochistic person is a *pursuit* of failure in one or several areas of psychological function that goes beyond the ordinary accompaniments of maladaptation. These are individuals who unfailingly succeed in snatching defeat from the jaws of victory and seem unable to recognize occasions for enjoyment or self-reward.

Self-defeating personality disorder is distinguished from the accidental consequences of psychological maladaptation by an unconsciously determined *desire* for defeat, shame, self-pity, humiliation, and secondary righteous indignation. Masochists *arrange* their lives for unhappiness. A man who loves sex marries a frigid woman, setting the stage for decades of bitter complaint. A woman is told that Mr. A. is a womanizer, and she meets him, falls in love, and he *is* a womanizer and she suffers.

Masochists exaggerate their defeats and minimize their successes. A patient who had just won a significant prize in his field found himself far more concerned with the nastiness of the cab driver who took him to the award ceremony than he was with the award. Incidentally, this little vignette points up that masochistic patients may do very well in some sectors of their lives, but if they do, they will drain their success of much of its pleasurable quality. The pursuit of pain in these patients leads them to avoid usually pleasurable experiences, or at least to not acknowledge the pleasure that would seem to be in order.

The self and object representations of the masochist deserve note. These individuals assume that all objects close to them exist as a source of frustration and malice. In effect, they use their relationships in the external world to produce endless duplications of the refusing, cruel preoedipal mother that dominates their internal world. Some masochistic patients will acknowledge that there are good, giving persons in the world, but it is part of the special bad luck with which the patient is cursed that these good people are not part of *his* (or *her*) world. Internally, the masochist simultaneously or alternately maintains a double fantasy; one of himself as controlling and extracting secret pleasure from the actions of malignant others who wish to harm him, and another of himself as innocent child victim of malicious parents who might love him if he is submissive. These internal representations of objects are matched by a self representation that includes the disagreeable knowledge that one is incapable of the self-esteem that comes from the inner conviction that one is able to give oneself the pleasures that one craves. The masochistic patient does not regard himself or herself as a reliable provider of satisfaction. The patient lacks the capacity for adequate appropriate assertion in the world, and his or her aggression is generally confined to inner anger or self-defeating expressions of aggression in the wrong place, at the wrong time, against the wrong people.

Masochistic patients are also great blamers, and while they are capable of wallowing in self-pity and debasing *themselves* with an excess of self-blame, when you examine more carefully, they are always blaming someone else. For example, an isolated man who believed he was unlovable because his body was so unappealing that he could not blame anyone for running from him, at a slightly deeper level held his mother to blame for having cursed him with his unacceptable body. Incidentally, this was all part of an inner fantasy; his body was in no way abnormal.

As one would expect of a group of severely narcissistic patients, self-defeating patients may be extremely self-centered. Some masochistic patients who seem overtly self-sacrificing, unassertive, empathic, and nice, will, on closer examination, prove to be interested primarily in their own special suffering and resentment, and their empathy is limited. A man who was regarded by his friends as the most understanding and "nicest" person in their circle confessed to his utter boredom with his friends' troubles, but he was too passive and frightened to try to shut anyone up. He did, however, enjoy the reputation he had of being a special person in his group. Masochistic patients are convinced of the special quality of their suffering—no one else endures as much as they do.

The covert narcissism of masochistic patients is often disguised behind their passive depressive stance, and Walter Mitty–type fantasies of greatness, specialness, and revenge are revealed after one gets to know the person better. They frequently have fantasies of being specially victimized in ways that will bring them finally to the attention of the cold, uncaring outside world. These patients may have fantasies of suicide, or of being prey to a deadly disease, but the major content of these fantasies is that finally others will know how much they have suffered. They are in general not at risk for suicide.

Finally, a word about the operations of conscience in the masochistic patient. As with all narcissistic patients, the superego in masochistic patients is deformed—it is both excessively harsh and corrupt. These individuals suffer severe pangs of guilt for every shortcoming and failure to achieve perfection, as well as for the anger they feel against those to whom they are close, and this guilt leads them toward further self-punitive actions. Because these self-punishments are accompanied by some degree of secret satisfaction, these patients further incur the wrath of conscience for indulging in such forbidden pleasures. While some self-defeating characters torture themselves with hyperscrupulosity—a technique that allows them to make hidden fun of their educators, proving that all rules are ridiculous and designed to prevent any pleasure—another group may flout the rules of society, but in ways that guarantee their being caught and punished, further adding to their burden of suffering. In both cases, it is as if inner conscience does not act to prevent the damaging action, but appears on the scene only for the sake of punishment. Self-reward and self-soothing do not seem to be in the repertoire of the severely masochistic patient.

Edmund Bergler (1949, 1952) suggested some years ago that the clinical sequence that he labeled the mechanism of "injustice collecting" is paradigmatic for the masochistic character (or SDPD personality) and that understanding the mechanism of injustice collecting is the key to recognizing the masochistic character. There are three steps to this sequence of injustice collecting:

1. Either through their own provocation or by their misuse of an available opportunity to personalize one of life's regularly ex-

pectable unfairnesses, masochistic persons arrange to experience disappointment, rejection, and humiliation. They experience a great deal of pain but are totally unaware of their role in engineering the misfortune.

2. Having garnered the unconsciously sought-after injustice, masochistic persons respond with righteous indignation and defensive rage against the refusing or humiliating object. Close examination, however, reveals that the rage is not genuinely intended to right a wrong or to gain a victory; rather, its purpose is to demonstrate to their own accusing inner conscience that they were not guilty of the charge of having wished for and provoked the injury and of the even worse accusation that they enjoy the injury. "How can anyone believe that I enjoy defeat? Look how furious I am at my enemies." Because the motivation of this rage is the desire to quiet conscience, rather than to achieve positive goals in the external world, the expression of the anger is often inappropriate in timing and dosage, thus leading to further actual defeats.

3. After the defensive aggression peters out, masochistic persons succumb to depression and self-pitying feelings characterized by the thought "This only happens to me."

Consider the following minor example of injustice collecting:

> A man tells his wife that he is not sure what time he is coming home that evening. He arrives earlier than usual, and he feels disappointed that his wife is not home. When she arrives a half hour later he berates her for not having been there. She feels unjustly accused and is angry in turn; meanwhile, another evening is ruined and the husband mopes through the evening obsessing about how he could have made such a bad marriage.

Masochistic persons often take personally what less neurotic individuals accept as ordinary, thus lending a certain paranoid flavor to masochistic patients' behavior. The following case provides a more substantial example:

Case 1

A lawyer who has been warned repeatedly because he is late with briefs and documents receives a smaller bonus at the end of the year than some of his colleagues. He is enraged and indignant and conveys this to the senior partner, who tells him that if he is not happy at the firm perhaps he should leave. He quits on the spot—in the middle of a recession—and lapses into a self-pitying depression over his bad luck, realizing the mess he now is in.

My clinical experience would indicate that this three-step mechanism of "injustice collecting" that Bergler described is indeed paradigmatic for those patients with SDPD. All of us engage in this technique at some time or other, to some degree, but the masochist makes it his or her life's work. The mechanism of injustice collecting serves not only as a marker for SDPD but also as an indicator of the powerful narcissistic component that enters into self-defeating behaviors. The mixture of narcissistic and masochistic defenses complicates the treatment, because the patient perceives even the need for help as a blow to his or her fragile self-esteem. Every interpretation of the patient's self-defeating behavior, no matter how carefully phrased, will arouse in the patient a feeling of wounded pride and personal injury, either because the interpretation means that the therapist figured something out that the patient could not, and the patient is being "one-upped," or because the interpretation, no matter how gently it is phrased, implies that the patient's behavior has been both irrational and infantile, and the patient is being humiliated. These narcissistic injuries in response to interpretation form one aspect of the negative therapeutic reaction discussed below. While interpretation of masochistic behaviors elicits narcissistic defenses, interpretation of narcissistic defenses elicits masochistic defensive behavior. Helping these patients to understand the secret pride and pleasure in their suffering may lead them to create new defeats and new heights of suffering in their effort to prove that they cannot be accused of wanting to be the victim that they seem always to be. This alternation of masochistic and narcissistic defenses contributes greatly to the complexity and unavoidable lengthiness of therapy with these patients.

As in all personality disorders, there is every gradation from mild to severe. The severe cases give the impression of a relentless pursuit of self-destruction from which the patients cannot be deflected—even by psychotherapy or analysis. The milder cases are compatible with considerable success in life, with some sectors of these patients' personalities being relatively immune to the effects of their disorder. However, even when aspects of life are outwardly successful, there is a damaged inner capacity for pleasure in the accomplishment. Like all narcissistic patients, masochistic patients often have little capacity for self-reward, but require the applause and admiration of others to make their achievements meaningful to themselves. But because others are basically always the depriving enemy, these rewards are never large enough.

When treating masochistic patients, it is necessary to be aware that their suffering is no less authentic despite its being unconsciously pursued and used as a source of narcissistic inflation. The provocation and sometimes barely hidden relish of their self-pity may tempt one to forget the genuine misery of these patients.

Treatment

Self-defeating patients often present initially with an acute depression or anxiety related to a crisis they have created—for example, provoking a spouse to threaten to leave or creating difficulties at work—and they seek rapid help in solving a reality situation or getting some relief from their symptoms. Crisis interventions can be extremely effective in relieving these patients of temporary peaks of illness, especially at the beginning of treatment. Reassurance and preliminary interpretation may bring very rapid relief. Usually, however, this relief is quite temporary. This positive response is in part a tribute to the better-adapted health-seeking aspect of the patient, but it also represents a defense and later resistance in the therapy, as the patient demonstrates that there was never anything wrong with him or her that kindness could not cure. Therapists can be lured into believing that they have an "easy" case on their hands when they see how quickly the patient responds to therapeutic interventions. However, when there is a history of significant self-defeating behavior and injustice collecting, one can be reasonably certain that the "honeymoon" will not last and treatment will be prolonged and taxing.

These treatments may be especially painful for both patient and therapist. I will try to give examples of some of the kinds of behavior that are common in the treatment of these patients.

The Negative Therapeutic Reaction

In 1923 Freud noted that

> there are certain people who behave in a quite peculiar fashion during the work of analysis. When one speaks hopefully to them or expresses satisfaction with the progress of the treatment, they show signs of discontent and their condition invariably becomes worse. One begins by regarding this as defiance and as an attempt to prove their superiority to the physician, but later one comes to take a deeper and juster view. One becomes convinced, not only that such people cannot endure any praise or appreciation, but that they react inversely to the progress of the treatment. Every partial solution that ought to result, and in other people does result, in an improvement or a temporary suspension of symptoms produces in them for the time being an exacerbation of their illness; they get worse during the treatment instead of getting better. They exhibit what is known as a "negative therapeutic reaction." (Freud 1923/1961, p. 49)

Freud ascribed this negative therapeutic reaction to an unconscious sense of guilt.

Case 2

> A 29-year old banker entered treatment because of his increasing realization that although he is unusually able and competent, he manages to make a bad impression at critical moments, displaying himself as anxious and uncertain and spoiling his chances for

promotion to a more responsible position within the firm. He complained bitterly that he worked harder than anyone else and was on the brink of exhaustion, and was unappreciated. As we explored these behaviors and feelings he became more aware of his angry competitiveness with peers, its relation to his feelings toward his siblings during his childhood, and the degree to which this anger frightened him and made him feel guilty. After a brief moment of relief and gratitude that he could now more comfortably face something that he had to some degree already known, he became depressed and angry at me, convinced that I had called him a bad person for being so full of anger, and that I must now hate him. Furthermore, I had misunderstood the problem: he did not work harder than anyone else; in fact, he did not work hard at all. He was convinced that it was hopeless for us to continue to work together because I so totally failed to understand him. Episodes such as this were repeated innumerable times in the treatment, often having the intended effect of leaving me feeling confused and helpless.

Case 3

Another patient, in response to every interpretation or clarification, would respond with initial interest ("I never thought of that before"), would begin to elaborate how that view helped him to understand some of his behavior, and then would appear the next day looking depressed and would say, "I was thinking about what you said. It doesn't help me. And it wasn't very nice to hear that I have yet one more fault."

Negative therapeutic reactions tempt the therapist to angry retaliation, bullying, feelings of confusion, and a sense of being deskilled. It is of enormous help to recognize the use and unconscious meanings of negative therapeutic reactions and that these meanings can be brought within the patient's coping capacities as they begin to be understood. The therapist's sympathetic but dogged persistence is essential in helping the patient to begin to gradually side with the therapist and accept the aid that is being offered.

It is important to make every effort to interpret the occurrence of negative therapeutic reactions, bringing them into the transference. This enables the patient to begin to see that the sense of hopelessness and depression is occurring in relation to positive events in the treatment and, especially, in response to helpful interactions with the therapist. The mere fact that the therapist persistently regards the patient's negative reactions as something that can be understood helps to begin to modify the internal qualities of the harsh superego that previously demanded punishment whenever pleasurable possibilities arose. The patient can begin to grasp that it is possible to carry on an inner argument with that portion of his or her superego that flatly denies the patient his or her rights to pleasure. The therapist's attitude also brings to the patient's attention the angry, hating components of the negative therapeutic reaction—the demands for reparation and vengeance before pleasurable capacities can be admitted.

Finally, a word of caution. Patients can respond with what seems like a negative therapeutic reaction to the therapist's faulty understanding of them. Simply the fact that a patient has a regressive reaction to an interpretation does not justify labeling it a negative therapeutic reaction. One must first be reasonably sure that the patient is not responding to countertransferential insensitivity, empathic failure, or unconscious attack on the part of the therapist. A therapeutic attitude of considerable self-scrutiny is highly desirable when treating masochistic patients, because their provocative capacities tend to bring out the worst in their therapists.

Damaged Capacity for Positive Identification

It is a crucial component of all psychotherapy that the patient has some ability to form a positive attachment (i.e., a positive transference) to the therapist. All forms of psychotherapy, from behavioral to psychoanalytic, probably depend significantly upon the capacity to internalize some aspects of the therapist as a figure who is loving, and as one who can be loved, idealized, or emulated. One of Kohut's (1971) major contributions was to recognize the hidden elements of positive transference in those severely narcissistic patients who seemed detached from the therapist and the therapeutic process. Many masochistic patients are equally detached because of their narcissistic pathology, and in addition they use almost all interpersonal transactions for the purpose of demonstrating that they are perpetually frustrated, refused, and unappreciated. This inner need to prove their victimization within the treatment situation can dominate the transference and is a significant deterrent to the formation of positive attachment to the therapist or to the treatment situation, as in the following example:

Case 4

A patient describes that she had been very bothered by my greeting her in the hallway and holding the office door open for her rather than waiting for her to come into my waiting room. She said, "We were fighting over who was going to get to the door first and who was going to get in first." My ordinary politeness, an opportunity for her to feel that I respected her and that we shared a mutual regard, was interpreted by her as a sign of competitive aggression against her. She could not permit herself to be the beneficiary of even trivial demonstrations of kindness or respect that would bring us closer together, and she therefore reinterpreted my motives as hostile and controlling.

Some patients with SDPD report that the impending vacation of the therapist is a financial relief and a convenience and nothing more. Moreover, they do not remember favors done them, and any therapeutic progress is regarded as entirely their own achievement, made in spite of the obstructions of the therapist. One patient said to me, "It gives me a creepy feeling, it makes my skin crawl to think that you are involved in my life. I'm in this by myself." Furthermore, these patients can be relentlessly denigrating and devaluing toward the therapist, reflecting their narcissistic need to eradicate all traces of superior or enviable traits in the therapist, as well as the masochistic need to deny that anyone can help them with their suffering. This inability to identify with the strengths and benign intentions of the therapist deprives the patient of a source of ego support that forms an important part of any successful treatment. Some analyses are unusually painful for the masochistic patient because of his or her inability to form a positive identification with the analyst (Cooper 1984).

Masochistic patients fight against their budding positive identifications because such responses undercut their conviction that
all interpersonal contacts result in victimization. The challenge to
the therapist is to maintain his general benevolence, i.e., therapeutic neutrality, neither going to excessive lengths to prove his good
intentions and that he is a "nice guy," nor openly or covertly berat-
ing the patient for his or her one-sided inability to see the therapist
in any positive way. In time, the patient's own inner conscience
becomes a source of conflict as the patient stands inwardly accused
of falsifying the relationship and insisting on feeling aggrieved. As
inner conscience becomes an ally of the therapist, at least temporarily, the patient can begin to experience the therapist as helper
and model for identification, thus beginning to soften some of his
or her own harsh self-condemnation.

Provocation—Conscious and Unconscious

Provocation is the stock in trade of the masochistic patient, and the
therapist is often astonished by the extent and ingeniousness of the
patient's provocative capacities. These are the patients who regularly pay their bills late, forcing the therapist to ask for the money,
which proves that the therapist is only a money-grubber. Or after
the therapist, at considerable inconvenience, changes an appointment time because the patient explained that the change was essential, the patient casually says that the old time was just as good
but that she is willing to accommodate the therapist if he wants this
new time. A chronically late patient once comes on time and instantly pounds on the shut office door while the therapist is still
with another patient, feeling indignant that the therapist is a minute late beginning the session. A patient makes his therapy the
topic of cocktail-party conversation, wildly misquoting or fabricat-
ing his therapist's remarks.

These provocations are all preludes to injustice collecting, intended to elicit aggression from the therapist, whereupon the patient will overlook his or her provocation and perceive himself or
herself as being victimized. Patience and a sense of humor are essential in dealing with patients in these situations. It is an error to

let these situations go unnoticed, because this usually leads the patient to up the ante in his or her desire to justify the grievance. On the other hand, scolding, moralizing, or making pleas for understanding only convince the patient that the therapist has his or her own, and not the patient's, interests at heart. It is often helpful to use interpretations of situations outside the transference, where the self-damage of the patient's endless provocation may be more apparent.

Frequently, the patient becomes aware of his or her disappointment in having been unable fully to engage the therapist in punitive behaviors toward him or her, and begins to realize the unconscious intent of the provocations. For example, a chronically late patient who began each session with a set of somewhat hypocritical apologies for the lateness and sorrow for the distress that his lateness undoubtedly caused the therapist was taken aback—and helped—by the therapist's explanation that while he was sorry that the patient was not getting the full benefit of the treatment, he, the therapist, enjoyed the extra free time, and thus no apology was required. Of course, the patient seized on this to say that he always knew that the therapist didn't really want to see him. While it is essential to avoid retaliation in the face of provocation, reality testing should not be sacrificed, and patients need to understand that provocations beyond a certain point cannot be tolerated.

There is also a group of masochistic patients who are excessively compliant—seemingly the opposite of provocative. Every interpretation is savored, bills are paid instantly, the attitude is always friendly, but the patient gets no better. These patients' good behavior turns out to be part of an inner demonstration that, in spite of their doing everything that is asked of them, they get nothing in return. They are not specially loved and given special treatment. Eventually, if this is not interpreted, these patients become overtly angry and hurt, and leave treatment.

Unconscious Demand for Reparation and Vengeance

One of the greatest obstacles to change in self-defeating patients is their unwillingness to make peace with their perceived torturers until they are convinced that those unconsciously maintained malicious internal figures from the past have made amends for the suffering that these patients feel has been inflicted on them. For many of these patients, giving up the painful life that they lead means admitting that the harm done them by parents and educators was less massive than they claim; they are not damaged beyond repair as they have insisted and partly believed. They cannot bear the thought that no one will be punished for the terrible things that were done to a poor innocent child—the patient—and no one will now make up for the suffering they have endured. These patients refuse to accept that there is no court of appeal and there is no choice but to call it a day.

The self-pitying aspects of the self-defeating character come to the fore around the conviction that "I deserve to be given special privilege and sympathy because no one has suffered as I have at the hands of my cruel parent." All of the aggression that these patients feel toward parents, and all the fury they retain over the fantasy of the parent (usually the mother) as all-powerful and capable of making the child entirely happy if only she wanted to, lead them to insist that they should not be forced to "forgive and forget." Someone should pay for the crimes that were committed. This demand usually falls upon the therapist in some form—often with the bitter complaint that the therapist is insufficiently sympathetic to how miserable the patient has been and does not share the patient's view that he or she has been innocently victimized by cruel parents. These patients, unconsciously and sometimes consciously, deny themselves pleasurable experiences because they do not want to feel well until someone—a parent or more usually a parent surrogate, such as a spouse—has paid the price for their suffering. At the same time, of course, there is no reparation that would be large enough to soothe these patients' grievances. When patients do receive some form of apology or a gesture of reconciliation, they respond with a bitter sense of too little and too late. In fact, the gesture of appeasement from parent or spouse often serves only to prove that the patient is right in feeling injured; if the other person were not guilty, he or she would not try to "buy off" the patient with conciliatory gestures.

Case 5

A patient, late in an analysis, described a visit to his parents' home and said, "They were genuinely glad to see me, and they can tell that I am now a much happier person than I used to be. They take great pride in my successes. And it never occurs to them that they owe me an apology for what they put me through. I know this is stupid, but I can't bear the thought that they are getting away with it. They don't even feel guilty. It made me very depressed and I ended up moping around. I could tell it bothered them and I was glad. But they didn't seem as unhappy as I was. Finally, I picked a fight over what my mother served for lunch—the same crap that she knows I don't like to eat. I knew I was behaving stupidly, but I couldn't help it. It was worth it to me to ruin the visit if it hurt them. But they were feeling fine when we spoke on the phone the next day, and I still feel like shit. I guess that's a pretty good example of my masochism in action."

This vignette also reveals one aspect of the so-called sadistic component to many self-defeating behaviors. What is significant in this regard is that the aggression is not enjoyed for itself; rather, it is a part of the patient's continuing self-pity and secretly enjoyed suffering, and the harm done to the other is a by-product of the patient's continued pursuit of his own lack of pleasure. Furthermore, the patient usually suffers far more than his victim.

A further example is the shy, lonely man who meets an attractive woman who clearly likes him. He is about to ask for a date and has the thought, "I won't give my analyst the satisfaction."

The demand for reparation and vengeance, and the unwillingness to give up one's self-defeating behaviors until that impossibly unrealistic demand has been met, are often particularly difficult impediments in the treatment. These patients' inability to take pleasure in what would ordinarily be gratifying achievements includes their unwillingness to admit their psychological intactness, as well as their unwillingness to let parents, spouses, or therapists "cash in" on the pleasure of their success when they ought to be making up for what they did to the patient. Patients with SDPD often feel a moral fervor—for example, "Simple justice," "An eye for an eye," "It's only fair," "People should apologize when they have hurt someone," "One should pay for damage that one did"— that harkens back to the moral teachings of the nursery and lends a tone of self-righteousness to what is at bottom one more defense against having to give up the secret pleasures of self-defeat. Persistence in one's therapeutic attitude of helping the patient to see his or her motives for retaining feelings of victimization; appropriate sympathy and empathy over the unremediable reality of past suffering; and helping the patient to begin to accept the fact of his or her current adult autonomous status—all help the patient to overcome the temptations to get stuck in vengeance and self-pity. As patients begin to improve, and as they experience increasing satisfaction in their lives, it becomes increasingly difficult for them to fall back into this more neurotic mode.

Denial of Pleasure

It is implicit in all that has been said above that self-defeating patients have a need to deny ordinary conscious sources of pleasure and to insist on their miserable lot in life. When this quality is prominent, it can lend a depressive air to the patient and to the treatment situation that may lead the therapist to consider antidepressant medication. Some of these patients may fit criteria for dysthymic disorder, and a trial of medication may be indicated. However, a large group of these patients are not medication-responsive but do respond to psychotherapy or psychoanalysis. Successful treatment requires that the therapist retain appropriate neutrality—that is, while sympathetic to the real suffering of the patient and empathic to the patient's enchainment by unconscious conflicts, the therapist is also insistent that the continued disorder of the now-adult patient is the patient's responsibility and that remedy lies with the patient. It is easy to become angry, bored, and depressed in dealing with what is often a monotonous litany of childlike whinings and feelings of injury, or a persistent stream of aggressive provocations. It is here that the therapist's professional education and experience, his or her theoretical understanding of the disorder and appreciation of the havoc it is causing in the patient's life, help the therapist to maintain a therapeutic stance and enjoy his or her work. Helping the masochistic patient to reduce his or her pain, contrary to the joke about sadists treating masochists, is ultimately a source of great satisfaction for both patient and therapist.

Conclusions

The treatment of SDPD, although always difficult, is most likely to succeed when the therapist is prepared with an adequate theory of the disorder that enables him or her to weather the severe stresses that the treatment of these patients can elicit. Without an understanding of the unconscious roots of the disorder, the therapist is prone to respond to the provocation and negativity of these patients with aggressive attempts to convince the patient to change such obviously maladaptive behavior. The therapist will then quickly find himself or herself involved in power struggles that are doomed to failure.

I believe that a clear recognition of the narcissistic aspects of the masochistic behavior and the ability to interpret both the narcissism and the masochism greatly facilitate the treatment. The concept of the *narcissistic-masochistic personality* can be helpful. The experienced therapist of patients with SDPD is also aware that in spite of his or her best efforts, even patients who will eventually do well are liable to go through difficult periods of treatment in which the patients' self-damaging tendencies and overt suffering are carried to lengths greater than those experienced before treatment. Nonetheless, the persistence of the therapist's efforts, a consistent therapeutic stance, and his or her benevolence combined with a willingness to present reality to the patient, will in most instances yield therapeutic results that are gratifying to both the patient and the therapist.

References

American Psychiatric Association: Diagnostic and Statistical Manual of Mental Disorders, 3rd Edition, Revised. Washington, DC, American Psychiatric Association, 1987

Bergler E: The Basic Neurosis, Oral Regression and Psychic Masochism. New York, Grune & Stratton, 1949

Bergler E: The Superego. New York, Grune & Stratton, 1952

Cooper AM: The unusually painful analysis: a group of narcissistic-masochistic characters, in Psychoanalysis: The Vital Issues, Vol 2. New York, International Universities Press, 1984, pp 45–67

Cooper AM: The narcissistic-masochistic character, in Masochism: Current Psychoanalytic Perspectives. Edited by Glick RA, Meyers DI. Hillsdale, NJ, Analytic Press, 1988, pp 117–138

Cooper AM: Narcissism and masochism: the narcissistic-masochistic character. Psychiatr Clin North Am 12:541–552, 1989

Deutsch H: Psychology of Women. New York, Grune & Stratton, 1944

Dizmang LH, Cheatham CF: The Lesch-Nyhan Syndrome. Am J Psychiatry 127:671–677, 1970

Fiester SJ: Self-defeating personality disorder: a review of data and recommendations for DSM-IV. Journal of Personality Disorders 5:194–209, 1991

Freud S: Three essays on the theory on sexuality (1905), in The Standard Edition of the Complete Psychological Works of Sigmund Freud, Vol 7. Translated and edited by Strachey J. London, Hogarth Press, 1953, pp 123–245

Freud S: The ego and the id (1923), in The Standard Edition of the Complete Psychological Works of Sigmund Freud, Vol 19. Translated and edited by Strachey J. London, Hogarth Press, 1961, pp 1–66

Freud S: The economic problem of masochism (1924), in The Standard Edition of the Complete Psychological Works of Sigmund Freud, Vol 19. Translated and edited by Strachey J. London, Hogarth Press, 1961, pp 155–170

Kohut H: The Analysis of the Self. New York, International Universities Press, 1971

Kraft-Ebbing RF von: Psychopathia Sexualis. London, FA Davis, 1895

Rado S: An adaptational view of sexual behavior, in Psychoanalysis of Behavior: The Collected Papers of Sandor Rado. New York, Grune & Stratton, 1956, pp 186–213

Sacher-Masoch L von: Sacher-Masoch: An Interpretation by Gilles Deleuze (1870), together with the entire text of "Venus in Furs." Translated by McNeil JM. London, Faber & Faber, 1971

Van der Kolk BA: Psychological Trauma. Washington DC, American Psychiatric Press, 1987

Chapter 7

Management Approaches for the Repetitively Aggressive Patient

Gary J. Maier, M.D.

We live in an aggressive era. Evidence of this aggression can be seen in nearly all aspects of our society, including our hospitals and prisons (Carmel and Hunter 1989; Lion and Reid 1983). The Veterans Administration hospital system reported more than 12,000 assaults by patients in a recent 5-year period. Many chronically mentally ill patients remain hospitalized because of assaultive behavior. Increasingly, clinicians working in inpatient hospital settings, forensic facilities, outpatient clinics dealing with impulse disorders, and even general practice cannot avoid treating patients for whom aggressive behavior is the primary reason for therapy.

With the increase in the treatment of aggressive patients has come a disturbing increase in the incidents of aggression against therapists, as well as line staff in hospital and prison facilities. Learning to manage the aggressive patient has become an increas-

The author thanks the following colleagues for their collaborative involvement in developing aspects of the clinical model and developing techniques to manage the aggressive patient: R. Althouse, Ph.D.; K. Bauman, Ph.D.; M. Bernstein, Ph.D.; D. Doren, Ph.D.; L. Goldapske, RT; T. Kuhlman, Ph.D.; J. LeClair, Ph.D.; R. Miller, M.D., Ph.D.; C. Monroe, Ph.D.; B. Morrow, R.N.; E. Musholt, Ph.D.; L. Stava, Ph.D.; G. Van Rybroek, Ph.D.; J. Whitman, M.D.; and the staff at the Mendota Forensic Center, Madison, Wisconsin.

ingly important skill. The American Psychiatric Association (APA) finally acknowledged the need to train psychiatrists in management and treatment skills and to raise their own consciousness about safety in the clinical workplace (American Psychiatric Association Task Force on Clinician Safety 1991).

Human aggression is an interactive process. An approach to the sequence and cycles of aggression has been presented elsewhere (Maier et al. 1987, 1988; Van Rybroek and Maier 1987) and will be the focus of this chapter. Understanding these processes has led to the development of specific and strategically placed intervention strategies. However, for interventions to be effective they must occur in a rational context, one that will give direction to prevention, management, and treatment. Further, while it is true that specific principles guide specific interventions, general principles underpin a rational, comprehensive approach to managing aggression *as it is encountered in process.* The principle thrust of this chapter will be to outline the process of aggression so that clinicians can rationally apply the growing range of management and treatment techniques. Shining a light on the process of aggression will help bring the subject out of the shadow of psychiatry (Lion 1987).

Managing human aggression is the responsibility of individuals and institutions. Individual clinicians must interact to talk down and take down aggressors. Specialized institutions have the global responsibility of developing programs to manage and treat such patients, inmates, and so forth. Nevertheless, because the processes of human aggression are the same for drunk persons fighting in a bar or patients fighting in a day room, general principles of management apply in both situations. Further, because human aggression is usually a high-intensity, low-frequency event, the affect aroused at the time of aggression can preclude rational management at the time, and for a significant period after, when corrective measures should be discovered and implemented. The low behavioral base rate and high intensity of the aroused affect make it difficult to develop or raise individual or group consciousness about the need to be prepared to manage aggression and to continue to be vigilant. All too often the only thing learned from a traumatic aggressive event is that it is desirable to avoid such intense, frightening, and painful situations. Learned avoidance can in turn become unconscious denial (Maier and Van Rybroek 1990). Because aggression is traumatic and to be avoided and then denied, clinicians must make a conscious commitment to overcome the countertransference issues that fuel their unconscious defense mechanisms.

The Process of Aggression

The model presented below consists of two parts, the linear *aggression sequence* and *aggression cycles*.

The Aggression Sequence

The linear process of aggression can be divided into three general phases: preaggression, aggression, and postaggression. Further breaking down these phases can help clarify the different factors that are involved (see Figure 7–1). These more definable stages contrast the differences between the medical/psychiatric aspects of the behavior, for which clinicians have expertise because of training, and the characterological aspects of the behavior, for which clinicians have assumed responsibility because of proximity, but for which they have not yet developed expertise. Aggression occurring in a medical setting can be regarded as a linear process that may be broken down into six phases: 1) preaggression, 2) aggression, 3) control, 4) diagnosis and assessment, 5) treatment and management, and 6) postaggression.

Because the first three phases of the aggressive sequence can follow each other in rapid succession and can cause physiological stress in the observer, they are often difficult to discern. Because these phases are not clearly separated and must be addressed as they happen, clinicians can also become confused and interventions can become misplaced. In order to clarify these phases, a brief description of the characteristics and boundaries of each phase is presented below.

Preaggression phase.   Monahan (1981) has begun to identify the complex relationship that exists among the various factors that determine the emergence of aggressive behavior. At present, describing the origins of this phase can be directly related to the theoretical orientation of the clinician. For a Freudian, the preaggression phase can begin as early as the emergence of dental aggression in infancy (Perls 1947). At the other end of the spectrum, a behaviorist may limit the origins of the phase to the various contingencies in operation moments before the aggression erupted. While Tanke and Yesavage (1985) have demonstrated that the Brief Psychiatric Rating Scale (BPRS) can be used to identify patients who will aggress but who do not give verbal cues prior to their aggression, research of this type has not yet resulted in the development of a reliable etiological classification for preaggressive patients.

Nevertheless, Harris and Varney (1983) have reported that patient-patient aggression is usually the product of direct interaction between patients. Patients report a number of reasons they aggress against each other, ranging from a simple "payback" for a previous transgression, to acting out a command hallucination. Whatever

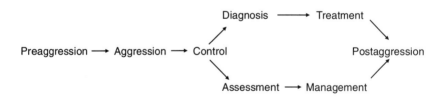

Figure 7–1. The linear aggression sequence. In an inpatient setting this sequence consists of six phases. In medical settings the difference between the two tracks of the latter phases is often a source of confusion. Individuals from a number of disciplines—security guards, prison guards, police, SWAT members, and military teams—are charged with the responsibility of controlling and managing aggressive persons. Staff who work in medical settings share this responsibility, and they use similar interventions. They are also able to diagnose and treat these patients, and to the degree that aggressive behavior is part of the illness, treatment reduces aggression. The postaggression phase recognizes the need to document and even research each aggressive event, unfettered by incipient countertransference feelings that often contaminate fact finding that can lead to better management and treatment techniques.

the origins, the preaggression phase typically ends with either a verbal threat or with a physically aggressive act.

Aggression phase. Dubin (1985) has pointed out that verbal threats often precede physical aggression. Verbal threats are a serious warning that physical aggression is ripe. Verbal abuse and verbal threats are reliable precursors to physical aggression, and for this reason they tell the person who is the object of the threat to reduce his or her profile and get help. Understanding the relationship between verbal and physical aggression can be lifesaving.

The aggression phase begins with a verbal threat or an act of physical aggression (Thackrey 1987). Although neither medical nor psychiatric dictionaries define the word "fight," common sense tells us that this phase consists of punches, kicks, bites, and scratches. Often one patient is the manifest aggressor and a patient or clinician is the manifest victim. The phase continues until the aggressor dominates, regains self-control, or is subdued. When clinicians witness the onset of this phase, they must intervene, either by talking down or taking down the aggressor patient. This phase involves engaging the patient until clinicians have established sufficient control.

During the emergency constituted by the aggression phase, clinicians must physically restrain the patient while they continue to respect his or her rights as a person. At the same time, because the patient may continue to act in an uncontrolled manner, some of the patient's rights are suspended (e.g., in an emergency, medications can be given against a patient's will). Once the patient is controlled, however, individual rights are reinstated.

During the aggression phase, the alliance that exists between clinician and patient breaks down. The aggressive act disrupts the trust necessary for the maintenance of a therapeutic alliance and requires staff to use aggression management techniques to regain control of the patient. During this process, clinicians must utilize police authority, and, conversely, the patient loses rights until control is achieved. It is for this obvious reason that it is important to distinguish between the concepts of *control* and *management*, which are not based on trust, and *treatment* or *therapy*, which is based on

trust. This fundamental, basic difference is many times not sufficiently understood by administrators, training directors, or patient
advocates.

Control phase.   During the control phase the aggressive behavior
is stopped, either because the patient develops self-control or because the clinical staff intervene (Roth 1985). When clinicians arrive after the patient has stopped his or her aggressive act, the
control phase is synonymous with the development of self-control
by the patient and his or her resulting ability to demonstrate responsibility. In other situations the clinicians must actively intervene to stop the aggression, which often means they must physically
control the patient. In these situations, control is initiated and
maintained through physical and/or chemical restraint and, as appropriate, seclusion.

When the patient has finally regained self-control, the clinician
may impose a probationary period during which the patient must
demonstrate that he or she can and will accept verbal direction.
This period often occurs while the patient is secluded. The control
phase ends when the clinicians give the patient the responsibility
for self-control in the open milieu.

Diagnosis and assessment phase.   There is a difference between
diagnosis and assessment. Using the medical model, diagnosis is
reserved for the process of determining the presence of medical
or psychiatric illness. Unfortunately, medical and psychiatric diagnoses are usually of little value in determining the probability of
future aggression because aggressive behavior is seldom pathognomonic of any specific disorder, and worse, aggression can be associated with any medical or psychiatric disorder, as well as no
disorder.

Diagnosis follows the traditional medical and psychiatric process and is based on history, physical examination, laboratory tests,
the patient's mental status, neurological examination, psychological tests, and other special medical procedures, such as computed
tomography scan, X-ray, electroencephalogram (EEG), and so
forth. The process can take from a few days to several weeks and

may include clinical trials on medication. Diagnoses are stated in the DSM-III-R format (American Psychiatric Association 1987).

The term *assessment* is reserved for the process of determining the probability that a patient will become aggressive in the immediate future (hours, days, or weeks) (Tardiff 1989). Assessment for aggression potential is accomplished by reviewing the patient's history of aggressive behavior at home, at school, and at work; in hospitals; in correctional facilities; or in the armed services. The relationship between the aggressive behavior and environmental/situational factors is important. The outline of aggressive behaviors in the Overt Aggression Scale (OAS; Yudofsky et al. 1986)—aggression against others, aggression against property, threats toward others, and aggression against self—is useful in establishing meaningful clinical categories. These categories can be utilized to detect patterns that can then be used to help determine the long-term management plan. While past behavior is still the most reliable predictor of future behavior, patients who manifest behavior from more than one category are often more dangerous than those who act out with only one pattern (Depp 1976).

Treatment and management phase.   The term *treatment* is used in the classic medical sense and refers to all the traditional approaches used to help mentally ill persons, including psychotherapy, psychopharmacology, and some behavioral approaches based on learning theory. When aggressive behaviors are closely associated with the psychiatric illness (e.g., paranoid schizophrenia), treating the illness will often significantly reduce the aggression. In this paradigm the aggressive behavior is considered to be a sign of illness because the treatment does, or appears to, correct the primary pathology. Frequently, however, the aggressive behavior is characterological or only coincidentally associated with the psychiatric condition. In these cases the terms *manage* and *management* are used to refer to the interventions. These terms refer to approaches used to exert external control over aggressive behavior. Talk-down and take-down procedures, seclusion, and ambulatory restraints are good examples. Clinicians may need to continue specific treatment and/or management techniques to help a patient maintain behavioral control for short periods of time, or for the indefinite future.

Postaggression phase: aggression postmortems. Following each aggression of any significance, an independent fact-finder should review all aspects of the aggressive event and then meet with the principals involved in order to fully understand from their perspectives what happened, what might have prevented it, and, once started, what would have brought it under control more quickly and with less trauma. Following this procedure will allow each aggressive event to become a learning event, not just a traumatic event. A report should follow in which the incident and the outcomes are described and recommendations made to senior clinicians and administrators that will result in greater safety. These can range from a review of the staffing pattern, to the need for audio or video surveillance in a particular area, or the need for referral to an employee victim program (Dawson et al. 1988). Not only can careful review of these data over time suggest new ways to intervene, but such review can also identify patterns of aggression unique to the specific unit or facility, which will suggest alternate ways of responding. Following staff who have been injured as they return to duty is another function of these postmortems.

It's About Feelings: How Do You "Fight"?

The model described above can best be understood if it is personalized. See if this process does not apply to the last argument or "fight" you had with a significant other. The process is often first recognized when it is clear there is an escalating disagreement that no solutions or compromises appear to be able to resolve (i.e., aggression phase). Moreover, the emotional intensity slowly becomes the most dominant aspect of the argument. To the degree emotion is aroused, logic recedes. The argument continues until some crisis, ultimatum, or, in the best cases, resolution is achieved. When there is no resolution there is a period when further good-faith efforts to problem-solve will fail. This is because the emotion has not subsided in both parties. Good-faith attempts to readdress the issues when emotion is still labile simply reactivate an adversarial response. A refractory period then follows the argument (i.e., control phase). As both parties regain self-control, they not only review their arguments, issues, and feelings, but they make some attempt to see the issues raised by the opponent (i.e., assessment phase). This self-assessment is extremely important because out of it comes the sense of compromise. Further, the assessment often includes a review of the issues that led up to the argument. What we naturally do is go back to some reference point in the relationship when things seemed to be on an even keel and let that act as a baseline (i.e., preaggression phase). Although this process may be idiosyncratic, the process of *this* argument will need some common historical context. In the renegotiating phase, emotion having cooled, the opportunity arises for the issues, now circumscribed, to be resolved (i.e., management phase).

In summary, conflict-laden interpersonal interactions occur that strain relationships (i.e., preaggression). When they are excessive, they result in an argument (i.e., aggression). The argument continues until the emotion is dissipated and one or both parties regain self-control (i.e., control). Separately both parties review the content and dynamics of the argument and try to account for its origins, the demands, the resentments, and so forth (i.e., assessment). Then, when the time is right, the parties recontact each other and bring the issues and process to a more satisfactory resolution (i.e., management). Even though all of the stages identified in this process do not occur in all arguments, in general this process underlies argument. It also applies to the significant and dangerous process of physical aggression.

Managing Repetitive Aggression in an Inpatient Setting

The Physical Aggression Cycle: Clinicians' Perspective

The second part of the model consists of identifying the processes that occur when aggression becomes repetitive. Although several authors (Kaplan and Wheeler 1983; McGee 1985; Rada 1981; P. Smith, unpublished manuscript, California Department of Developmental Services, Sacramento, CA) have described cyclic patterns of aggression, these patterns have not been incorporated into a general model, nor have the authors focused on the critical role that clinician countertransference plays in maintaining the cyclic process. The following, then, will describe these processes from the perspective of the clinician, with specific reference to the need to identify and resolve feelings. The description of the physical aggression cycle from the patients' perspective will then be described.

Description of the cycle.   Physical aggression often results in the chain of events illustrated in Figure 7–2. The clinicians respond rapidly to the patient-aggressor. If the aggressor is not imminently dangerous, the clinicians may try to talk him or her out of further action (i.e., talk down). If that option seems unsafe, they hold or restrain the patient (i.e., take down). If the patient continues to struggle and if he or she has psychotic symptoms, psychotropic medication may be administered. In some facilities the patient is often secluded after this kind of aggression.

After the aggression is controlled, the clinicians spontaneously

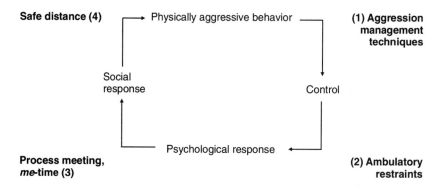

Figure 7–2. The physical aggression cycle: clinicians' perspective. The cardinal points of the cycle—physically aggressive behavior, control, psychological response, and social response—represent the normal progression of clinician-patient dynamics that can result from an aggressive episode. The midpoints 1–4 represent those points at which patients and staff can make the most effective interventions.

inquire about physical injuries that they may have received. They usually do not ask whether co-workers were frightened by the aggression or were angry that the patient put them in such jeopardy, and they usually do not recognize that they have these feelings themselves. The "normal" process of dealing with aggression often does not provide staff with an opportunity to discuss their feelings, and thus fear, anger (Lion and Pasternak 1973), rage (Madden and Lion 1976), or a sense of helplessness may go undetected and unresolved (Adler 1972).

If the patient has been put in seclusion or transferred to a more secure ward, he or she is usually returned to the original ward after a short time. Clinicians and other patients will prepare for his or her return with undiscussed and unresolved feelings. As a result, when the patient returns, some clinicians and patient peers may try to avoid him or her, thereby minimizing any further interaction. The distrust and anger clinicians and other patients feel may be evident to the aggressor and cause him or her to feel alienated and become defensive. Given this response, the likelihood is high that a small incident will evoke another act of aggression and begin the cycle again.

Physical aggression is usually public and observable, and because there is sound and fury, clinicians will usually agree about the patient's behavior and the actual physical acts that they observed. If clinicians are given the opportunity to discuss their feelings about the aggressor and the aggressive behavior, they will be open about them, even though they may disagree about the feelings the scene aroused.

Interventions. As the description of the cycle suggests, the administrator of the facility has responsibility for preparing clinicians to deal with physical aggression and to resolve their feelings about it. Clinicians must be equipped with effective aggression management skills (Infantino and Musingo 1985), both through pre-employment training sessions and through regular in-service training. Aggression management skills include the ability to identify the early warning signs of aggressive behavior, to verbally interact with the patient in order to de-escalate emotional intensity or prevent repeat aggression (i.e., talk down), to defend oneself if attacked, and to use physical holds that secure the patient but do not put pressure on joints. These components of aggression management can be taught, but because they are not used frequently, refresher courses are needed. Clinicians must feel safe and know that if they are attacked, they will be quickly supported.

Seclusion and restraint should be options for dealing with serious and persistent aggression (Tardiff 1984). Ambulatory restraints can be effective in liberating a patient from seclusion in a safe manner (Van Rybroek et al. 1987). Clinicians must also have the option of using chemical restraint (Eichelman 1988; Tardiff 1983; Yudofsky et al. 1981), both short-term and long-term, to calm severely agitated patients (see below).

Countertransference issues must be addressed. Clinicians should be encouraged to discuss the feelings of fear and anger they may have toward selected patients. Clinicians should be prompted to identify and share these feelings, privately or in team meetings. Awareness of the physical aggression cycle and implementation of the measures described make it easier to approach the previously aggressive patient and to refocus on the patient's humanity. As a result, social distancing will decrease and the possibility that the cycle will be reactivated is diminished.

The Physical Aggression Cycle: Patient's Perspective

Description of the cycle.   The first two points of the patient's perspective of the physical aggression cycle are the same as in the clinical perspective (i.e., physical aggression leads to control). The patient has an emotional response and, when released from seclusion, experiences social distress if there has been no effective intervention among the patient, his or her peers, and the staff. From the patient's perspective the cycle has four cardinal points: physically aggressive behavior, control, psychological response, and social response (see Figure 7–3). Developing effective interventions between the events of the cycle has been difficult because little research exists on the patient's reaction to his or her aggression or to seclusion, or on the patient's own feelings and perception of how his or her social role is affected by the aggression.

Binder and McCoy (1983) reported that the four most common reasons for seclusion on an inpatient crisis intervention unit are 1) agitation, 2) uncooperativeness, 3) anger, and 4) a history of violence. Mattson and Sacks (1978) reported the maintenance of a therapeutic environment as the most frequent reason. Several authors (Binder 1979; Wadeson and Carpenter 1976) have reported seclusion as an effective means of controlling the destructive behavior of schizophrenic, hypomanic, organically impaired, and depressed patients. These diagnostic groups account for the vast majority of seclusions in all types of hospitals. The problem one can see, then, when trying to understand patients who require seclusion is that they are not a homogeneous group.

Interventions.   Given the diagnostic mix, clinicians should first attempt to give patients true asylum while in seclusion. This means that clinicians should empathically test reality for patients during the secluded period. Because of the long-term negative effects of seclusion, every effort should be made to liberate patients from this condition. Ambulatory restraints were in fact designed for that purpose (Van Rybroek et al. 1987). Ambulatory restraints are ac-

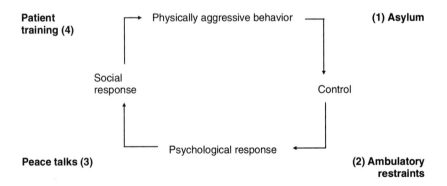

Figure 7–3.   The physical aggression cycle: patient's perspective. The cardinal points of the cycle—physically aggressive behavior, control, psychological response, and social response—represent the normal progression of clinician-patient dynamics that can result from an aggressive episode. The midpoints 1–4 represent those points at which patients and staff can make the most effective interventions.

cepted by patients because they allow them more freedom and greater privileges (e.g., ability to smoke, watch television, etc.) in a manner safe for them and others.

It is important to discuss the aggressive episode with the patient as soon as possible. This includes a review of antecedent behavior, the aggressive act itself, feelings toward the victim, feelings about the consequences of seclusion, and loss of privilege and/or increase in medication. In order to help resolve the feelings of both aggressor and victim, a *peace talk* is arranged between them (see Figure 7–3). A peace talk is an interactive discussion between aggressor and victim that is mediated by a clinician and designed to resolve conflict. Such an intervention allows them to "discuss" the situation and to either agree or disagree about responsibility, or to make appropriate apologies and verbal commitments to respect each other. If significant progress is made, the aggressor and victim discuss the episode in a ward meeting with patients and staff. Peace talks and follow-up with staff and other patients are techniques that can be used to reintegrate the aggressor into the unit community as a nonthreatening, productive member.

Repetitively aggressive patients found in the inpatient setting, in general, have three skill deficiencies. These patients require anger identification/management skills, assertiveness training, and social skills training. When these patients are trained in these skills, aggressive behavior can be prevented. There is nothing unique about these programs. Feeling-identification groups that are already part of treatment must focus on the specific feelings aroused by aggression. Fear, anger, depression, and anxiety are included. It is also important to remember that many repetitively aggressive patients are as frightened by their behavior as are those around them. Most facilities and many clinicians have expertise in training patients to be constructively assertive and in helping them to develop social skills.

Other Management Issues

The aggression dynamics described above can be more easily observed in the laboratory of a closed setting. The interventions identified can be placed in a meaningful context because the pathogenic processes of aggression are understood. Nevertheless, there are other important elements that must be considered when managing repetitively aggressive patients. These include leadership (Heider 1985), staffing patterns (Maier 1986), architectural security (Infantino and Musingo 1985), seclusion and restraint (Tardiff 1984), ambulatory restraints (Van Rybroek et al. 1987), gallows humor (Kuhlman 1984), and prosecution of willful aggression (Hoge and Gutheil 1987; Maier 1989; Miller and Maier 1987). Each of these areas has become progressively sophisticated. The references will be useful to those interested in more information.

Managing Repetitive Aggression in an Outpatient Setting

The principal differences between the inpatient setting and the outpatient setting are the loss of control of important parameters, including unpredictable stress, availability of alcohol and other substances of abuse, and the lack of a support system. The focus of this section will be on two important areas: 1) teaching patients to identify and manage stress, especially stress that leads to frustration and anger, and 2) the relatively new field of antiaggression psychopharmacology. These approaches depend on the development of a management and treatment plan based on a clear review of past aggression. The focus must be on identifying the antecedent conditions that predispose to aggression. Identifying the stressors that predispose the aggressive behavior and then finding alternate ways to manage the stress are critical.

Anger/Stress Management Techniques

The approach to be described is a cognitive-behavioral intervention that follows a more general therapeutic model that Novaco (1976) calls "stress inoculation." To paraphrase Novaco, this approach is a coping-skills therapy by which the trained clinician aims to provide the patient with the cognitive and behavioral resources for managing stressful situations and for regulating personal stress reactions (Novaco 1976).

The stress inoculation procedures constitute a therapy that is based upon developing coping skills in the patient and then exposing the patient to manageable doses of a stressor that arouse, but do not overwhelm, his or her defenses. The procedures are designed to help the patient learn to cope with stressful events that have a high probability of occurrence. Additionally, in learning how to regulate thoughts, emotions, and behavior and to optimize environmental conditions so as to reduce exposure to stressors, the patient achieves management of his or her anger by preventive means as well as by coping activities.

According to Novaco, the treatment approach involves three basic steps or phases: 1) cognitive preparation, 2) skill acquisition, and 3) application training. The *cognitive preparation* phase educates patients about the functions of anger and about their personal anger patterns. It also provides a shared language system between patient and clinician and introduces the rationale of treatment. An instructional manual for patients is used to facilitate these tasks. Patients are also asked to maintain a self-monitoring record or diary that serves as a data base for discussion of therapeutic principles and goals. The anger control components of the cognitive preparation phase consist of a) identifying the persons and situations that trigger anger, b) distinguishing anger from aggression, c) understanding the multiple determinants of anger, d) understanding provocation in terms of interaction sequences, and e) introducing the anger management techniques as coping strategies to handle conflict and stress.

The *skill acquisition* phase teaches cognitive awareness, arousal reduction, and behavioral coping skills that follow from the mode of anger. At the cognitive level, the patient is taught to view provocative circumstances and to modify the exaggerated importance often attached to events. The ability "not to take things personally" is a fundamental skill. This is accomplished by fostering a task orientation to provocation, which involves a focus on desired outcomes and the implementation of a behavioral strategy to produce those outcomes. The cognitive modification goals are facilitated by the use of self-instructions in the form of coping self-statements designed for specific provocation events. Applied to various stages of a provocation sequence, these self-statements serve as instructional cues that guide the patient's thoughts, feelings, and behavior toward effective coping.

For arousal reduction, the patient is taught relaxation skills and is also encouraged to begin a personally suited program that is explicitly directed at reducing arousal as monitored by the patient and clinician. This may involve continued use of deep-muscle relaxation techniques and/or alternative strategies such as hypnosis, meditation, or even yoga. The behavioral coping skills concern the effective communication of feelings, assertiveness, and implementation of task-oriented, problem-solving action. The patient is helped to maximize the adaptive functions of anger and to minimize its maladaptive functions. When arousal is activated, the patient is taught to recognize anger on the basis of internal and external cues and then to communicate that anger in a nonhostile form or use it to energize problem-solving action, keeping the arousal at moderate levels of intensity. The task-oriented responses gear the person to engage in behavior that is instrumental to producing desired outcomes. Anger then becomes a signal that problem-solving strategies are to be implemented, which requires a focus on issues and objectives. This keeps anger from accumulating and prevents aggressive overreaction by imposing thought between impulse and action.

Finally, the various coping skills are modeled by the therapist, who then gives the patient the opportunity to practice them in the *application training* phase. The anger control procedures are designed to build personal competence, and therefore the patient's proficiency must be tested. The practice is conducted by means of imaginal and role-play inductions of anger. The context of these simulated provocations is constructed in collaboration with the patient. The provocations are presented in a hierarchical sequence, as in systematic desensitization. The scenarios involve anger situations that the patient is likely to encounter in real life. The coping skills that have been rehearsed with the clinician are then applied to these simulated provocations beginning with the mildest and progressing to the most anger arousing. This process continues throughout the course of treatment and enables both patient and clinician to gauge the patient's proficiency.

This promising procedure is particularly effective for outpatients with average intelligence. Patients with posttraumatic stress disorder, spouses that batter, and even persons whose aggression is associated with alcohol or substance abuse are excellent candidates. This approach, accompanied by aerobic exercise and the use of low doses of a benzodiazepine, can attenuate years of aggressive behavior.

Antiaggression Psychopharmacology

A substantial body of research has demonstrated that pharmacological modulation of three neurotransmitter systems (the GABAergic, the noradrenergic, and the serotonergic) can produce marked alterations in aggressive behavior. Four basic principles of clinical application that can enhance trials of pharmacological treatment of the violent patient have been identified. Evidence suggests that behavioral and social learning approaches to the management of aggression can be more effective when implemented after the patient has been stabilized through pharmacological intervention (Eichelman 1988).

Principles of the clinical application

Because many of these medications have not been specifically approved by the FDA for use in managing aggression, it is suggested that the clinician consider each trial on one of the following medications an "N = 1" research project. The strategy can be simplified if one uses as a guide the following four principles:

1. Diagnose and treat the primary illness.
2. Measure the aggressive behaviors (using, e.g., the OAS).
3. Use single-variable manipulation.
4. Start with the most benign medication.

First, the primary illness must be identified and treated with the most appropriate conventional methods. If the patient has paranoid schizophrenia, then a neuroleptic should be started and increased to a dose that reduces the signs and symptoms of the psychosis. While this is in process, the undesirable aggressive behaviors must be identified. Then, using an assessment instrument such as the OAS, the aggressive behavior must be documented so that a baseline for assessing change can be established.

Once a meaningful baseline is set, only one treatment variable should be changed at a time. The antiaggression medication should be the only variable once it is started. Finally, the medication with the most benign potential for harm should be given the initial trial. The four major medication types are presented in increasing order of potential harm.

Benzodiazepines. These medications have been found to be quite effective in helping patients manage the early stages of irritability and frustration that can escalate to anger and then aggressive behavior (Boyle and Tobin 1961; Lion 1979). The mechanism of therapeutic action seems to be through the GABAergic system (Costa et al. 1976). These agents are indicated for the management of the prodromal or preaggression phase, for acute chemical restraint, for control of a patient who has aggressed, for patients with intermittent explosive disorder, and for patients with a diagnosis of major psychosis in the acute phase (Bick and Hannah 1986; Kalina 1964; Monroe 1975).

No workup prior to benzodiazepine is usually necessary because these medications are generally safe and have a low side-effect profile. The dosage schedule varies with the specific drug and based on whether it is given on an "as needed" (i.e., prn) or a scheduled basis. Once the baselines for the aggressive behaviors are noted, medications like oxazepam, 10 mg, can be given on a one-, two-, or three-times-a-day basis, or 10 to 20 mg can be given on a prn basis up to four times a day. Patients are instructed to take a prn when they can identify the signs of frustration, and/or when they know that certain stressors are likely to challenge their ability to cope.

The trial is run for a 2- to 8-week period depending on the frequency of the aggressive behavior. If the medication is only given on a prn basis, a series of 20 doses is often sufficient to help establish whether there is any change in the aggressive behavior. Once the patient either has received 20 doses of prn medication or has run a trial from 2 to 8 weeks on a regularly scheduled dose, the aggressive behaviors pre- and posttrial are compared. From this the efficacy of the medication can be determined. If improvement is noted, the successful regimen can be continued until new habits are formed.

After a period of 6 months the medication should be reviewed because of the potential for addiction. The clinician is reminded that some patients have a paradoxical reaction to these medications, which can lower inhibition and appear to increase aggressive outbursts. Should this occur or if there is no change in aggressive outbursts associated with the trial period, the medication should be discontinued, and the clinician can move on to a second trial on a different medication.

Lithium.   The DSM-III-R definition of mania for bipolar disorder includes a description of irritability, which, therefore, is a legitimate precursor feeling of a major affective disorder that could lead to anger and aggression. Accordingly, patients who have an atypical bipolar disorder or are repetitively aggressive and dysthymic deserve a trial on this medication. Its use should also be considered when a patient presents with an atypical cyclic pattern to aggression (Sheard 1971; Sheard et al. 1976). Lithium works by both decreasing noradrenaline and increasing serotonin in different areas of the central nervous system.

Prior to initiation of lithium, the workup used with the patient who has manifested aggressive behavior is the same as that for a typical bipolar patient. This workup includes an electrocardiogram (ECG), a thyroid panel, BUN, and determination of serum creatinine and serum electrolytes. Assuming that all of these are within the norm, then the patient can be started on a dose of lithium carbonate, 600 mg po bid, with lithium levels monitored on a weekly basis. The therapeutic range to manage aggression is 0.5 to 0.7 meq/liter level of lithium. The serum levels do not need to be as high to be effective in modulating irritability or preaggressive feelings as those expected for effective control of acute mania. Once a therapeutic level is established, it takes 6 to 8 weeks to determine if lithium is having an antiaggression effect, by comparing the number of aggressions during the trial with the base rate. Again, if a reduction is noted, maintenance lithium with monthly serum levels is indicated. If not, the clinician can move to another medication.

Beta-blockers. When one considers the "fight-flight" response, it makes theoretical sense that some patients, especially those with organic disorders, may have their noradrenergic system hyperstimulated. Beta-blockers are therefore indicated in patients who have organic brain syndromes (Sheard et al. 1976; Yudofsky et al. 1981) and in those selected patients with a major psychosis.

Prior to the initiation of a beta-blocker, the workup includes an ECG and determination of serum electrolytes. The orthostatic blood pressure and pulse should be taken daily for 1 week prior to the implementation to establish a baseline. These measurements should be taken before each dose of beta-blocker is given, and the dose must be held if the systolic blood pressure is below 90 or the diastolic blood pressure is below 60, or if the pulse is below 30.

While metoprolol (Mattes 1985), pindolol (Greendyke and Kanter 1986), and nadolol (Yudofsky et al. 1981) have all been reported to have antiaggression properties, the following dosage schedule for propranolol (Yudofsky et al. 1981) is becoming established in the literature. Propranolol is started at 20 mg po bid times five days. It is then increased by 40 mg bid for one day, then 60 mg in the A.M. and 40 mg in the P.M. for one day, and then it is further increased by 20 mg per day until the dose of 300 mg po bid is reached. If there is no antiaggression response, this medication can be increased to as much as 1,000 mg per day. Yudofsky has reported using doses of up to 1,500 mg. Again, a period of up to 6 to 8 weeks is often required to establish whether the medication has an antiaggression effect.

Anticonvulsants. These medications are left for last principally because they have the potential for depressing the bone marrow, which is one of the more serious potential side effects. These agents are indicated for aggressive patients who appear to have a seizure variant and have EEG abnormalities. Patients with episodic dyscontrol syndrome appear to benefit (Maletzky 1973). Even aggressive patients with a major psychosis have responded to anticonvulsants (Hakola and Laulamas 1982). Phenytoin and carbamazepine (Tegretol) have been most effective. The carbamazepine level workup includes a CBC and platelet count.

The dosage schedule for carbamazepine is as follows. The patient is placed on carbamazepine 300 mg po bid. Weekly carbamazepine levels are drawn until the serum levels reach 8 to 12 mg %. The dosage is adjusted up until that serum level is reached. The carbamazepine must be given before 7:30 A.M. on the day of the blood work. Once stabilized between 8 and 12 mg %, monthly carbamazepine levels and CBCs with platelets are determined. It takes up to 2 months to establish whether the carbamazepine has an antiaggression effect.

Patients who are seriously repetitively aggressive should be given a trial on each of these medications in the suggested order, because there is a growing body of research that shows that these medications can be specifically helpful for individual patients. Whether the clinician works with inpatients or outpatients, teaching patients anger identification and control and the skillful use of antiaggression medication can aid the clinician in helping to diminish the morbidity and help the patient resume a high level of social functioning. But even these powerful interventions can be misused if the clinician is motivated to manage the patient out of fear. The following section is one of the most important because of the denied feelings governing managing aggression, for it is the repetitively aggressive patient that arouses the most feeling.

Denial and Countertransference Issues

The psychiatric literature clearly demonstrates that fear and anger are the most common countertransference reactions that are aroused in clinicians who work with aggressive patients (Colson et al. 1986; Lanza 1983)[1]. In fact, for clinicians who work with repetitively aggressive inpatients, fear and anger are the principal long-term occupational hazards of their work (Lanza 1985). Denial is a frequently used defense mechanism for clinicians to tolerate feelings of fear, anger, helplessness, and frustration (Sandler et al. 1970). It is therefore important to bring back into focus the psychodynamics of personal and group processes and apply them to the clinicians who are expected to control, manage, and treat the aggressive patient. Understanding how these feelings are developed and how they can become the driving force governing clinical decision making with repetitively aggressive patients is especially important. In the following subsections the process of transference and then the stages of development of countertransference are described.

The Process of Transference

The process that an aggressive person may go through when escalating toward physical aggression can be conceived of as having five stages (see Table 7–1). The five behavioral stages, which consecutively include minor motor changes, verbal abuse/threats, major motor changes, physical aggression, and relaxation, are commonly associated with a range of patient feelings. Not every patient experiences these feelings, and the feelings do not proceed in this order for every case. Nonetheless, the process of the behavioral stages and their associated feelings, as presented in Table 7–1, is common enough to be identified as the typical order of escalation that results in physical aggression and control (Tardiff 1989; Yudofsky et al. 1986).

Physical aggression against a clinician can cause significant physiological arousal. The analytic concept of *transference* (Sandler et al. 1970) has traditionally referred to unconscious feelings that

---

[1]Countertransference reactions in this chapter refer to any clinician feelings, conscious or unconscious, derived from the clinician relationship. In this chapter I deal only with the fear, anger, hate, and rage spectrum of feelings because they are specifically aroused by aggression.

originate from relationships that were significant to the patient's earlier life and that are then transferred onto the therapist or other people who are important to the patient. Aggressive patients transfer their feelings (usually anger or rage) in a physical manner onto their victims. The escalating process of psychological arousal results in the physical projection, or transference, of the feelings onto the actual body of the victim.

With the above as a foundation, consider the typical reaction of a clinician to the five stages of escalation experienced by the patient. When the clinician observes minor motor changes that may indicate feelings of anxiety and frustration, he or she will empathically approach the patient. When the patient surprises the clinician by responding with verbal abuse or threats of physical harm, the response is one of anxiety. Next, as the patient escalates to major motor behavior, the clinician most typically feels fearful and in retrospect will identify that it was at this stage that he or she began to feel anger. The fact that the patient in this stage is pacing rapidly, invading other people's space, and making verbally abusive and threatening comments is alarming and frightening. If the patient escalates to actual physical aggression, the clinician is empowered to contact that patient and subdue him or her if necessary. Feelings of self-preservation can be typical during this stage.

The counteraggression required to subdue a person who is in the process of injuring or attempting to injure may jolt the clinician into the shocking awareness that he or she could become a killer in self-defense. The average mental health professional finds it very difficult to maintain this awareness. Nevertheless, aggression, if severe enough, can arouse murderous impulses in the cli-

Table 7–1. Stages of escalation of aggression

Behavioral states	Associated feelings	Clinicians' responses
Minor motor	Anxiety	Empathy
Verbal abuse/threats	Hostility	Anxiety
Major motor	Anger	Fear/anger
Aggression	Rage	Counteraggression
Exhaustion	Relaxation	Frustration

nician. The extreme discomfort that accompanies the realization that one could transform into a killer, given the right circumstances, may account for the fact that staff members often have such strong, intense denial around the whole issue of managing patient aggression.

Once the aggressor is sufficiently controlled and is exhausted and perhaps beginning to relax, the clinician is also able to physically relax. However, following aggression the clinician will not be able to release the intense feelings aroused in him or her as the result of the physical experience. Typically the clinician feels frustrated. He or she therefore goes through a series of feeling changes as the stages of escalation progress, except that he or she ends where the patient began, frustrated.

The clinician in his or her responses goes through the feeling processes that start with empathy and then move to anxiety, fear, anger, counteraggression, and, finally, frustration (see Table 7–1). In a real sense the clinician's reactions, in their sequence, trail behind the patients' feelings, making it plausible to postulate that the patients' feelings are transferred to the clinician when the clinician becomes the target of their aggression. Clinicians who experience this chain of feelings repeatedly without a means of support will in turn develop chronic countertransference reactions. All too often the clinicians' psychological reactions to each single aggression are minimized. By minimizing the impact of aggression on clinicians, a subtle denial takes place that ultimately will handicap the clinicians in their development of effective approaches to the prevention, management, and treatment of aggressive behavior. If clinicians are consumed with unresolved feelings of fear and anger toward patients, they will not be able to see clearly how to develop more humane and effective interventions.

Countertransference Reactions: Stages of Development

The stages of escalation describe the feeling process of an individual episode of aggression. When individual aggression multiplies to repeated aggressions, a different intrapsychic countertransference process evolves. The evolution of countertransference feelings as they move from acceptable conscious awareness to unconscious denial and acting out can be conceived of as involving six stages (see Figure 7–4). These stages are discernibly different and indicate a growing intensity of feeling that progressively challenges the clinician's psychological defenses.

The means by which the visible signs of each stage are assessed by the individual clinician and others are shown in Figure 7–4. It can be seen that in the initial stages simple personal assessment or awareness of the development of negative feelings is sufficient to manage these feelings. But as the feelings intensify and strain the individual's psychological defense system, peers and other staff, as well as the supervisor, may be required to assist in managing feelings too weighty to be handled alone. Finally, if the above interventions fail and the feelings grow in intensity and complexity, personal therapy may be in order as a means to offer resolution and holistic self-acceptance (Maier et al. 1989).

Me-Time: A Structure to Resolve Countertransference Issues

Every effort must be made to allow clinicians to learn how to understand and attenuate the process of escalation, and to work through the stages of countertransference. The process of resolution begins with a conscious awareness that countertransference exists. This is tantamount to saying that the denial generally associated with this process has been consciously acknowledged and that a full-faced attempt to prevent and resolve countertransference feelings through ongoing discussion is expected and valued. The discussions are sanctioned to occur on an informal and formal basis.

The informal discussion occurs throughout the day by all levels of staff and includes dialogues that occur in the corridor, nursing station, staff breakroom (but away from the patients), at lunch, and after work. In these discussions the staff simply acknowledge how they feel toward individual patients or all of the patients as a group. These discussions are invaluable and establish a general cli-

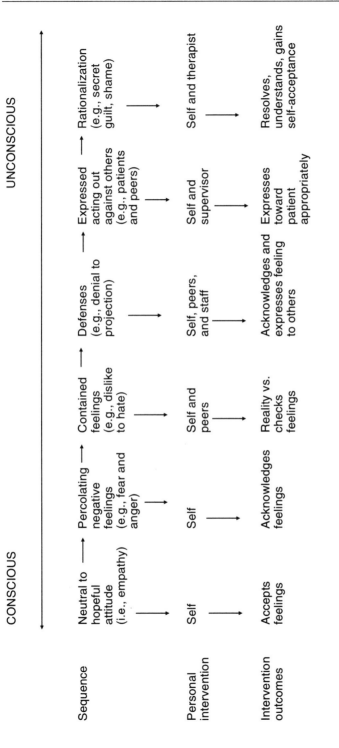

Figure 7–4.   Stages in the development of countertransference feelings. Staff countertransference reactions, if left unchecked, will proceed through the six-stage sequence shown. For each staff member, there is a personal intervention that if successful will lead to predictable, healthy outcomes.

mate that will legitimize all types of feelings, good and bad, from hate to love. However, as informal discussions, they can hardly be effective in bringing entrenched countertransference reactions into awareness so that these reactions can be resolved. Their worth, instead, is in laying the groundwork for a semiformal process called *me*-time.

Me-time is a regularly scheduled semisupervisory session that occurs among all levels of staff under the direction of the unit supervisor(s). *Me*-time is recommended to take place a minimum of 1 hour per week, but it may occur up to 1 hour per day on units with a high rate of aggression. In general, the goal of *me*-time is to consciously tune into the feeling processes of staff. This may be a difficult process in itself and will likely be met with the typical resistances such as silence, anger, projection, and rationalization. When staff are allowed to meet in a confidential manner on a regular basis, however, a process will evolve in which staff will come to trust each other enough to share their real feelings.

There are only a few simple rules. First, all nursing and clinical staff must attend. Past the attendance rule and the fact that racist and sexist comments are not acceptable, staff are encouraged to express themselves in language that is meaningful and satisfying to them. They may talk about individual patients, the current patient group, their peers, their own idiosyncratic issues, or anything else that may be on their minds. The process of encouraging free expression and working through staff differences when life and death are at stake is beyond the scope of this chapter (see Binder and McCoy 1983).

Aggression: A Process in the Service of Transcendence

This chapter was written before, during, and after the Persian Gulf War. Like many at that time, I felt a sense of failure that nonviolent interventions were not sufficiently developed to preclude war as a method of solving the dispute. Although much was said about diplomacy and sanctions, the fact is we went to war. As a clinician who has worked for nearly 20 years with aggressive patients, who has read transcripts of horrible crimes, who has witnessed vicious attacks and been threatened and attacked enough to wonder about my own vocation, individual aggression and war seem a misguided part of the plan. Senseless aggression is especially hard to accept.

But we all need rationalizations. In the belief that there are some things that are bad, stopping aggression seems a noble goal. Yet time and experience show that no matter how horrible aggression and war are, they appear to be part of the human process. Death is a passage all life must experience. Violent death is one form. So while I personally believe war will become an outmoded form of international problem solving, meditating on the reality of the Gulf War I came to conclude that beyond active protest, honoring one's duty is the path that will lead to a greater understanding and even acceptance of the role alleged evil plays in the divine dance. As Krishna said to Arjuna on the battlefield in the Bhagavad Gita, when one approaches a test with a dutiful attitude, the struggle can result in growth and even transcendence. Whatever war you struggle with, the Gulf War helped me discover that the greatest personal contribution I could make to a more peaceful world was to practice peace by becoming more accepting and tolerant of my adversaries, and to "turn over" the responsibility for those things I want to control, but cannot, to some other authority. In the worst-case (best-case?) scenarios the authority may become spiritual, and the life-and-death struggle, the seed of faith. It is this process that the murderers I have worked with wish they had had available to them during the buildup to their crimes.

References

Adler G: Helplessness in the helpers. Br J Med Psychol 45:315–326, 1972

American Psychiatric Association: Diagnostic and Statistical Manual of Mental Disorders, 3rd Edition, Revised. Washington, DC, American Psychiatric Association, 1987

American Psychiatric Association Task Force on Clinician Safety (Dubin WR, Chairperson): Unpublished report submitted to Council, May 1991

Bick PA, Hannah AL: Intramuscular lorazepam to restrain violent patients. Lancet 1:206, 1986

Binder RL: The use of seclusion on an inpatient intervention unit. Hosp Community Psychiatry 30:266–269, 1979

Binder RL, McCoy SM: A study of patients' attitudes toward placement in seclusion. Hosp Community Psychiatry 34:1052–1054, 1983

Boyle D, Tobin JM: Pharmaceutical management of behavior disorders: chlordiazepoxide in covert and overt expressions of aggression. Journal of the Medical Society of New Jersey 58:427–429, 1961

Carmel H, Hunter M: Staff injuries from inpatient violence. Hosp Community Psychiatry 40:41–46, 1989

Colson DB, Allen JG, Coyne L, et al: An anatomy of countertransference: staff reactions to difficult psychiatric hospital patients. Hosp Community Psychiatry 37:923–928, 1986

Costa E, Guidotti A, Mso CC: A GABA hypothesis for action of benzodiazepines, in GABA in Nervous System Function. Edited by Roberts E, Chase VN, Tower DB. New York, Raven, 1976

Dawson J, Johnson M, Kehiayan N, et al: Response to patient assault: a peer support program for nurses. J Psychosoc Nurs Ment Health Serv 26:8–15, 1988

Depp FC: Violent behavior patterns on psychiatric wards. Aggressive Behavior 2:395–306, 1976

Dubin WR: Emergency Psychiatry for the House Officer. Jamaica, NY, Spectrum, 1985

Eichelman B: Toward a rational pharmacotherapy for aggressive and violent behavior. Hosp Community Psychiatry 39:31–39, 1988

Greendyke RM, Kanter DR: Therapeutic effects of pindolol on behavioral disturbances associated with organic brain disease: a double-blind study. J Clin Psychiatry 47:423–426, 1986

Hakola HP, Laulamas VA: Carbamazepine in treatment of violent schizophrenics (letter). Lancet 1:1358, 1982

Harris GT, Varney GW: Assaults and Assaulters in Psychiatric Facilities. New York, Grune & Stratton, 1983

Heider J: The Tao of Leadership. New York, Bantam, 1985

Hoge SK, Gutheil TG: The prosecution of psychiatric patients for assaults on staff: a preliminary empirical study. Hosp Community Psychiatry 38:44–49, 1987

Infantino JA Jr, Musingo S-Y: Assaults and injuries among staff with and without training in aggression control techniques. Hosp Community Psychiatry 36:1312–1314, 1985

Kalina RK: Diazepam: its role in a prison setting. Diseases of the Nervous System 25:101–107, 1964

Kaplan SG, Wheeler EG: Survival skills for working with potentially violent clients. Social Casework: The Journal of Contemporary Social Work, June 1983, pp 339–346

Kuhlman TL: Humor and Psychotherapy. Homewood, IL, Dow Jones-Irwin (Dorsey Professional Book), 1984

Lanza ML: The reactions of nursing staff to physical assault by a patient. Hosp Community Psychiatry 34:44–47, 1983

Lanza ML: How nurses react to patient assault. J Psychosoc Nurs Ment Health Serv 23:7–11, 1985

Lion JR: Benzodiazepines in the treatment of aggressive patients. J Clin Psychiatry 40:70–71, 1979

Lion JR: Training for battle: thoughts on managing aggressive patients. Hosp Community Psychiatry 38:882–884, 1987

Lion JR, Pasternak SA: Countertransference reactions to violent patients. Am J Psychiatry 130:207–210, 1973

Lion JR, Reid WH (eds): Assaults Within Psychiatric Facilities. New York, Grune & Stratton, 1983

Madden DJ, Lion JR: Rage, Hate, Assault and Other Forms of Violence. New York, Spectrum, 1976

Maier GJ: Relationship security: the dynamics of keepers and kept. Journal of Forensic Science 31:603–608, 1986

Maier GJ: The successful prosecution of a "not guilty by reason of insanity" patient for the willful assault of a hospital staff. Psychiatric Residents Newsletter 9:1–2, 1989

Maier GJ, Van Rybroek GJ: Offensive images: managing aggression isn't pretty (editorial). Hosp Community Psychiatry 41:357, 1990

Maier GJ, Stava LJ, Morrow BR, et al: A model for understanding and managing cycles of aggression among psychiatric patients. Hosp Community Psychiatry 38:520–524, 1987

Maier GJ, Van Rybroek GJ, Doren DM, et al: A comprehensive model for understanding and managing aggressive inpatients. American Journal of Continuing Education in Nursing, Section C, 1988, pp 1–16

Maier GJ, Bernstein MJ, Musholt EA: Personal coping mechanisms for prison clinicians. Journal of Prison and Jail Health 7:29–39, 1989

Maletzky BM: The episodic dyscontrol syndrome. Diseases of the Nervous System 34:178–185, 1973

Mattes JA: Metoprolol for intermittent explosive disorder. Am J Psychiatry 142:1108–1109, 1985

Mattson MR, Sacks MH: Seclusion: uses and complications. Am J Psychiatry 135:1210–1213, 1978

McGee JJ: Gentle teaching. New Zealand Journal of Mental Retardation 40:13–24, 1985

Miller RD, Maier GJ: Factors affecting the decision to prosecute mental patients for criminal behavior. Hosp Community Psychiatry 38:50–55, 1987

Monahan J: The Clinical Prediction of Violent Behavior (DHHS Publ No (ADM)81-921). Rockville, MD, National Institute of Mental Health, 1981

Monroe RR: Anticonvulsants in the treatment of aggression. J Nerv Ment Dis 160:119–126, 1975

Novaco RW: Treatment of chronic anger through cognitive and relaxation controls. J Consult Clin Psychol 44:681, 1976

Perls FS: Ego, Hunger and Aggression. New York, Vintage Books, 1947

Rada RT: The violent patient: rapid assessment and management. Psychosomatics 22:101–109, 1981

Roth L: Clinical Treatment of the Violent Person (DHHS Publ No (ADM)85-1425). Rockville, MD, National Institute of Mental Health, 1985

Sandler J, Dare C, Holder A: Basic psychoanalytic concepts, III: transference. Br J Psychiatry 116:667–672, 1970

Sheard MH: Effect of lithium on human aggression. Nature 230:113–114, 1971

Sheard MH, Marini JL, Bridges CI, et al: The effect of lithium on impulsive aggressive behavior in man. Am J Psychiatry 133:1409–1413, 1976

Tanke ED, Yesavage JA: Characteristics of assaultive patients who do and do not provide visible cues of potential violence. Am J Psychiatry 142:1409–1413, 1985

Tardiff K: A survey of drugs used in the management of assaultive inpatients. Bull Am Acad Psychiatry Law 11:215–222, 1983

Tardiff K (ed): The Psychiatric Uses of Seclusion and Restraint. Washington, DC, American Psychiatric Press, 1984

Tardiff K: Concise Guide to Assessment and Management of Violent Patients. Washington, DC, American Psychiatric Press, 1989

Thackrey M: Therapeutics for Aggression: Psychological/Physical Crisis Intervention. New York, Human Sciences Press, 1987

Van Rybroek GJ, Maier GJ: Aggressive inmates: hitting critical components of management. Correct Care 1:7, 1987

Van Rybroek GJ, Kuhlman TL, Maier GJ, et al: Preventive aggression devices (PADS): ambulatory restraints as an alternate to seclusion. J Clin Psychiatry 38:1081–1085, 1987

Wadeson H, Carpenter WT Jr: Impact of the seclusion room experience. J Nerv Ment Dis 163:318–328, 1976

Yudofsky S, Williams D, Gorman J: Propranolol in the treatment of rage and violent behavior in patients with chronic brain syndromes. Am J Psychiatry 138:218–220, 1981

Yudofsky SC, Silver JM, Jackson W, et al: The Overt Aggression Scale for the objective rating of verbal and physical aggression. Am J Psychiatry 143:35–39, 1986

Chapter 8

Compliance Problems and Their Management

Douglas A. Puryear, M.D.

Compliance problems are a major source of difficulty for the psychiatrist, whether in the private office, clinic, emergency room, or hospital. In fact, problems of compliance are ubiquitous and frustrating in all of health care; few reading this require a definition such as "Compliance refers to the patient's following of the physician's recommendations for his or her treatment." Considering noncompliance, one probably thinks of failure to take medication as prescribed, such as in a patient with hypertension, but there are other examples, such as a diabetic patient's failure to follow a necessary diet or a cigarette addict's failure to stop smoking.

Previous writers have studied compliance problems both clinically and scientifically, and have devised many ingenious and partially effective approaches. A review of the literature would more than fill this volume, let alone this chapter, and shall not be attempted here. Rather, I shall draw the reader's attention to the many forms in which compliance problems may appear in psychiatry (see Table 8–1), the many reasons for them, and some approaches that may help. These forms, reasons, and approaches are interwoven in each case example. Readers desiring more extensive information are referred to Meichenbaum and Turk's *Facilitating Treatment Adherence* (1987) and the other references.

Table 8–1. Common forms of compliance problems

Medication problems	Refusing hospitalization
Missing appointments	Failing to perform assignments
Dropping out of or refusing therapy	

Forms of Noncompliance

Failure to maintain a medication regimen and dropping out of therapy are probably the most common of the many forms in which compliance problems can manifest in psychiatry.

Medications

Case 1: The Negotiator

A 24-year-old graduate student came to see me dissatisfied with his current psychiatrist who had him stabilized on 50 mg of haloperidol daily following a second psychotic break. They had been arguing bitterly about the need for medication. When I called, the doctor seemed happy for me to take over. The patient, angry and guarded, minimized and avoided discussing details of his illness and focused on his feeling that he did not need medication. I explained that my goal was to use the minimal effective dose of medication, sometimes none at all, but that I was very conservative; that we could work together to avoid any more hospitalizations and to use minimal medication; and that because of the risk of another costly breakdown, and because I'd just met him and I'm conservative, I preferred lowering the dose slowly; then we could assess how he was doing and consider lowering it further.

He reluctantly accepted this. I suggested an initial decrease to 45 mg a day; he angrily suggested dropping to only 10 mg. We discussed and negotiated; he resentfully agreed to try 40 mg, but only if we negotiated a written schedule for further reductions. We followed this plan, although often renegotiating the schedule and discussing whether or not he needed any medication at all.

The patient slowly became calmer and less angry, but still guarded and defensive. Over a year's time he began to trust me, to accept the illness, and to work more collaboratively, although continuing negotiations about medication and how often he needed to see me. He then revealed that his family, who lived out of town, had been opposed to his taking medication, and he also discussed some delusions that he had not shared with me. During our second year two brief breaks were handled smoothly by reducing stress and briefly raising his medication, although never as much as I suggested. He eventually accepted a maintenance low dose, raising it slightly at any warning signals, such as tension or insomnia.

He is now usually off medication but reinstitutes it briefly when indicated. We meet quarterly. During our 10 years of work he has had three brief breaks and one short hospitalization. He has maintained and advanced in his job, improved his social relationships, and developed an active recreational life. For 3 years he has shown no evidence of psychosis.

One approach to compliance is to develop a respectful, collaborative relationship between physician and patient, with both collaborators dedicated to dealing with the illness to optimize the quality of the patient's life. This team effort requires information exchange, discussion, suggestions and recommendations, and negotiation. For many schizophrenic patients, autonomy is a particularly sensitive major concern. Problems of trust and self-esteem also may lead to denial of problems and treatment avoidance.

Missed Appointments

Missed appointments often are a form of resistance. The therapist needs to review the preceding session and consider both his or her actions (or lack thereof) and the issues the patient is struggling with (Langs 1973a, 1973b). The overall therapy, its progress, and the therapeutic contract must also be considered. While using a working hypothesis that missed appointments are due to resistance, the therapist must realize that they may be due to life circumstances, as the patient often maintains. The therapist cannot argue the point, but can suggest that other factors might also be involved. This lays the groundwork for further exploration in the event of a recurrence.

Dropping Out or Refusal of Therapy

A patient's dropping out or refusal of therapy is usually a major resistance. Major resistances must be addressed promptly, especially when seen in the first session (Langs 1973a, 1973b). There can, however, be many reasons for dropping out or refusal other than resistance, such as major errors by the therapist, an inadequate therapeutic contract, the offering of the wrong type of therapy for the patient, the provision of therapy in a way that the patient cannot accept, or simply a patient-therapist mismatch (Weiner 1982). On the other hand, most therapists have experienced having a patient "drop out" of therapy and later learning that the patient had made a great deal of progress and was doing very well, of which the following case is an extreme example.

Case 2: The One-Timer

A patient came to me complaining bitterly about his unhappiness, which he primarily blamed on his overbearing boss. Initially in the interview, I listened, wondering about oedipal conflict, father transference, passivity, and so forth. I made a few gently supportive comments. Later, gathering past history and medical information, I asked, "Why do you stay in the job?" The patient thought a minute and said, "I really don't know." At the end of the interview I told him I would be happy to see him in therapy and that we could explore further to understand more the roots of his unhappiness. He said he wanted to think about it and would call if he wanted a second appointment. My heart sank: I wondered what error had caused me to lose this patient.

Months later I saw him in an office building. He gave me a friendly greeting and thanked me for my help. I asked him what kind of help I had given. He replied that my question, "Why do you stay in the job?" had stayed on his mind, and the more he thought about it, the less he was able to answer it. He quit his job, opened an office of his own, and had never felt better. I wished him luck.

Sometimes apparent noncompliance may indicate that the physician's recommendation is wrong (Talmon 1990, p. 9; see Case 5 below).

Refusal of Recommended Hospitalization

Occasionally when a patient refuses a recommendation of hospitalization (or sometimes other recommendations), the psychiatrist refuses to treat him or her anymore. The explanation often is that "I [the psychiatrist] have to refuse to treat him as an outpatient, or else I'm giving a mixed message and he thinks I don't really believe he needs hospitalization." I believe that this is usually an erroneous approach and that the psychiatrist should take means, such as written informed consent and family meetings, to protect himself or herself, but continue working with the patient in the ways available. The psychiatrist should try to understand the reasons behind the refusal, reconsider the appropriateness of the recommendation, and attempt to maintain and improve the alliance. Partial compliance is usually superior to no treatment and may improve with time (Schwartz 1990).

The AMA Emergency Patient

Occasionally in the emergency room, the family opposes our recommendation to hospitalize a patient for whom we think it is indicated, and who we feel is possibly dangerous but not sufficiently so to legally qualify him or her for involuntary hospitalization. Further, we feel that there are serious legal risks in involuntarily hospitalizing a patient against the wishes of the family. If the family refuses, we explain our reasoning. Then if the family still refuses, we ask them to sign the patient out against medical advice (AMA). We handwrite the document, an example of which is given below, and ask them to sign it:

> We have been advised that our son and brother, Mr. A., is at high risk of killing himself. We have been advised that he will likely shoot himself, probably in the head, but might also hang himself, jump off a building, swallow pills, or use some other method. We have been advised to constantly keep him in sight, including the bathroom and sleeping, until assured by medical authority that he is no longer dangerous. Hospitalization has been strongly recommended for his safety, but we have refused. We accept full and

total responsibility for whatever happens and relieve Dr. —— and —— Hospital from any responsibility.

Additional details may be added as necessary. After asking all family members present to read the document, we then read it out loud to them and ask each of them to sign it. Sometimes they sign it and take the patient home; sometimes they refuse to sign it and take the patient home. Sometimes they change their minds and accept our recommendation. By going through this rather formal ritual, we avoid arguing with the family, a procedure that usually causes people to become more set in their position; instead, we go along with them, in a way that might cause them to change their minds.

Failure to Perform Assignments

Sometimes in therapy, especially family therapy, a task is assigned to assess the patient's motivation. Exploring the reasons a task was not performed can, as in the following example, provide insight into the larger meanings of the patient's problems and suggest more effective ways to work with the patient (Hanley 1982).

Case 3: The Insecure Student

I consulted with a resident and his patient, a minority graduate student having difficulty passing examinations. As I questioned the student, I learned she had done well in some difficult undergraduate courses. She described her sense of shock the first time she failed an examination in graduate school. This failure became a preoccupation that caused her difficulty on further examinations and increasing agitation. The resident requested consultation partly because of the patient's adamant refusal of psychological testing to clarify the problem. I carefully explained to the patient that I was not advocating the testing, but was interested in understanding her reasons for refusing. She described her fear that the testing would reveal that she actually was not intellectually capable of handling graduate school. I supportively referred to the evidence of her achievement in college, but emphasized that her fear was a strong and genuine feeling. Later, I suggested to the resident that this issue might in fact offer an effective entry into understanding more about his patient's sense of inadequacy.

Efforts to understand the reasons for patients' noncompliance sometimes pay off more than efforts to gain compliance. Often, once the physician understands the basis for noncompliance, the patient becomes more compliant. At other times, once the basis for the reluctance is understood, the physician alters what he or she asks the patient to do.

Other Forms of Noncompliance

There are many ways in which a patient cannot comply with what the physician wants from him or her.

Case 4: The "Kinda Did It" Man

One of a young man's reasons for therapy was difficulty on jobs. Early in his therapy, I recommended a book I thought might be helpful to him. When he made no comment about the book after several sessions, I inquired. He said that it had been helpful and that he had "kinda read around in it." His handling of this advice helped clarify some of his employment difficulties. Rather than trying to achieve the compliance of having him read the book, the issue became understanding how and why the patient did not comply, his attitude and way of approaching a task, and how this might apply to other areas in his life.

Sometimes one can make use of the noncompliance, working with it to achieve a therapeutic outcome rather than specifically trying to resolve it.

Reasons for Noncompliance

Many of the numerous possible reasons for compliance problems arise from the patient-therapist relationship (see Table 8–2). These could be considered transference/countertransference problems in the broadest sense of those terms. Patients bring many

Table 8–2.   Common reasons for compliance problems

Lack of alliance	Lapses in physician's responsibilities
Resistance	Medication side effects
Acting out	Life circumstances
Autonomy conflict	Systems problems
Misunderstandings or ignorance	

issues to their treatment, including autonomy, dependency, and passivity conflicts; self-esteem and ego boundary problems; classical resistance; and the need to save face. Therapists' issues include narcissism, a sense of omnipotence, self-esteem, and the need to save face. Intertwining of the therapist and patient issues can lead to severe interpersonal conflict, which may either be overt or played out over compliance.

Other, nonrelationship reasons for compliance problems could be categorized under medication side effects, life circumstance problems, and systems problems. These various reasons are usually interrelated, operating in self-reinforcing feedback; the noncompliance in each case is usually due to more than one factor (Meichenbaum and Turk 1987). Some of the myriad possible reasons for noncompliance will be explored in the subsections and case examples below.

Lack of Alliance

Alliance must come from both sides. There is a common tendency to label the patient "unmotivated," when actually the physician has failed in his or her primary task of developing and maintaining alliance. There are indeed unmotivated patients, but aside from conserving the physician's time and ego, there is very little benefit in assuming that lack of motivation is the problem.

Case 5: The Unhappy Wife

I practice a variety of therapies, but am primarily a psychodynamic psychotherapist. A young woman came complaining bitterly about her husband. Some of her psychodynamic difficulties were fairly apparent. She was reluctantly persuaded to undertake individual psychotherapy. During the first few sessions she continued to complain about her husband while I began to confront her resistance of talking about her husband rather than about herself and her own internal problems. She then dropped out.

I believe that by the textbook my approach was proper and that I am entitled to label the patient "unmotivated." However, I believe I lost a patient who had real potential for individual psychotherapy and who apparently was motivated enough to come to my office several times even when clearly not being offered what she wanted. Had I worked with her initially on her marital problems, and perhaps even seen her and her husband together, they might have benefited, and she very well might have later entered productive individual psychotherapy. Patients often must be "induced" into treatment in one way or another, and it may be the psychiatrist's failure to recognize, accept, and deal with a patient's "request" that leads to the noncompliance (Lazare et al. 1975).

Resistance

Classical resistance is a common underlying reason for compliance problems. In psychotherapy, the patient is resistant to the psychotherapeutic process because of reluctance to face unpleasant material. More broadly, the term might apply to all noncompliance arising from the doctor-patient relationship in any type of treatment, even if simply pharmacotherapy. The classic technique of understanding and then interpreting, rather than trying to exhort, coerce, persuade, or otherwise push through the resistance, is often the most useful approach. It is not, however, the only useful approach, nor is it always sufficient in itself.

Case 6: The Frugal Buyer

A narcissistic patient in therapy became less angry and demanding but continued to be extremely sensitive to every perceived slight. Although her life was better and she was more comfortable and enjoying more, she frequently complained that therapy was not helping her. She called to cancel an appointment and to say that she was terminating. I had some ideas how this related to resistance. I called and asked her to come discuss the situation before terminating. She said there was no reason to, that therapy was too expensive, and that it would be a waste of money to come in just to satisfy me. I said that if she would come, I would let her determine payment. She could pay me what she felt the session was worth, and if it was worthless she could pay nothing, but I thought it important that we discuss termination. She agreed. The session was productive, and the patient paid the full fee and continued in therapy.

This patient seemed ready to drop out of therapy as a major resistance to dealing with certain painful narcissistic issues. This required interpretation, but the narcissism had to be respected and protected in order to have that opportunity.

Sometimes, especially with borderline or narcissistic patients, the psychiatrist must lean over backward to enable the patient to "comply" and continue therapy. The psychiatrist must also protect himself or herself. For example, I may be able to tolerate one night call a week for a month from a new borderline patient; this gives us a month to develop a new strategy for the patient's coping with his dysphoric episodes. I may prescribe a benzodiazepine against my better judgment for 2 weeks if a patient clearly would drop out of therapy without it. I may be willing to stay 30 minutes late each Tuesday for a month until a patient feels able to leave a new job half an hour early for her sessions. Each of these concessions has a limit, determined by my degree of comfort. The experience of someone (in this case the therapist) responding to the patients' needs while still protecting his or her self-interest is usually a new one for borderline patients. If the psychiatrist bends too far, he or she may get into an untenable position, or his or her resentment may interfere with the therapy. Patients may eventually become compliant if the psychiatrist complies enough with their wishes and meets enough of their needs to allow them to comply.

Acting Out

Acting out, referring to dealing with inner turmoil or conflict through behavior rather than memory, reflection, and discussion in therapy, is by definition a resistance and an interference with compliance. In the broader sense of acting out, a patient's inner turmoil and conflicts expressed in behavior can interfere with any form of treatment. Limits often need to be set to deal with acting out, but other means may be more effective. Again, one tries to deal with acting out primarily by understanding and interpreting it. Beyond that, one often must collaboratively work out such issues with the patient.

Case 7: The Tardy Patient

A patient with narcissistic problems was always late to his appointment. It became clear that he was consistently 5 minutes late. We began to explore the meanings of this. The patient always had excuses for his tardiness: red lights, construction, accidents, last-minute telephone calls, and so forth. I suggested he seemed to time his leaving as though there would never be any problems. He suddenly had an "Aha" experience, "If I plan to leave 5 minutes earlier, I would usually make it on time!" Later, he revealed that he occasionally arrived early and would sit outside in his car so as to arrive promptly 5 minutes late. He explained that he was uncomfortable sitting in the waiting room waiting for me, because it made him feel that I was too important and that he was too dependent on me. He preferred his own imaginary picture of my sitting waiting for him. We worked on understanding these issues and he began arriving on time.

The noncompliance in this example seemed primarily a defense of the patient's narcissism, as well as a transference and a real relationship issue. Limit setting would probably have been disruptive in this case, whereas exploring and understanding led the therapy far beyond the issue of the 5 minutes tardiness.

Autonomy Conflict

The patient's sense of autonomy frequently affects his or her level of compliance; this is, perhaps, especially the case in adolescents, schizophrenic patients, and paranoid patients (see especially Cases 1 and 11).

Case 8: The Adolescent Protester

> For many months, an adolescent patient began each therapy ses-
> sion with a protest about his parents forcing him to attend ther-
> apy, which he found absolutely worthless. As he improved, I
> became increasingly frustrated with his deriding of therapy and
> his *apparent* lack of commitment to it [see discussion of counter-
> transference and therapist's narcissism in "The Physician's Re-
> sponsibilities" subsection below]. I finally confronted him: "You
> are 17 years old, pretty husky, have your own car and a part time
> job. How on earth can your parents '*force*' you to come here?"
> The patient never returned.

Some patients are able to comply with treatment only so long
as they can fly a banner of defiant noncompliance and deny their
need for treatment. This manner of noncompliance may relate to
difficulties with self-esteem, passivity, autonomy, and so forth, and
perhaps may eventually be confronted, interpreted, and worked
through. However, it may not always be necessary to do so, and the
timing is particularly crucial. The patient's sense of autonomy may
need protecting, which will be promoted by a collaborative therapeutic relationship.

Misunderstandings or Ignorance

Noncompliance can arise from misunderstanding or ignorance either in the patient or in the psychiatrist. In supervising residents,
I find that when a patient says he or she wants to drop out of therapy, often the resident immediately tries to talk him or her out of
it. Usually this should be taken as an expression of a feeling or an
urge and explored therapeutically, as with any other material. An
inexperienced therapist may not hear the statement as therapeutic
material and, especially if his or her self-esteem is threatened, may
panic. This lapse may in itself push the patient out of therapy.

There is an increasing tendency to call all medications, including our psychoactive medications, "drugs." This is unfortunate,
particularly in dealing with schizophrenic patients, who have some
tendency to be concrete. "Whatever you do, don't take any drugs,

but whatever you do, be sure and take your drugs." I have had patients refuse to take medications in the emergency room on the basis of, "I just say 'no' to drugs."

The Physician's Responsibilities

Throughout this chapter, the attitude is maintained that it is the physician's responsibility to foster compliance, and many examples of noncompliance illustrate physicians' errors in approach, misunderstanding, ignorance, countertransference, narcissism, sense of omnipotence, excessive expectations, or rigidity. These are major sources of compliance problems. Thus, the physician must continually be aware of such tendencies within himself or herself and of the ever present danger of their intrusion into the treatment process (see Cases 2, 5, and 9).

Related problems involve the psychiatrist's expecting something of the patient that the patient simply cannot do. This inability to comply may be due to emotional problems such as delusions, conflicts, hopelessness, or inability to handle family opposition; to problems of other internal resources, such as organic memory impairment, psychotic disorganization, depressive anergia, or religious or cultural beliefs; or to lack of external resources, such as money, time, transportation, baby sitter, and so forth.

In crisis intervention, if the patient does not do an assigned task, the crisis intervener assumes responsibility, indicating that he had done a poor job of selecting the task, most often by assigning one that was too difficult. It is the crisis intervener's job to select and define a task in such a way that it is certain that the patient will do it and will be successful at it (Puryear 1979).

Medication Side Effects

Side effects are a common reason for medication noncompliance. Sometimes these side effects are mild and may not be apparent to the physician; furthermore, they may not be brought to the physician's attention unless he or she specifically inquires. Physicians sometimes tell patients that they simply must endure side effects because of the benefits of the medications. This counsel is rarely effective. Occasionally patients complain of side effects that seem minimal, or not apparent, or unlikely to be due to the medication. These complaints must be taken seriously and investigated. In spite of the physician's belief or the statements in the *Physicians' Desk Reference*, the symptoms must be considered possibly due to the medication and bothersome to the patient. Sometimes it will seem that the patient is complaining about side effects, cost, inability to swallow pills, and so forth, when in fact he or she has other reasons for reluctance to take the medication. This can be gently inquired about, but it is difficult to dissect out the true underlying reasons from the complaints and possible genuine side effects. The physician must seriously work on the complaints with the patient until the resistance becomes obvious. Then it may be dealt with directly.

When prescribing, it is worthwhile asking patients whether they are particularly sensitive or particularly invulnerable to medications in general. A patient who reports that he or she is sensitive will almost always experience severe side effects unless cautiously started on the lowest possible dose of any medication.

Medications can be quite expensive; often physicians do not know the cost of the medicines they are prescribing and sometimes are not aware of the patient's financial circumstances. The more the physician knows about the patient, the better compliance will tend to be (Brand et al. 1977).

Overall, to gain and sustain compliance with any medications, the physician must listen to the patient and be quite concerned about side effects. The physician must be willing to try various strategies of medication reduction, side-effect medications, or medication change. The physician must make it clear to the patient that the side effects are being taken seriously and that the physician will work hard to minimize them (Bartko et al. 1988; Corrigan 1990; Van Putten 1974, 1976).

Life Circumstances

At times, compliance problems truly have little to do with resistance. Residents sometimes complain that their clinic patient is "not motivated" when the patient misses appointments. A patient might miss an appointment because of an inappropriate type of therapy incongruent with his or her life circumstances (Acosta 1982), lack of a clear contract (Weiner 1982), or many other reasons. I often ask the resident to ask the patient, when next she appears, how she gets to the clinic. Sometimes the resident sheepishly reports that to get to the appointment his "unmotivated" patient has to get up at 5:00 A.M., wait in the dark at the bus stop in a dangerous neighborhood for a bus on an unreliable schedule, and stand in line 30 minutes to get into the clinic. She then sits in a waiting room clearly labeled "Psychiatry" where her name is publicly called out when she is finally summoned in to see the doctor. Given such an ordeal, and the life circumstances of many of these patients, it is a feat of strength and courage that they ever keep any clinic appointment.

Case 9: The Clinic Patient

> In a mental health clinic I saw a middle-aged black woman, poorly educated, whose mild depression seemed largely situational. She was working two jobs and taking care of her husband, who had also been working two jobs until he fell and fractured a vertebra. The family could not make ends meet, and she was having great difficulty obtaining food stamps or disability for her husband. I urged her to contact the appropriate agencies and be assertive. She seemed to me unduly passive, pessimistic, and somewhat resistant to my encouragement. I thought about the difficulties an uneducated middle-aged black woman might have, particularly in the South, dealing with bureaucracies. I decided to intervene, both to help her and to serve as a model. After some hours on the telephone, carefully introducing myself as "*Doctor* Puryear," I still had not been able to even contact the appropriate person in either agency. I had learned a great deal.

Sometimes the apparently noncompliant patient knows things the physician does not (Acosta 1982; Lazare et al. 1975).

Systems Problems

We have discussed problems that might arise from transportation and clinic systems. It is difficult for most people to have a loved one enter psychotherapy. They do not know how the patient might change; they may feel the threat of losing him or her. They do not know what portrait of themselves might be painted; they may feel excluded, fear the patient's attachment to another person, and so forth. They may discourage the therapy and have negative reactions to any changes the patient begins to make. It takes courage and strength for a patient to persist.

Classical individual psychotherapy is a closed dyadic relationship, but I find that patients often need assistance in dealing with their significant others, and occasionally I have to meet with these individuals. In working with an adolescent, or with a psychotic, potentially psychotic, or severely depressed patient, I almost always meet with the family to form an allliance and sometimes to offer help. Otherwise, if the family is not with you, they usually wind up against you. Also, with unstable patients, I may eventually need help from the family.

The Negotiator (continued from p. 217)

> As mentioned above in the case of the graduate student with schizophrenia and medication reluctance, I learned late that his parents had discouraged his use of medication. One of his breaks occurred while visiting them, and they called me, quite upset. On the phone the patient told me he was off his medication. I persuaded him to resume at least a low dose. He cleared quickly, and the parents never discouraged medication again. On his next break, his father flew in and stayed with him to provide structure and support. We met together. The break again cleared in a few days and another hospitalization was avoided. When dealing with a seriously ill patient, one needs an alliance with significant others, and confidentiality must be carefully titrated.

Other Reasons for Noncompliance

Many other reasons for compliance problems overlap with those already discussed. One example is use of massive denial—characteristic of alcoholic persons, but frequently seen in other patients—which serves as a resistance as well as perhaps protecting self-esteem and/or autonomy.

Case 10: The Good Son

A psychotic young man who seemed schizophrenic was brought in by his mother. He took two doses of haloperidol willingly and reintegrated fairly well. He refused, however, to take the fluphenazine decanoate shot ordered before discharge. My explanations that it would help him avoid the hospital, think clearly, and sleep, only met protests that he had no illness and no problems and did not need medication. I had noted his courtesy toward his mother. When I said that it would make his mother feel better, he willingly took the shot.

Some patients seem unable to acknowledge their illness, although they may have at least an unconscious awareness. This is common in persons with schizophrenia as well as those with diabetes, hypertension, and alcoholism. The problem may be related to self-esteem, another major sensitivity for many people with schizophrenia. The young man in the vignette above could take the medication altruistically when he could not from the position of a mentally ill patient. Confrontation can be useful; at other times it is better to acknowledge (although not necessarily endorse) the patient's viewpoint and to find a way that the patient can collaborate within his or her own framework while maintaining self-esteem and autonomy—that is, "save face" without having to "give in" to the physician's perceptions. The physician needs to enable the patient to be compliant. A noncompliant patient may be ambivalent, rather than simply unmotivated or resistant.

Case 11: The Refuser

A psychotic young woman was seen involuntarily in the emergency room. She was hostile and defensive. She denied that anything was wrong or that she needed any help. By history and presentation she appeared bipolar manic. I told her that the nurse would bring her some medicine and that after she was calmer we could talk. She angrily replied, "I don't need any of your damn medicine! Do I have to take it?" I replied, "Yes," and walked away. She took the medication and eventually calmed down.

A psychotic patient may be too disorganized and burdened with overstimulation to adequately attend to decision making, and thus may be relieved when someone takes over. Some patients simply prefer their doctor to tell them what to do; these patients would rather not think about it or make decisions themselves. This may work well, but I have concern about the long-term course of such treatment. It is not clear what the manic young lady meant by her question, "Do I have to take it?" There was no legal reason that she had to. I chose to interpret it as her saying, "I think I need medication, but can only accept it under protest, so please tell me that I have to take it and then I can." I learned from raising adolescent children that sometimes one must respond only to the affect, and sometimes only to the words. I heard in the patient's question a suggestion of a potential willingness to take the medication. Sometimes physicians can respond to the positive side of the patient's ambivalence and avoid entanglement with the negative side.

Efforts to gain compliance will never be uniformly successful. Especially in the emergency room, the physician needs a hierarchy of approaches to gain quick compliance. Although guessing the treatment that is most likely to be effective with a given patient, the physician also orders options such that if the treatment fails, the physician has not painted himself or herself into a corner but still can try another. For instance, ultimatums—"No, we can't force you to take medicine, but we will be forced to hospitalize you if you don't try it"—are a last resort.

These examples show resistance as a multifactor phenomenon that may be dealt with by addressing its components (Kelly et al. 1987; Meichenbaum and Turk 1987).

Approaches to Compliance Problems

Approaches to compliance problems obviously should be individualized. One underlying principle is to try to understand the reasons behind the problem and then to devise strategies to address them. In practice, this is not always possible, and there are many avenues toward increased compliance (see Table 8–3).

Preventative

We strive to establish a collaborative relationship with a mutually agreed-upon treatment contract, mutual understanding, and good communication. Usually this involves some education for the patient and perhaps the family (see Case 1).

The Family Coping Project.   When we see a schizophrenic patient in the emergency room we offer the family the Family Coping Project, a free six-session program educating the family about schizophrenia, medications, the mental health system, problem solving, communication, and community resources, based on the work of McGill, Falloon, and others (McGill and Falloon 1984). Many of the families who take this program report that it made significant difference in the quality of life and in "compliance." We find many of these families have never been told a diagnosis, have not had the purpose of the medication explained, or have not received the most elementary information to assist them in dealing with their family member's illness (Cain 1986).

Medication compliance will be enhanced if the physician can 1) understand and address the patient's concerns, 2) understand the patient's goals and use the medication to help the patient achieve these goals, and 3) understand the patient's life and behavioral patterns and integrate the medication taking based on that understanding (Corrigan et al. 1990; Diamond 1983; Falloon 1984).

Clarify Misunderstandings

Case 12: The Sensitive Patient

I explained to a schizophrenic patient that I saw schizophrenia as similar to alcoholism, both painful and troubling illnesses that

Table 8–3.   Some approaches to compliance problems

Prevention	Interpretation
Clarification of misunderstandings	Change in treatment approaches
Mechanical methods	Redefinition of "compliance"
Use of outside resources	Paradox

no one asks for or deserves, but that once having them, one has responsibility to learn all he or she can about the illnesses and try to deal with them. The patient became withdrawn. At the following meeting he was still somewhat withdrawn and angry. When I inquired, he explained that he disliked being called an "alcoholic." He clarified that he had "heard" me say that he was like an alcoholic, and in fact heard nothing that I said after that. I thanked him for explaining, apologized, and then clarified my intention, and now use diabetes for the analogy rather than alcoholism.

Mechanical Methods

Patients may be truly forgetful or disorganized. For medication compliance, they can be helped by plastic boxes divided into compartments to hold each day's pills, by fluorescent signs on the refrigerator, by keeping their pills next to their toothbrush, or by any method tailored to their life-style.

One study found that when state hospital patients were met in the hospital by their aftercare worker and given a clinic appointment, compliance rates for that first appointment rose to 68% from the 22% achieved by simply telling patients to call the clinic (Stickney et al. 1980).

Outside Resources

Family members can be harmful or helpful in compliance issues, which they may find difficult. In general, patients need to develop autonomy and handle their medications and appointments themselves, and they tend to resist family monitoring. However, if the family does not monitor, often the patient will fail in compliance. The family can be educated, supported, and encouraged in their attempts to facilitate compliance. They can be taught approaches to decrease conflict around compliance while moving toward patient autonomy. For example, family members can be taught to give positive reinforcement for medication and appointment compliance, rather than make these issues arenas for stress and conflict. Sometimes getting less intensely involved people to take over working with the patient on compliance can reduce the friction attached to those issues and the general stress level in the home. In our Family Coping Project, families are taught problem-solving approaches, noncritical communication, and the different ways to avoid escalations.

Sometimes patients who fail to keep clinic appointments will comply with a nurse who delivers a long-acting injection at home. Social "clubs" have been used instead of clinics to monitor medication in a more facilitative informal setting (Bartko et al. 1988; Frances and Weiden 1987; Olarte and Masnick 1981).

Interpretation

Interpretation is the standard therapeutic approach to dealing with resistance and with related noncompliance.

Case 13: The Talker

A woman in therapy persistently complained that there was simply not enough time; she had too much to tell me. She filled each session with details about troubling situations in her life, without discussing feelings, fantasies, or memories. She often wanted advice on how to deal with these situations, which I sometimes gave. Otherwise, most of my comments were brushed aside, seeming to be experienced simply as interruptions of her pressured rush to get every detail in before time was up. Eventually, she explained her view of therapy: that if only she could tell me everything that was troubling her, then I could give her the answer, and everything would be alright. She connected this with her childhood idea that her father knew all the answers but never seemed to have the time or interest to give them to her. After this insight, her participation in therapy improved. Later, the patient described her mother's habit of presenting problems to be addressed but always leaving out critical details, and connected this with her own driven need to include every possible detail. Therapy developed into a truly collaborative dialogue, and the patient began to experience the painful feelings that had been avoided by this transference resistance and negative identification.

Negotiation

The physician frequently cannot get all of the compliance he or she wishes. For example, a common problem is the alcoholic patient who cannot be moved beyond denial. If rapport is maintained, a compromise written contract may be negotiated. The contract might state that the patient denies that he has a problem (or is an alcoholic, or needs Alcoholics Anonymous), but that if he cannot stay dry for 3 months (or winds up in the emergency room again, or loses his job) he agrees to then attend three AA meetings a week for 6 months. Sometimes the patient actually lives up to the contract. The approach can be tried with other patients; for example, a resistant schizophrenic patient may agree to resume medication if his voices return (see Case 1).

Change of Treatment Approach

When patients are not compliant, the physician needs to rethink the situation to see if he or she is in error and/or needs to become more compliant with the patients' wishes or needs. Sometimes the problem exists not in the patients, but rather in the viewpoint of the physician.

Case 14: Dr. Alma's Patient

Ms. B. had a borderline personality with severe compulsions, obsessions, anxiety, and depressive features. She had been in therapy with Dr. Alma for many years. When Dr. Alma moved to another city, the patient transferred to Dr. Bone. However, she kept referring to Dr. Alma and comparing Dr. Bone's interventions unfavorably with those of Dr. Alma. Dr. Bone regarded this as resistance. Finally, in exasperation, Dr. Bone confronted the resistance; "I am not Dr. Alma; I am Dr. Bone! Dr. Alma is not your therapist anymore; I am your therapist now!" Ms. B. did not return for further sessions. She then came to see me. I empathized with her feelings and with how difficult it had been to give up Dr. Alma, whom she had known for so many years and who had been so helpful. I told her that while I considered myself a good therapist, clearly I was not as good as Dr. Alma and it would be painful and difficult for her to work with me after her better experience with him, but that I would do my best.

Versions of the following occurred repeatedly:

Ms. B.: "This is awful! I feel terrible! I can't go on this way! What am I to do? Can't you help me? Tell me what to do!"
Dr. P.: "You are really feeling awful and you're very upset. What would Dr. Alma have said?"
Ms. B. [*after reflection*]: "Oh! He would have said [*etc. etc.*]."
Dr. P.: "Does that make sense to you?"
Ms. B.: "Yes, that helps."

On occasion, I urged Ms. B. to call Dr. Alma when she was in a crisis. Instead of seeing Ms. B.'s preoccupation with Dr. Alma as a resistance, I thought that Dr. Alma had been becoming a much needed internal soothing object for her. I viewed my task as furthering this process so that he became more internalized and available to her. Ms. B. made progress. She gradually became more able to use me and my interventions, and was increasingly able to turn to her internal representation of Dr. Alma for help. If the patient is not complying with the physician's wishes, the physician can change his or her approach, treatment plan, or recommendation so that it is congruent with what the patient will do.

Redefinition of Compliance

The physician can get entangled with the ways that the patient is not complying, and miss important areas of compliance. Sometimes it is simpler to change expectations or perceptions, or simply to define whatever the patient is doing as "compliance." A long-term time frame can be utilized, so it may be helpful to think of a patient as "not fully compliant at this particular time," rather than as "noncompliant" (see Cases 2 and 14).

Case 15: The Elective Mute

An adolescent began his therapy, and each subsequent session for a while, by stating that he absolutely refused to talk to me. We had many long and productive discussions about why he would not talk to me, and eventually about his related feelings.

Paradox

Paradox is a useful technique that sometimes gains compliance. It works partly by avoiding an opportunity for resistance (Haley 1976). In the emergency room, sometimes a patient in seclusion begins to hit the door. This is disruptive in the area, and there is some danger the patient will hurt himself or herself. Telling or asking the patient to stop is rarely effective. There are many ways to try to deal with this, including straitjackets, forcing intramuscular medication, and so forth, which are assaultive and not entirely satisfactory. I have about 50% success with the following approach. At the window of the seclusion room, I order the patient to hit the door again. Sometimes the patient refuses, but often he or she complies. I then order, "Hit it again," and then, "Okay, one more time." Often the patient refuses. Sometimes he or she hits it again. I then may say, "Okay, that's three. Do you want to hit it once more?" They frequently decline.

This tells the patient that hitting the door will not provide him or her with much leverage because we do not mind. The opportunity to resist the order to hit the door offers a different and less painful way to be negative and hostile. This may be viewed as a "hypnotic" technique, gaining the patient's attention, gaining "control" over some behavior, and then using suggestion (i.e., "once more" implies stopping). It probably works in different ways with different patients (Hanley 1982).

Case 16: The Hopeless Case

A despondent 41-year-old woman came to see me with somatic problems, insomnia, and dysphoria. She quickly related a lengthy list of internists and psychiatrists who had been unable to help her and of medications that had not worked. Although she had no energy or motivation and was unable to work, she did not fully meet the criteria for major depression. Whenever I made a gentle suggestion or raised a hypothesis, she tended to not agree. At session's end she urgently asked for help in getting more sleep. Nothing the other doctors had tried had helped. I told her I did not think I could help her with that. I then made a couple of suggestions she might try, but expressed doubt that they would help or that any medications could help with her particular problems. I said that it seemed to me she really felt very badly and had been having difficulty for quite a while, and that I really did not feel I could be of much help to her. I then set a fee and made an appointment for the following week. The next week, she said she had tried *some* of my suggestions and had slept "maybe a little better." I expressed surprise that she had noticed any improvement.

In our weekly meetings, she often urgently requested help for some problem, and I always assured her that I could not really help. Eventually learning that she had never grieved her mother's death, I interpreted her guilt, telling her that she needed to suffer and nothing would help her much until she thought she had paid off that guilt. I tried to facilitate her grieving, but she was very resistant; she had never been to the cemetery—could not even drive by it. I asked about hypnosis. She said several doctors had failed to put her into a trance. I said I certainly could not, and asked if she had ever been in a trance. She said she had found school very boring and unrewarding, and learned to put herself into a trance during class. I asked how she had done this. As she described in detail her procedure of imagining herself window-shopping in a mall, she went into a trance. Thereafter, when I would mention her wonderful trance technique she would go into a trance. Using this, she was able, in her imagination, to visit her mother's grave. In real life, she became able to drive to the cemetery and stand outside the gate.

The patient gradually improved, perhaps 80%, and found employment. She decided to stop therapy after a year, because it was inconvenient now and had not helped very much. I apologized for having been unable to help her and said she could call me in the future if she wished.

This patient seemed an example of a negativistic person who will tend to react *against* anything the physician does. She also did seem to need suffering. I felt that if I ever tried to help her or point out improvement, she would be forced to get worse or to discontinue. It seemed clear she would resist any therapeutic efforts, suggestions or medications, or proclaim them failures. Because I took the stance that I could not be of any use, she could defeat me only by getting better. Within that carefully maintained framework, we were able to accomplish some psychodynamic therapy and some appropriate grieving. This case presented many *potentials* for noncompliance. The paradoxical approach was used in hopes of avoiding these potentials (Rohrbaugh et al. 1981).

Other Approaches to Compliance Problems

Physicians need to be flexible and to have the ability to take more than one approach, offer more than one type of treatment, and perhaps assume more than one role (see Cases 6 and 11).

Case 17: Ms. C.

Ms. C., a young girl medically cleared in the emergency room after an overdose, refused to speak to me except to say that I could not call her mother. Fortunately, a girlfriend was with her. I said that I did not have to call her mother yet and that she could figure out who I might call instead, and then I left the room. The friend came out in a few moments to tell me to call the aunt. She explained that Ms. C. thought she was pregnant and so could not face her parents, especially her stepfather. I asked the friend to call the aunt. When the aunt arrived, I met with them all. Ms. C. would not talk to me. We discussed the situation briefly. I asked them to figure out what to do and left the room. The aunt called the mother. The mother came and was more supportive than Ms. C. had expected. Together, except for Ms. C.'s not talking to me, we developed a list of problems and options, and I left them to work out their approaches. The aunt, mother, and friend presented me with a plan of how to deal with the stepfather, the boyfriend, and the possible pregnancy. Ms. C. was in agreement, having participated in the planning while I was out of the room. I helped them polish the plans a little, and they left, with Ms. C. looking much more cheerful, never having talked to me.

Physicians generally need to avoid power struggles and arguments with their patients (see subsection "The AMA Emergency Patient" above).

Sometimes an emergency room patient refuses to take medication, stating that God will heal him or her. We point out that God moves in mysterious ways his wonders to perform, and that in his benevolence he has provided physicians and medication. Sometimes after these suggestions the patient takes the medication.

Case 18: The Hexed Medication

A paranoid patient had been stabilized on trifluoperazine, but discontinued it, saying the neighbors had put a hex upon it. A new prescription was filled in the pharmacy, and the hospital chaplain and the patient took the new pills to the chapel. The chaplain placed the pills on the altar and blessed them for protection from the hex. The patient was then able to take them and restabilized.

Discussion

Our case examples illustrate the widely variable forms of, reasons for, and possible approaches to compliance problems and how these aspects interweave in multiple combinations in each case. Certain principles underlying the approaches to compliance run through the cases:

1. The physician is highly responsible for the degree of compliance. He or she may need to "induce" treatment, for example, by helping patients see that they are experiencing discomfort, are contributing to that discomfort, and have the potential for doing something about it. The physician must also explain how treatment may help them reach their own goals. The physician must make compliance easy for patients and offer treatment in ways that patients can accept. With some patients, particularly those with borderline and narcissistic disorders, the physician must meet the patients more than halfway, taking more than

his or her share of the responsibility for maintaining treatment, but at the same time setting limits for his or her own protection.

2. The therapeutic alliance is the foundation for any treatment and for compliance. The physician bears much responsibility for helping patients form this alliance and for maintaining it. The task in any treatment is forming a collaborative team, both parties sharing responsibility for the treatment and its progress. The physician enhances this process by treating patients with respect, taking their concerns seriously, being flexible and willing to negotiate a treatment contract and compliance issues, and taking pains to educate patients and at times their families.

3. The physician must attempt to understand patients' concerns and viewpoints, and what the particular compliance issue means to them. It is important to attend to the needs of the family and their effect on the patient, and to be aware of other external factors that may affect the patient's compliance.

4. The physician, using a flexible approach, needs to meet patients' needs within the framework of the patients' concepts. If a particular approach to foster compliance does not work, another approach needs to be tried. Often these alternatives need to be arranged in a hierarchy so that the failure of one does not preclude the use of another. It is important to consider patients' capabilities, internally, interpersonally, and situationally, and to not try for compliance behaviors that patients cannot achieve.

5. We may speak of compliance issues or compliance problems rather than "noncompliance," preferring to view compliance as a process. Compliance is initiated, fostered, and developed. It waxes and wanes. Patients may be ambivalent. Compliance may be partial, and while patients are noncompliant on one issue, they may be quite compliant on others. This attitude assists the physician to flexibly explore the issues and try different approaches, rather than effect premature closure by labeling patients "noncompliant."

6. The use of medication is perhaps the most common and obvi-

ous area for compliance problems, and all of the principles discussed apply in this area. The psychiatrist needs to educate patients, and usually their families, about both the illness and the medications. Side effects should be inquired about and taken seriously. Patients' beliefs, values, conflicts, goals, and situation all need to be considered.

Overall, the relationship between the patient and the physician is the primary factor involved in compliance, and attending to the relationship sets the stage for all other measures of dealing with compliance issues.

References

Acosta F: Effective Psychotherapy for Low Income and Minority Patients. New York, Plenum, 1982, pp 12–18, 22, 40

Bartko G, Herczeg I, Zador G: Clinical symptomatology and drug compliance in schizophrenic patients. Acta Psychiatr Scand 77:74–76, 1988

Brand FN, Smith RT, Brand PA: Effect of economic barriers to medical care on patient's noncompliance. Public Health Rep 92(1):72–78, 1977

Cain JM: Prevention and treatment of neuroleptic noncompliance. Psychiatric Annals 16:577, 1986

Corrigan PW, Liberman PR, Engel JD: From noncompliance to collaboration in the treatment of schizophrenia. Hosp Community Psychiatry 41:1203–1209, 1990

Diamond RJ: Enhancing medication use in schizophrenic patients. J Clin Psychiatry 44 (no 6, sec 2):7–14, 1983

Falloon I: Developing and maintaining adherence to long-term drug-taking regimens. Schizophr Bull 10:412, 1984

Frances A, Weiden P: Promoting compliance with outpatient drug treatment. Hosp Community Psychiatry 38:1158–1160, 1987

Haley J: Problem Solving Therapy. San Francisco, CA, Jossey-Bass, 1976 pp 67–80

Hanley WF: Erickson's contribution to change in psychotherapy, in Ericsonian Approaches to Hypnosis and Psychotherapy. Edited by Zeig JK. New York, Brunner/Mazel, 1982, pp 29–36

Kelly GR, Mamon JA, Scott JE: Utility of the health belief model and examining medication compliance among psychiatric outpatients. Soc Sci Med 25:1205–1211, 1987

Langs RJ: The Technique of Psychoanalytic Psychotherapy, Vol 1. New York, Jason Aronson, 1973a, p 108

Langs RJ: The Technique of Psychoanalytic Psychotherapy, Vol 2. New York, Jason Aronson, 1973b, p 381

Lazare A, Eisenthal S, Wasserman L: The customer approach to patienthood. Arch Gen Psychiatry 32:553–558, 1975

McGill C, Falloon I: Family Care of Schizophrenia: A Problem Solving Approach to the Treatment of Mental Illness. New York, Guilford, 1984, pp 178–179

Meichenbaum D, Turk DC: Facilitating Treatment Adherence: A Practitioner's Guide Book. New York, Plenum, 1987, pp 41–68

Olarte SW, Masnick R: Enhancing medication compliance in coffee groups. Hosp Community Psychiatry 32:417–419, 1981

Puryear DA: Helping People in Crisis: A Family Oriented Approach to Crisis Intervention. San Francisco, CA, Jossey-Bass, 1979, p 143

Rohrbaugh M, Tennen H, Press S, et al: Compliance, defiance, and therapeutic paradox: guidelines for strategic use of paradoxical interventions. Am J Orthopsychiatry 51:454–466, 1981

Schwartz R: The use of ultimatums in psychiatric care. Hosp Community Psychiatry 41:1242–1244, 1990

Stickney SK, Hall CW, Gardner ER: The effect of referral procedures on after care compliance. Hosp Community Psychiatry 31:567–569, 1980

Talmon M: Single-Session Therapy. San Francisco, CA, Jossey-Bass, 1990

Van Putten T: Why do schizophrenic patients refuse to take their drugs? Arch Gen Psychiatry 31:67–72, 1974

Van Putten T: Drug refusal in schizophrenia and the wish to be crazy. Arch Gen Psychiatry 33:1443–1446, 1976

Weiner MF: The Psychotherapeutic Impasse. New York, Free Press, 1982, pp 42–43

Section II:

Situational Factors

Introduction to Section II

Problems often arise in treatment not only because of the nature or severity of the disorder itself, but because there is some situational factor confounding the disorder. In this section the authors address a representative sample of three such problems. In Chapter 9, Howard Zonana and Michael Norko explore the problems of patients who are in mandated treatment. The authors provide a practical and useful approach to understanding the specific issues that arise in mandated treatment. Familial considerations, while varying from patient to patient, provide a context for understanding every patient. Stuart Sugarman, in Chapter 10, presents a clinically useful conceptual framework for classifying difficult familial situations, and recommendations on how the clinician might approach these situations. Sara Charles, in Chapter 11, concludes this section by discussing the treatment of patients who are physicians who have been sued.

Chapter 9

Mandated Treatment

Howard Zonana, M.D.
Michael A. Norko, M.D.

The term *mandated treatment* on first examination seems rather straightforward: it is treatment that is commanded or obligatory, with the implication that the treatment is forced, coerced, and involuntary. However, many psychotherapists are uncomfortable accepting patients who do not come voluntarily. Treatment must be freely chosen if the patient is expected to be motivated and to reveal private, intimate thoughts and fantasies. Yet, upon further examination, in few cases is treatment the result of a perfectly voluntary choice. Most patients enter treatment under some form of coercion or duress.

Still, there would seem to be obvious differences between a patient who enters outpatient, insight-oriented psychotherapy and a patient who is ordered to undergo therapy as a condition of parole following incarceration for a criminal offense. On the surface, the former action would be considered voluntary and the latter involuntary. But what if a psychotherapy patient is seeking treatment because his employer is threatening to fire him or his wife is threatening divorce? What if a sexual offender is eager to receive antiandrogens and therapy so as to avoid any subsequent arrests? The relationship between voluntariness and coerced treatment is frequently not as simple as it appears. There are degrees of voluntariness, and we should more accurately ask if the choice is "voluntary enough," weighing the competing values.

In this chapter we define *mandated treatment* as a subcategory of coerced treatment: it is treatment institutionally prescribed or ordered with negative consequences as the alternative. Mandated treatment, by our definition, arises from authority that has substantial interests beyond the provision of appropriate health care. This treatment usually follows some transgression of acceptable behavior, either criminal or employment related. Formal mandates are issued by courts, probation officers, employers, administrative boards, and professional organizations. These referrals form a continuum of coercion, ranging from the threat of immediate incarceration in correctional facilities or loss of job or licensure, to those that may have little immediate consequence. The common sources of referral that are considered mandated, based on the above definition, are the subject of this chapter and are summarized in Table 9–1.

One further point should be clarified. Although coercion is clearly involved in civil commitment of mentally ill persons, we have not included this aspect of involuntary treatment among the mandated treatments that we will be examining. Although the result of civil commitment is the immediate loss of liberty, there is not the antecedent threat of another sanction such as incarceration or the loss of a job for failure to comply with the court order. Further, the commitment order is not an unlimited authorization

---

Table 9–1. Mandated sources of referral

Mandated treatment in the criminal justice system
    Insanity acquittees
    Probation and parole referrals
    Restoration of competency
      Competency to stand trial
      Competency to be executed
    Substance abuse diversion programs
Coerced treatment—outpatient commitment
Mandated treatment in the workplace
    Impaired physicians
    Employee assistance programs
    Disability evaluations

for treatment. Most states now require some form of judicial or nonjudicial review of treatment refusals. The assessment of competence and the appropriateness of the treatment usually make up the content of these reviews.

In the type of mandated treatment we are discussing, the patient generally agrees to the treatment even if that agreement is made to avoid what is considered to be more severe or less attractive consequences. In addition, most psychiatrists are familiar with treating civilly committed patients and do not regard them with the same negative attributes as they do mandated patients. Outpatient commitment, on the other hand, involves many issues similar to those in treating patients on parole or probation. Because this modality is relatively new, we devote some discussion to it, even though it is not strictly a mandated treatment by our definition.

In a similar fashion, the treatment of children is inherently coercive, because the child is generally not treated as competent and the parents' wishes predominate. We do not include the family as an institutional referral, although some of the same conflicts arise for clinicians in the context of the treatment of children as in the areas we will address.

Coercion in Mental Hospitals

Coercion has always been an integral part of inpatient psychiatric treatment. It was not until 1881 that the concept of a voluntary admission was first endorsed in Massachusetts. Prior to that time, mentally ill persons were seen as so globally incompetent that it made no sense to permit them to assent to hospitalization. In the United States, the majority of inpatients remained involuntary until the early 1970s (Stone 1975).

The routine use of civil commitment distinguishes and characterizes psychiatric care from that of other medical specialties. The appropriate boundaries and standards are continually debated in state legislatures and have undergone pendular swings during the past 100 years. Recent political and economic trends have resulted in a reduction of beds in the public sector, which has led to an increase in the proportion of involuntary certifications and commitments. Voluntary patients without health care coverage are more likely to be refused admission in state facilities that are filled to capacity unless they are extremely ill.

Psychiatrists and mental health professionals seem to find coercion (in the form of mandates) coming from agencies separate from departments of mental health quite troublesome. The incentives to avoid incarceration or other "punishment" cast doubt on a patient's motivation to an extent that seems very different from coercions that come from families, spouses, friends, or even employers. The substitution of treatment for what may seem a "deserved" punishment may also engender a negative reaction in clinicians. While some forms of coercion may intrude objectionably on individual rights, some types of coercion may enhance motivation or allow a treatment trial that would not have otherwise occurred (e.g., offering treatment as a first response to poor job performance rather than dismissal).

Dilemmas for Treating Clinicians

Clinicians who evaluate and treat patients who are mandated for treatment are faced with a number of difficulties in all phases of the process. During the evaluation phase many mandated patients will present with hostility, suspiciousness, and denial. It may not be easy to discern to what extent these symptoms are pathological, characterological, manipulative, or a consequence of these patients being placed on probation and (from their point of view) forced into treatment with someone whom they see as being primarily interested in issues of public safety. Real paranoia may be dismissed as manipulative, and situational suspiciousness may be diagnosed as paranoia (Schottenfeld 1989).

Many patients, voluntary or involuntary, are frequently defensive in their initial presentations. They will deny symptoms and their need for treatment. Especially in understaffed clinics, clinicians often will dismiss mandated patients, or any patient with pending legal issues, with comments like "Come back when all your legal difficulties are over" or "Come back when you are really interested in treatment." These patients will not be offered the same opportunity to become engaged in treatment as someone who enters without a legal mandate. Whether this initial presentation is assessed as the usual anxiety and defensiveness of a new patient or as the actions of someone who is trying to beat the system and waste the valuable time of the clinician can change the nature of the interaction and the ultimate result. Often an extended period of evaluation is the only way this assessment can be made.

This initial rejection is frequently fueled by powerful countertransference reactions of clinicians. Many of these patients have committed one or more violent or otherwise antisocial acts in the past or present, acts that frighten or terrify clinicians. These patients and their past may continue to directly or indirectly threaten the clinician. It is difficult for many clinicians to explore violent and sadistic fantasies and to become aware of their own wishes to see these patients suffer retribution. Clinicians often feel as sentenced to the treatment as the mandated patient and frequently feel they must continue treatment regardless of what the patient may do. This sense of entrapment may lead to feelings of resentment and subtle encouragement of antisocial behavior to get rid of the patient.

There are many aspects of treatment under these conditions that distinguish the tasks of the clinician from those encountered in ordinary clinical work. Before discussing the distinguishing features that can make the work more difficult and expansive, it would be useful to describe several advantages to doing this type of treatment. The presence of a strong external motivator (such as reincarceration) can increase the chances of successful treatment in patient populations that are traditionally difficult to treat (e.g., individuals with character disorders, persons with substance-use disorders, sex offenders). The probation order may permit significantly more aftercare following hospitalization or institutionalization than usually occurs with chronically ill long-term patients subjected to brief hospitalization and discharge (Gibbens et al. 1981). The "luxury" of enforced aftercare may thus facilitate a more successful social adjustment to the community in individuals who need substantial social rehabilitation. However, the legal authority that enforces the treatment and helps motivate the patient also imposes extra responsibilities—both clinical and legal—on the clinician.

General Clinical Principles

The treatment of mandated patients does carry some inevitable conflicts for clinicians in terms of reports to the mandating authority. Sometimes these reports are perfunctory and merely need to state that the patient is in treatment and in "good standing." (Even this degree of disclosure is more than some clinicians are comfortable accepting.) At the other extreme, all treatment notes and medical records may be requested and testimony before an administrative board or court may be required. Any limitations on, or the absence of, confidentiality should be clear to both the clinician and the patient at the beginning of any evaluation or treatment. In fact, several issues should be clarified and determined by clinicians prior to any evaluation or treatment contract:

1. Who is the mandating authority?
2. Is the referral governed by statute, regulation, court order, contract, etc.?
3. What are the reporting requirements?
4. What are the consequences of the patient's failure to comply with treatment?
5. What are the limitations on confidentiality?
6. Is the confidentiality surrounding the evaluation different from that surrounding treatment?
7. What responsibility is the treating clinician agreeing to accept?

The relationship between voluntariness and mandated treatment can have consequences for the nature of the treatment contract as well as for the obligations of the therapist who agrees to accept patients under some form of mandate. Some treatments are very dependent upon a patient's motivation for their effectiveness, whereas others are not. The effects of medication, such as lithium, are less dependent on a patient's attitude than the production of free associations to a dream. We do not question the ability of involuntarily committed patients to benefit from treatment even though we encourage patients to be voluntary. Appelbaum (1985) has noted that "many mental health professionals believe . . . that in the absence of judicious (but not necessarily judicial) coercion, patients will not receive needed care, their condition will deteriorate, and they will suffer psychological and perhaps physical distress" (p. 306). In fact, many involuntary or mandated patients do very well in treatment and seem to benefit from some external coercive pressure (Rappeport 1974). The threat of job loss, the threat of loss of a license (such as to practice medicine or to fly airplanes), or the threat of incarceration can be a powerful incentive to alter behavior.

Mandated Treatment in the Criminal Justice System

Insanity Acquittees

The treatment of insanity acquittees is, a priori, a difficult clinical situation because of the overt dual mandate to provide both treatment and security for these patients. Ignoring either of these mandates in favor of the other generates serious problems. Developing a model for integrating these concepts is critical to successful management of these patients (Scales et al. 1989). Such a collaborative forensic model requires proactive staff development, because security staff generally have little training or experience in clinical issues and clinical staff generally have little training or experience in security issues. Psychiatric training generally does not include clinical experience in maximum security treatment facilities where the role of security staff is a prominent and integral part of the treatment setting.

In some jurisdictions, this problem of training is managed by developing specialized forensic divisions that handle all insanity acquittees. Most jurisdictions, however, probably have some combination of specialized services and "mainstreaming" of acquittees with general psychiatric populations. Clinicians working in general treatment settings may have a difficult time appreciating the interplay of security and treatment issues and of their duties and accountability to the individual patient as well as to society.

Another common difficulty encountered in treating insanity acquittees is found in the clinical presentation of the patient. Although there is a large body of literature about the insanity defense and much public and professional debate about the use of the insanity defense, there is relatively little written about the acquittees or about what happens to them after acquittal. This is unfortunate, because while the pretrial and trial phases in insanity defense cases may last months to, at most, a few years, the result of that process may lead to lifelong treatment relationships between the acquittee and forensic mental health professionals (Norko 1990).

In most jurisdictions, a successful insanity defense usually leads to hospital commitment, often with a lower standard for commitment than civil commitment, a lower standard of proof, and consequently longer hospitalization. As summed up in the *Harvard Law Review*, "[A]cquittal by reason of insanity is rarely a ticket to freedom" ("Commitment Following an Insanity Acquittal" 1980–1981, p. 605). Acquittees who have been found to be dangerous and mentally ill must usually prove they are no longer dangerous and that their mental illness has substantially abated and is likely to remain so. Clinicians familiar with chronically mentally ill persons will recognize what a sizeable task this represents. The insanity acquittee is spared imprisonment, but nonetheless suffers a loss of liberty. In the years of scrutiny that follow, these individuals also experience significant loss of privacy.

The quid pro quo of treatment for loss of liberty assumes treatability. Yet many of these patients are mentally and emotionally "unavailable" for treatment upon acquittal and remain in that condition for months to years. These patients typically deny their illness, their insanity, and their dangerousness, despite the fact that they presumably gave their competent and voluntary consent to the use of an insanity defense. Many patients even deny the criminal act that formed the basis for the defense, although it is usually not possible to go forward with an insanity defense without acknowledging commission of the act in question.

These patients also exhibit significant fear and self-doubt. Many patients begin to see themselves in stereotyped images and labels. Being acquitted on the grounds of mental disease or mental defect is, in the reality of many patients, to be labeled "criminally insane" and to be painted with that broad brush of popular imagery. These patients often fear that perhaps they *are* deranged madmen, vicious beasts, or other such threatening entities.

Insanity acquittees never feel "acquitted"; instead they feel sentenced. Not vindicated, they do not view their hospitalization with hope or expectation of treatment and improvement. At best they are confused about their situation and condition. At worst they defend against their fears and anxiety by employing rigid and extensive denial.

The obstacles for the clinician, then, are formidable. Not only must he or she navigate through the murky waters of the security/treatment confluence, he or she must also find a way to protect the treatment from being sabotaged by all this turbulence.

Fortunately, there is a developmental process that the acquittee/patient eventually experiences in most cases. Treatment can be conceptualized as occurring in stages, each with characteristic treatment issues and treatment approaches.

Clinicians need to help patients in the initial stage with their feelings of denial, anger, fear, hopelessness, and stigmatization. Treatment approaches during this initial phase, then, center around supportive care. It is important not to attempt to pressure patients into rapid progress. Insanity acquittees in the early stages should never be given the message "If you get better, you will get out." They are not ready to hear such a message, and, more importantly, it may not be true. Social forces and lingering concerns about future violence may demand prolonged hospitalization, particularly in high-visibility cases when the patient/acquittee has been a source of great trauma to the community. This is part of the negotiation among clinical, legal, and sociopolitical issues that is intimately involved in treating insanity acquittees.

Within a period of several months to several years, most patients will develop out of this early stage. They will be able to discard stereotypes and see their situation more realistically. As this happens, they also can acknowledge their often more pervasive, violent past. With this recognition, patients often begin to see some possible benefits of their insanity acquittal and the offered treatment, and are thus available to do more therapeutic work. This insight may bring fear of losing control as they see more clearly what they have done in the past. They also sense more clearly the fear of the community and begin to realize that they will have to face rejection and hostility upon their eventual release.

Some patients, however, do not make this transition, and go into a holding pattern of denial, anger, and hopelessness. These patients are generally low-functioning and have poor insight and low motivation. Low motivation can be both an element of their illness and the result of a lengthy commitment/sentence. These patients often regret and resent their insanity defense. They tend to complain that they could have been released sooner if they had pleaded guilty and been imprisoned. Failing to recognize their illness, they fail to recognize their opportunity for improvement. Without improvement, an insanity acquittal can indeed become a life sentence.

Treatment for this group "on hold" can be very frustrating to the clinician. Often the best that can be accomplished is to offer "humane custody" and wait for a change. Fortunately, the transition that most of the patients eventually experience can lead to very exciting—but still challenging—therapeutic work.

The first part of this late stage involves work not dissimilar to that involved in the care of any chronically ill patient: stabilization, education, rehabilitation, and fostering of independence. As this work progresses, the patient discovers that he or she must deal with the lifelong effects of his or her insanity acquittal. Some of these effects are related to stigma, but others are very realistic. The patient is indeed being scrutinized more carefully than before. He or she is both the object and subject of the dual legal mandate to protect the public and treat the acquittee. Release decisions are more difficult, because the stakes are higher by history. (An individual is generally presumed to be capable in the future of at least the same level of violence he or she has demonstrated before.) It can be very difficult for the acquittee to prove that he or she is rehabilitated enough to be released and will continue with appropriate treatment.

Patients are faced with a choice of either directly confronting public opinion and fear or progressing no further. The clinician's task is to realistically frame public fears and expectations in a productive way that provides a realistic but still hopeful assessment of the task ahead.

Progression to the late stages of treatment is heralded by patients' realization that they must change, or perhaps by their ability to not feel insulted by this notion. The clinician must help patients adjust to the notion that an absence of aggressive or criminal behaviors is simply not enough. The patients will have to demonstrate significant and fundamental improvement in their ability to understand their illness, recognize its effects, and control its manifestations in cooperation with their clinicians. They will have to demonstrate an ability to identify and cope with expectable life stresses, particularly of the type that provoked their past criminal and/or violent behavior. Patients must be taught to deal with the stigma of their illness and insanity acquittal, with the scrutiny that will be brought to bear on their lives, and with the higher price they will pay for future freedom.

In order to accomplish this, the clinician must develop a relationship with the patient in which the patient can see the restrictions as coming from an understandable societal concern and not from a controlling or punitive attitude on the part of the clinician. This task is made somewhat easier in jurisdictions in which decisions about placement and release are made by an external judicial or quasi-judicial body (e.g., the psychiatric security review boards in Oregon and Connecticut). This is not because the clinician can then "blame" someone else, but rather because it is helpful for the patient to have abstract societal concerns embodied in a tangible entity, such as a court or board. This approach also can confirm that due process is being provided and that the patient's future is not solely in the hands of a single physician.

It is also helpful to the therapy to have an external third party to which the clinician and acquittee must both respond. This can lead to an enhancement of the therapeutic alliance if the clinician can help the patient see that they share the same goals and that they must work together to manage the demands of a shared external reality.

Another way in which such an external body is very helpful is in assuming legal responsibility for release decisions. The existence of some formal process with a decision-maker immunized from suit allows the clinician to stay closer to the clinical issues in recommending transfers, leaves, or releases of insanity acquittees. Still, it is important to make recommendations that are sound and that are based on progress that can be substantiated by the data. A clinician who makes clearly negligent or reckless recommendations could well be sued for injuries or harm resulting from a release decision that was predicated on misleading or erroneous information being provided to the board.

Concerns over release issues have prompted clinicians to devise various risk management methodologies in making release decisions. One approach is to carefully orchestrate the facility's administrative procedures for making release decisions, involving many clinicians (Blankstein 1988). Another approach is to prohibit the treating clinician from making the release decisions, for reasons of both objectivity and professional ethics (Miller 1987). Clinicians have been admonished not to make predictions about future behavior that are overly definitive and unwarranted by clinical knowledge (Miller et al. 1988). Eisner (1989) has developed a rating scale to determine a patient's readiness for the community. As in all risk-management activities, documentation of the clinical work and the decision-making process is critical. Some institutions have videotaped an evaluation of the patient just prior to release so as to have good documentation of the patient's mental status.

Once released from inpatient settings, most insanity acquittees will continue in monitored outpatient therapy. A few acquittees may begin their course of treatment in the community. The treatment of insanity acquittees in the community is usually accomplished through some form of outpatient commitment. If such commitment is statutorily sanctioned and mechanisms are provided for ongoing monitoring and an ability to rehospitalize patients when necessary, then such programs can be quite effective (Bloom et al. 1986, 1988; Lamb et al. 1988). It can also be quite rewarding for clinicians to treat such patients.

Difficulties can arise around monitoring, especially if the treating clinician mishandles boundaries between confidentiality and reporting responsibilities. It is critical for an outpatient provider to maintain the same kind of relationship with the patient as was discussed above for the inpatient provider. The clinician must readily acknowledge and frequently use the external reality of societal monitoring, without being drawn into the role of being the agent of that control. As in all therapy, it is helpful for the patient to see the therapist as an ally if there is to be any progress. The alliance is not obviated by reporting responsibilities. Clinicians who are uncomfortable or inexperienced with negotiating these clinical and legal responsibilities should probably not agree to engage in such therapies without supervision or consultation.

Probation / Parole

Psychiatric treatment is often mandated as a condition of probation or parole. Prisoners who have completed part of their sentence may be paroled on the basis of good behavior in prison and the promise of compliance with an order of parole. Their progress is monitored by a parole board. A trial court may also order a period of probation as a part of an offender's sentence, in lieu of incarceration or some portion of it. Psychiatric treatment may be a condition of such orders when the offender has a history of mental illness, substance abuse, or sexual offense and the proposed treatment is judged to reduce the risk of repeat offense. Offenders are said to "violate probation" (or parole) when they fail to comply with any conditions of the order at any point during the effective period of the order.

The specificity of an order for psychiatric treatment can be quite varied. Many orders are nonspecific and give broad discretion to the probation officer to determine the details of the probation and notify the offender of those details. The probation officer in turn may delegate decisions about the adequacy of a proposed program to the therapist(s).

The legal authority that enforces the treatment and helps motivate the patient also imposes extra responsibilities—both clinical and legal—on the clinician. The therapist is presented with the responsibility to simultaneously protect the public and faithfully attend to the needs and rights of the offender patient. The therapist must first be able to deal with strong countertransference feelings that are evoked when treating a patient who has committed horrible crimes. Second, the therapist must overcome his or her own denial about the "bad news" related to the patient. This denial is manifested in the therapist's desire to see the patient as nondangerous and doing well in the therapy. Such denial can lead to the therapist's missing important, and at times subtle, messages of dangerousness and pathology from the patient or others. Denial may also lead the therapist to miss opportunities to examine unpleasant and/or uncomfortable material that may be critical to the offender patient's future success and the public's safety (Prins 1990).

Another legal responsibility that falls to the therapist is a duty to report on the patient's treatment progress to the authorities (i.e., the probation officer and/or the court). This requires a delicate balancing of issues of confidentiality and adequate disclosure to protect the public. Often it will suffice for the therapist to report on the offender patient's level of attendance and performance and the adequacy of treatment progress. However, at times the patient will reveal material that indicates a danger of harm to others. The duties are no different in this situation whether the therapist is engaged in a probation treatment or a nonmandated treatment: the therapist must hospitalize or take other steps to fulfill *Tarasoff* duties to protect victims.

Prins (1990) has offered a number of suggestions for successfully managing therapy imposed as a condition of probation:

1. It is essential to have full details about the index offense, including the analysis of it by a variety of professionals. It is also

important to have details of prior offenses. Such details will describe the risks of failure and may provide useful data on patterns of behavior and warning signs of impending decompensation and legal trouble.

2. Take nothing at face value: avoid superficial assurances, investigate hidden meanings, and look for trends and patterns.

3. In order to gather sufficient data, it is sometimes necessary to intrude into the personal social environment of the patient. Home visits and interviews with family, friends, and employers may be indicated and helpful in gathering data that the patient may be unable to provide or is consciously or unconsciously hiding.

4. Assess the risk of "unfinished business" (Cox 1979). This includes assessing any continued risk to the original victim and risk to others who resemble the original victim in any number of static or dynamic ways (such as physical appearance or relationship to the patient). Having extensive knowledge of the past offenses will help identify such predictive factors.

5. Ask the uncomfortable questions (Prins 1988). "Have past precipitants and stresses been removed? How accurately can the offender patient's current capacity for coping with provocation be assessed? What clues are available as to the offender patient's self-image? Were the circumstances of the original offense the last straw in a series of stressful events, or does the offender patient see everyone in his or her environment as hostile? Was the behavior "person specific" or a means of getting back at society in general? Does the person still feel threatened or persecuted? Has the offender patient come to terms, in part if not in toto, with what he or she did? What importance should be given to the offender patient talking about his or her offenses in an apparently guilt-free and callous manner?"

Harris and Watkins (1987) suggest, among other strategies, 1) providing structure and setting expectations; 2) providing as much choice to the patient as possible; 3) letting the client save face; 4) creating optimum anxiety for self-examination; and 5) allowing various styles of learning and change. Larke (1985) recommends using multiple models such as cognitive methods, behavioral methods, and support groups.

These issues of mandate, motivation, and treatment success are not mere subjects of theoretical debate but can become thorny clinical-legal problems. A recent appellate court decision illustrates some of the potential difficulties. In *State of Vermont v. Mace* (1990), the defendant was charged with sexually assaulting his 14 year-old stepdaughter. In a plea agreement he pleaded guilty to the amended charge of lewd or lascivious conduct with a child and received a suspended 1- to 5-year sentence with an order of probation. The order included the provision that he "attend, participate and complete" an identified sexual therapy program as directed by his therapist and as approved by his probation officer. Seven months later, the therapist reported to the probation officer that Mace was continuing to deny having had sexual intercourse with his stepdaughter and that this was interfering with the successful completion of his therapy. After a hearing on the matter, the trial court found that Mace had violated his probation. The decision was appealed to the Supreme Court of Vermont, which affirmed the trial court's decision.

From a clinical perspective, the supreme court decision was notable for several findings. The court supported the therapist's viewpoint that the defendant's denial of what had taken place would prevent him from benefiting fully from the treatment program. It also agreed that both the therapist and the probation officer had the authority to insist on such frank disclosure from the offender patient in order to satisfy the probation order. Because he had been given fair and repeated notice that his continued denial would result in a violation of probation, the court found no due-process violation in the actions taken.

The therapist should clearly know the parameters of the treatment order and ask for necessary clarification or modifications before accepting such a case. The therapist must be extraordinarily candid with the offender patient about issues of confidentiality, reporting, and treatment expectations. Fair notice to the patient of anticipated failure with compliance is essential, including repeated efforts to help the patient correct the problems leading to failure. The therapist should not be reluctant to notify authorities when the patient is failing to meet these expectations.

Therapists who know they will have difficulties with reporting responsibilities should proceed cautiously. Some therapists have strong feelings about the need for absolute confidentiality of psychiatric treatment. Because this is no longer possible in the current era, these therapists may need to review their stance toward this type of patient.

Restoration of Competency

Competency to stand trial.   In order for almost any criminal proceedings or a trial to occur, the defendant must be competent to stand trial. This means that defendants must be able to understand the legal proceedings against them and be able to participate in their own defense. When these abilities are questioned, the court will usually request an evaluation by mental health professionals of the defendant's competence to stand trial. The mental health professionals make their report and recommendations to the court, which then must render a finding on the defendant's competence. If the court finds the defendant competent, the trial proceeds. If the court finds the defendant incompetent on the basis of mental illness or mental defect (mental retardation), the court must decide further, based on the clinical report, if the individual's competence is restorable with appropriate treatment interventions. It is when the court finds that the individual's competence is potentially restorable and therefore orders a course of treatment that the mental health system becomes involved.

A defendant may be ordered into outpatient or inpatient treatment to restore competency, but the latter is far more common. This is so because the defendants are usually individuals whose mental health has deteriorated while they are out in the community and efforts to provide outpatient treatment have failed. Thus, the defendant becomes an involuntarily committed inpatient under a court mandate for treatment.

As with other forms of mandated treatment, special attention must be paid to issues of confidentiality and reporting. Because the treatment is ordered for the sole purpose of allowing the criminal justice system to go forward, virtually every aspect of the course of treatment will be subject to direct and cross-examination in court. Any reports may be deemed public information if introduced as evidence. Not only is it important to give the patient fair notice of the lack of confidentiality of the entire treatment process, it is also important for the reporting clinician to be circumspect about what is included in the report. Extraneous material that has no bearing on the issue of competency is best left out. For example, it might not be necessary to report the presence of a venereal disease in an individual whose incompetence was the result of an untreated mania. On the other hand, it may be necessary to describe even such highly sensitive information as an individual's HIV status if the incompetence is based on an AIDS dementia. Such data may require special releases in states where the confidentiality of HIV-related records is protected.

Treatment to restore competency to stand trial usually entails stabilization of the major psychiatric disorder and a psychoeducational approach to restoring the defendant patient's ability to understand the legal proceedings and participate in his or her defense. Clinicians must distinguish their role in this type of treatment from their more customary role in other clinical work. First, it is not the purpose in competency restoration to take a holistic approach to clinical care. The purpose is to identify and treat the main psychiatric disturbance that prevents the patient's understanding of, and participation in, his or her own defense.

Second, the psychoeducational techniques are the mainstay of treatment once the main mental disturbance is resolved. Clinicians may not feel comfortable teaching legal proceedings to defendant patients, particularly if they are not that familiar with the proceedings themselves. In a facility that does a fair number of these restorations, it is often a good practice to identify a particular staff member(s) whose responsibility is to run didactic groups for this purpose. Having identified staff for this purpose also relieves the other staff of the burden of having to become familiar with statutes, legal proceedings, criminal sentencing, and so forth.

The treating facility is also usually responsible for reporting back to the court when the defendant patient's competence has been restored. This requires formal reevaluation of competency during the hospitalization. It is best to have a separate team conduct such evaluations, rather than leave this function to the treatment team. Again, such a system places the burden for mastering the legal material on a small identifiable number of staff members who can then be properly trained in this work. Also, it is often better for purposes of objectivity, clarity of purpose, and ethical considerations to have an evaluation team distinct from the treatment team (Miller 1987).

The ultimate goal of treatment is restoration of competency, and when that is accomplished, the patient is discharged back to the court. This creates more problems than just the discomfort of the clinicians in taking such a narrow approach.

Lamb (1987) has described the systems problems that occur in the restoration-of-competency approach—problems that most clinicians who have done this kind of work have experienced. Once the mental health system has done its job and the legal proceedings go forward, mental health intervention often falters. Frequently, no follow-up psychiatric care is arranged for the defendant patient, whether he or she is released or imprisoned. Thus, patients with serious mental illness and histories of severe violence may be more likely to repeat their behaviors. Symptom resolution achieved during the restoration treatment is often wasted. Frequently, the mental health system, the criminal justice system, and the correctional system do not work together to provide coordinated care for this group of individuals, responsibility for whom is shared by all three systems.

Systemic solutions to these problems are generally found wanting. It is possible for clinicians to create individual solutions for individual cases when indicated or necessary. However, such interventions are usually costly in terms of investment of time and effort. Overworked clinicians, particularly those in the public sector who most often assume this type of work, will not be able to effect long-term solutions for more than a small handful of such clients. Lamb (1987) has recommended a comprehensive systemic approach to this group of very challenging defendant patients, including assertive case management; therapeutic supervised housing; an array of direct mental health services, including crisis services; and a close monitoring system involving cooperation between the mental health system and the courts. In the current absence of these services, clinicians doing this work will continue to be placed in the difficult position of providing a function that is legally necessary but clinically inadequate.

Competency to be executed.   Restoration of competency to be executed is an extremely narrow area of clinical concern. Very few clinicians have been exposed to this clinical situation, but the potential for exposure is growing. In the United States, 37 states have death penalties, and over 2,000 individuals now reside on death row. The controversies surrounding this highly circumscribed area of practice are intense. This issue generates intense feelings, raises profound ethical questions, and has a high potential for clinicians to act out their personal feelings about the death penalty in their professional practice. For these reasons it is worth describing the terrain of this difficult clinical situation.

In capital cases in which the defendant has any history of mental illness or any suggestion of current mental health problems, issues of competency may arise at many points throughout the legal process. At each stage, the pressures on the clinician will be more intense and always palpable. Defense attorneys struggle to find reasons to delay or avoid their client's execution. Prosecutors and public forces usually apply pressure in the opposite directions. It is therefore crucial for clinicians to be firmly grounded in their understanding of their role(s) and their responsibilities.

Issues of competency before and during trial are essentially the same as described above in the previous subsection. Once a defendant is convicted, a long series of various legal proceedings ensues: pre-sentence investigations, capital sentencing hearings, many levels of appeal, and various motions for postconviction relief. The convict's competency to participate in each of these stages can be questioned, with the possibility of evaluation and restoration if necessary. In the final stages of the process, when possible avenues of appeal have been exhausted, the issue of competency to be executed may arise.

The issue arises in contemporary practice because of the U.S. Supreme Court decision in 1986 in the case of *Ford v. Wainwright.* The Court held that the Eighth Amendment prohibits states from executing a prisoner who is "insane." In issuing their opinion, the Court justices reviewed the historical reasons for not permitting the execution of the insane: "such an execution has questionable retributive value, presents no example to others and thus has no deterrence value, and simply offends humanity" (*Ford v. Wainwright* 1986).

One further distinction is necessary before discussing the clinical difficulties presented in these cases: that between evaluation and treatment. There are many issues surrounding these evaluations in capital cases that are the subject of great controversy, debate, and explication. Full discussion of these issues surrounding evaluation would be tangential to the focus of this text. The reader should be aware, however, that a literature exists that reviews the legal, clinical, and ethical issues of performing these forensic evaluations (American Psychiatric Association 1986; Appelbaum 1986; Bonnie 1990; Heilbrun 1987; Heilbrun and McClaren 1988; Mossman 1987; Radelet and Barnard 1986; Ward 1986).

Treatment to restore competency in capital cases is also a highly charged subject. Those who oppose professional involvement in this treatment feel that it subverts the ethics and purposes of the medical profession by employing doctors to aid in the execution of criminals.

Another viewpoint gives predominance to the timing of the restoration within the legal process. If restoration is ordered at a time when further appeals can potentially be made, it is possible for clinicians to view this no differently from a trial-level competency restoration (Bonnie 1990). The possibility that an individual may be innocent or may have a legitimate motion on appeal that would only come to light were the individual to regain competence seems to open an ethical door that allows the clinician to serve both the interests of the criminal justice system and those of the defendant patient by offering treatment.

Most authors seem to argue that to provide treatment whose sole purpose is to allow the execution of a condemned prisoner (whose expressed preference is to live in an untreated condition) is to violate the ethics of the medical profession and its fundamental dictum: *primum non nocere* (Bonnie 1990; Radelet and Barnard 1986; Salguero 1986). These authors believe participation in the infliction of punishment is unethical in this instance. Clear professional guidelines do not, however, exist.

There may be some ethical relief in situations in which the clinician could reliably determine that the prisoner would have wanted treatment in such cases, but such reliability is hard to realistically imagine (Bonnie 1990). The passage by the U.S. Congress of the Patient Self-Determination Act (Omnibus Budget Reconciliation Act of 1990) and increasing use and awareness of advance directives may gradually make such knowledge more available. There is an opposing viewpoint that the punishment enacted as a function of societal law is not within the purview of the clinician; the clinician's responsibility is instead to provide adequate treatment under all circumstances out of respect for the patient's autonomy and rationality (Mossman 1987; National Medical Association, undated).

The clinical-ethical issues become even more complex when the prisoner is incompetent and refuses medication that would restore competence. This was the situation in the case of Michael Perry, a condemned prisoner in Louisiana whose case was argued before the U.S. Supreme Court in 1989 (*Perry v. Louisiana* 1990). The American Psychiatric Association (APA) and the American Medical Association (AMA) joined in taking the position that involuntary medication for the sole purpose of restoring competence to be executed violates the rights of the prisoner because it is not in the medical interest of the prisoner and is not necessary for another legitimate purpose, such as preventing danger to others (American Psychiatric Association/American Medical Association 1989). The organizations further argued that because such prisoners could not be medicated, nor could they be allowed to languish in a permanent psychotic state, their death sentences should be commuted to life imprisonment so that treatment could then be provided. The Supreme Court remanded the case back to Louisiana without an opinion on the substantive issues. On remand, the Louisiana Supreme Court (*State v. Perry* 1992) concluded that "a physician's prescription and administration of antipsychotic drugs to a prisoner against his will, pursuant to the order of a state court or other government officials for the purpose of carrying out the death penalty, does not constitute medical treatment but forms part of the capital punishment sought to be executed by the state." Although not permitting the involuntary use of medication to restore competence on a number of state constitutional grounds, the court did not resolve all of the issues. They did not commute the sentence, so that he may be executed if his mental status improves without the use of medication. It also leaves Mr. Perry in a psychotic state whereby he cannot be treated with medication unless an emergency develops.

Radelet and Barnard (1986) have also advocated commutation to life imprisonment as a solution to the "ethical chaos" of treating prisoners who are judged incompetent to be executed, focusing their argument on the rights of the mental health professionals and the ethical codes of their professions. At least one legal analysis has reached a similar conclusion, emphasizing the state's interest in preserving the moral integrity of the medical profession, as well as the rights of medical professionals (Salguero 1986). As stated at the beginning of this subsection, this type of case will not present itself to many clinicians. Radelet and Barnard (1986) have documented one case of restoration of competency to be executed, demonstrating the practical realities of these ethical dilemmas. But for those clinicians who work in settings where the potential for receiving such a patient is high, this case report should be reviewed by the medical staff before the "crisis" of the first such admission, as there are many complicated issues to be explored.

In principle, physicians should be permitted to relieve suffering and provide appropriate medical care to death row inmates. Involuntary treatment solely to restore competency to be executed should be deemed unethical. Efforts to determine an inmate's wishes regarding how he would like to be treated in the event of future incompetence should be periodically reviewed so that timely and accurate information will be available to clinicians. This situation provides an important paradigm to explore a number of ethical issues for the individual clinician as well as the medical and allied professional associations.

Alcohol and Substance Abuse

Paralleling development of public institutions for mentally ill persons during the latter part of the 19th century, some states developed institutions for the involuntary treatment of alcoholic persons (i.e., inebriate asylums). In 1874, Connecticut enacted statutes allowing for involuntary commitment of "inebriates" to private institutions. This was followed by similar legislation in other states. Civil commitment of addicts has remained a consistent approach during the 20th century—from the development of morphine maintenance clinics in the 1920s to the establishment of federal narcotics treatment facilities in Lexington, Kentucky and Fort Worth, Texas (Inciardi 1988; Maddux 1986; Musto 1973).

One novel development in substance abuse treatments occurred in 1972. The Treatment Alternatives to Street Crime (TASC) program began a series of diversion programs that by 1988 involved 18 states (Cook et al. 1988). Diversion, which originally meant keeping individuals out of the criminal justice system, now implies transfer from the criminal justice system to treatment programs at any stage of the criminal justice process. Treatment often becomes the only sanction or a major component of the sanctions imposed. Diversions can be formal or informal and can be pre- or postadjudicatory. An example of preadjudicatory diversion occurs when police officers transport someone to an emergency treatment facility or give someone the "choice" to go to a treatment facility rather than be arrested. It also can occur at the prosecutor's discretion prior to or after arrest and filing of criminal charges. It can involve conditional release: holding the disposition pending the outcome of an evaluation or treatment, or accepting a guilty plea with the understanding that treatment will occur.

Postadjudicatory diversion can occur prior to or after sentencing. These postadjudicatory cases usually involve monitoring by the probation department as a condition of release. Each of these types of referrals may lead to very different requirements regarding the nature of treatment, reporting, and drug testing. The suspension of prosecution or incarceration, or the dismissal of criminal charges, acts as a major incentive for defendants to participate in these programs.

Alcohol treatment is now also the accepted treatment modality for handling DWI offenses (Weisner 1990). In some jurisdictions DWI drivers are given a choice of treatment or criminal sanctions; in others they are automatically referred to treatment programs. Policies are affected by the number of prior offenses as well as the jurisdiction. Some programs may have the authority to prescribe inpatient or outpatient treatment. The use of disulfiram may be coerced by the threat of referral back to the criminal justice system if the patient refuses.

Among persons with substance-use disorders, the distinction between those patients who are voluntary and those who are coerced into treatment is enormously vague. The great majority of individuals seeking treatment are under some form of coercion— by family, spouse, employer, or court, or even by the need to decrease tolerance levels and therefore the cost of the habit. This has made studies comparing the results of treating "involuntary" patients with those of treating "voluntary" patients particularly hard to interpret. Studies seem to indicate that involuntary patients do at least no worse than voluntary patients on a variety of measures (Schottenfeld 1989).

Coerced Treatment in the Mental Health System: Outpatient Commitment

Outpatient commitment is defined by a court order directing an individual to comply with specific treatment requirements outside of a residential setting. The requirements may include taking medication, reporting to a monitoring facility, or participating in therapy, educational, or vocational programs. The goals of such commitment are generally to alleviate/reduce the individual's illness or disability, and/or to maintain or prevent deterioration of function in the least restrictive setting (American Psychiatric Association 1987).

Outpatient commitment is a form of treatment that can be conceived of as an extension of inpatient civil commitment, although there are important differences between the two processes, which will be discussed below. Outpatient commitment may seem regressive—from a civil libertarian perspective—in the wake of the deinstitutionalization movement. However, many of the predicates of that movement were never realized, such as the widespread availability of community mental health centers, the ability of patients to recognize their need for treatment, and their willingness to voluntarily accept it. Thus, it may be the failure of deinstitutionalization to provide continuity of care for chronically mentally ill persons that has created an impetus to provide a mechanism for involuntary treatment of outpatients.

Outpatient commitment can be utilized as an alternative to involuntary hospitalization or as a form of conditional release from involuntary hospitalization. It is most useful for patients who respond well to medication but have a history of noncompliance in outpatient treatment; patients who need externally imposed structure in order to function in the community but are not capable of requesting or creating such structure on their own; or patients for whom outpatient commitment as a form of conditional release represents the only way in which they might be realistically released from an inpatient setting (American Psychiatric Association 1987).

Outpatient commitment occurs either as a statutorily based procedure or as a judicially sanctioned process. Twenty-six states and the District of Columbia have statutory provision for this process. (New York State expressly prohibits it.) The remainder of states' statutes are silent on this issue. There are two basic statutory alternatives that are utilized. In most states, the criteria and process for civil commitment to inpatient or outpatient treatment are identical; the choice is made on the basis of argued needs of the patient. In some states (e.g., North Carolina and Hawaii), the criteria for outpatient commitment are less stringent than those for inpatient commitment. In some states that do not provide statutory procedures (e.g., Massachusetts), outpatient commitment can occur through a process of court order (Schmidt and Geller 1989). In these situations, individual clinicians or facilities must take it upon themselves to petition the civil courts to undertake a course of mandated treatment with a given patient. The available data about the efficacy of outpatient commitment are mixed (American Psychiatric Association 1987; Bloom et al. 1986, 1988; Geller 1986; Miller and Fiddleman 1984; Miller et al. 1984).

Outpatient commitment entails a number of clinical difficulties that are particular to this type of treatment. These difficulties can be described under the separate headings of legal/ethical issues, staff/institutional resistance, inappropriate commitments, and noncompliant/refusing patients.

Legal / Ethical Issues

Perhaps the most immediate difficulty encountered in outpatient commitment situations is the ethical/philosophical argument that pits patient autonomy against treater's paternalism. The legislative guidelines proposed by the APA's Task Force on Involuntary Outpatient Commitment (American Psychiatric Association 1987) offer a proactive ethical framework for engaging in such treatment. This framework defines the indications for seeking outpatient commitment, and the requirements of a proposed treatment plan.

According to these recommendations, outpatient commitment is indicated for the person who is suffering from a severe mental disorder; *and,* without treatment, is likely to cause harm to self or others or to suffer substantial deterioration; *and* lacks capacity to make an informed decision regarding treatment; *and* has been hospitalized for a mental disorder within the previous 2 years; *and* has been noncompliant with prescribed treatment outside the hospital. Further, there must be a reasonable prospect that the patient's disorder will respond to the requested treatment. Finally, the responsible clinician(s) and/or facility have agreed to accept the patient under the proposed conditions and treatment plan.

These recommendations also specify that a detailed treatment plan be prepared in advance of the request for outpatient commitment. This plan should contain provisions for monitoring the patient's mental status and compliance with the conditions of treatment. It should also include a plan for performing a thorough medical examination so that possible medical conditions causing or contributing to the patient's impairment are not overlooked.

Staff / Institutional Resistance

Outpatient commitment can yield poor results when the staff or facility attitudes toward such commitment are negative (Miller et al. 1984). Whereas hospital staff are accustomed to dealing with involuntary and chronically ill patients, many community mental health centers are not. On the other hand, when outpatient clinicians are favorably disposed to such treatment, the results have been quite good. For example, at St. Elizabeths Hospital in Washington, D.C., the same clinicians treat patients both while the patients are hospitalized and after their discharge. This arrangement removes communication and attitudinal barriers, with the result that outpatient commitment has been quite effective (Zanni and de Veau 1986).

Inappropriate Commitments

Poor results have also been documented in cases in which patients are sent to outpatient commitment not as a result of clinicians' petition, but as a result of negotiation between a probate court and the patient's attorney (American Psychiatric Association 1987). The reasons for such poor results are obvious. When outpatient commitment is pursued as a legal compromise or plea bargain, relevant clinical issues may be ignored. There may be no reasonable prospect for successful treatment, no workable treatment plan, no way to adequately monitor and supervise the patient, and no willing clinician/facility to accept the responsibility for the patient. It is quite helpful, therefore, to have the indications for civil commitment detailed in statutory language in order to avoid such inappropriate commitments. In the absence of such statutory inclusion criteria, clinicians would have to develop a good working relationship with the courts in order to keep judges and attorneys informed about limitations as well as possible benefits of outpatient commitment.

The Noncompliant / Refusing Patient

In many cases, the mere process of pursuing outpatient commitment will increase patients' compliance. Many patients will respond to the fact that their clinician(s) feels strongly about the importance of treatment and is willing to invest time and effort in taking such a stance. The involvement of the court and an order by a judge can also be impressive enough to some patients to facilitate their cooperation, assuming that adequate clinical resources are available to provide the ordered treatment (American Psychiatric Association 1987; Schmidt and Geller 1989).

There will always be cases, however, in which patients fail to follow the prescribed and ordered treatment, and procedures must be available to deal with such situations. Such provisions might include the ability to have the patient brought to the treatment location by the police; the ability to involuntarily medicate the patient; and the ability to have the patient committed to an inpatient facility or to have the outpatient commitment modified (American Psychiatric Association 1987). A distinction should be made between involuntary medication and physically forced medication. The latter is best avoided because many outpatient settings lack a sufficient number of properly trained personnel to forcibly administer medication in a safe manner and because the prospect of physical force might be sufficiently controversial to produce opposition from clinicians and patient advocates to the entire process of outpatient commitment.

Legal Liability

One of the goals of outpatient commitment is to prevent patients from doing harm to themselves or others without having to hospitalize them. The corollary to this goal is that there might well be an expectation of a greater degree of control over the patient by a clinician accepting and providing treatment via outpatient commitment (American Psychiatric Association 1987). Unless some reasonable immunity is provided, clinicians will understandably be reluctant to offer such care. Even if immunity is provided, clinicians might well be expected to be more aggressive in monitoring their patients and following up on any noncompliance with the approved treatment plan.

Mandated Treatment in the Workplace

Impaired Physicians

> If the doctor is doctoring a doctor
> Does the doctor doing the doctoring
> Doctor the doctor being doctored
> The way the doctor being doctor
> Wants to be doctored?
> Or does the doctor doctoring the doctor
> Doctor the doctor being doctored
> The way the doctoring doctor
> Usually doctors? (Lipsitt 1975)

With the publication of final regulations for the National Practitioner Data Bank established by the Health Care Quality Improvement Act on October 17, 1989, we entered a new era in a national effort to identify incompetent physicians. In the past, many physicians under investigation by state boards would voluntarily surrender their licenses in one state prior to a formal hearing and then would continue practicing medicine by moving to another state where they also were licensed to practice. In a number of cases state boards seemed to be happy to avoid lengthy and costly due-process hearings and did not seem to be concerned about the "transfer" of the problem. With the new data bank, any substantial loss of privileges, loss or suspension of licensure, and adverse malpractice settlements must be reported. In addition, any hospital granting privileges to a physician must consult with the data bank as a part of the credentialing process. This may well have a negative impact, however, on referrals to impaired-physician programs.

Attempts to provide rehabilitation programs for impaired physicians have grown dramatically since the publication of the AMA's Council on Mental Health report "The Sick Physician" in 1973 (American Medical Association 1973). Currently, nine states have legislated impaired-physician programs by state medical boards, by independent agencies, or by medical societies through contracts with medical boards. All other state programs are administered by medical societies (Ikeda and Pelton 1990). Most states have mandatory reporting obligations for physicians, hospitals, and state societies when they have information that appears to show that a physician is or may be unable to practice medicine with reasonable skill or safety. Consequently, some addicted physicians choose to be hospitalized in a state other than where they are licensed so that reporting will not constitute a legal duty for the treating hospital or physicians.

Studies are beginning to report profiles of impaired physicians. A review of Oregon's experience seems typical. Between 1977 and 1985, 63 physicians were placed on probation by the Board of Medical Examiners. The referral sources were most commonly from hospital administration, medical staffs, or peers, although 29% of those impaired physicians with nonalcoholic drug dependence were referred by pharmacists, reflecting a pattern of inappropriate or illegal prescription practices. The mean age of the impaired physicians at the time of evaluation was 48 years—on average, 10 years after the time of onset of their addiction or other impairment. Alcohol dependence accounted for 14 (22%) of the 63 subjects. Combined alcohol and drug dependence affected 10 (16%). Other substance dependence accounted for 40%. Affective, schizophrenic, and organic disorders constituted 22%. The total improvement rate was about 75%, indicating only that the physicians were back in their original jobs or working as physicians in another setting (Shore 1987). These outcomes parallel those findings reported from Georgia, California, Colorado, Minnesota, and Wisconsin.

By 1983 the Oregon Board had adopted a program requiring monitored urine samples for all addicted physicians. Random urine screenings were done on a weekly basis. A dramatic improvement rate of 96% was found for those subjects who had been monitored, compared with a 64% improvement rate for those who had no monitoring. On the other hand, alcohol-dependent physicians placed on disulfiram showed no significant improvement over those not given the drug.

One critical issue for psychiatrists who undertake the treatment of impaired physicians is the critical importance of being explicit about the nature and degree of responsibility that is being accepted. Generally, psychiatrists should confine their monitoring to issues related to exacerbation or emergence of psychiatric symptomatology. The hospital or employing institution must maintain the responsibility to continually assess the physician's skill and practice.

Employee Assistance Programs

Employee assistance programs (EAPs), originally directed toward alcoholism, have expanded rapidly in both number and scope of treatments being offered. In 1917, Macy's Department Store in New York City established one of the first counseling programs for employees. With the developing view in the 1930s that alcoholism was an illness rather than merely a moral or spiritual defect, the first occupational alcoholism programs were started in such companies as New England Electric, Kaiser Shipbuilding, and New England Telephone. Current estimates find close to 10,000 EAPs in the public and private sectors (Stackel 1987). By 1985, 68 different federal agencies reported to the Office of Personnel Management (OPM) that they had EAPs for their 2.1 million federal civilian employees (Bureau of National Affairs 1987). These programs are usually part of the benefit packages provided for employees. The rapid growth in the number of EAPs began in the mid-1970s largely due to availability of increased federal funding, provision for EAPs in many collective bargaining agreements, and courts holding employers increasingly responsible for causing or exacerbating employees' mental health or substance abuse problems. Stress in the workplace was seen as a common precipitating factor.

There are two basic models for these programs: one internally and one externally based. The internal programs consist of in-house staff that provide assessments, brief treatment, referrals to external providers for long-term treatment, and manager training.

One of the problems with internal programs relates to issues of employee trust. In spite of assurances to the contrary, many employees have a difficult time accepting that a plan that is run and staffed by the company will keep information protected. A larger number of EAPs have moved toward external contracts with providers. Some impetus came with federal funding for the development of occupational alcohol programs, and smaller companies were attracted to external programs. The goal of both types of programs is to maintain the employee in the work environment while concomitantly providing the incentive for the worker to obtain necessary treatment.

Some studies have suggested that self-referral was associated with poor outcome and that employees forced into treatment did better (Beaumont and Allsop 1984). One additional motivating factor in EAPs has been the idea that threat of job loss coupled with availability of treatment would make treatment more effective than treatment following job loss. Kurtz et al. (1984), in reviewing outcome studies, felt that none met rigorous criteria such as adequate sampling, use of control groups, uniform definitions of success, sufficient follow-up, or good cost-effectiveness measures. The design of many evaluation studies is so problematic that true efficacy cannot be accurately assessed.

One of the more controversial issues for EAPs has been the issue of drug testing and screening in the workplace. A National Institute on Drug Abuse survey found that drug screening rose from 3% to 30% between 1982 and 1985 in Fortune 500 companies. More recent studies show rates of up to 35% to 38% (Reuborne 1990; Wrich 1988). This has become a major area of legal disputes, and clear principles have not yet emerged. There has been no absolute ban on testing, and testing has been permitted where issues of public safety (*National Treasury Employees Union v. von Raab* 1989; *Skinner v. Railway Labor Executives Assn.* 1989) and reasonable cause have been found.

It is clearly important for clinicians working or consulting with EAPs to be very clear about employer reporting obligations, especially when employees are referred by managers or when employment is specifically tied to treatment evaluation or outcome. It is usually helpful to have these agreements in writing and make them available to review with patients. It is also important to be clear about the availability of the mental health or substance abuse records. In federally supported substance abuse programs, confidentiality is governed by federal statutes and regulations that are quite restrictive. Confidentiality obligations can also be affected by program descriptions in company brochures and state statutes.

Mandated Disability Evaluations

There is another category of workplace referral that deserves some mention because of the potential for abuse and its notoriety. Although not treatment per se, "fitness for duty" evaluation requests have become increasingly commonplace. They have recently been the focus of attention in the military and among civilian employees of the military, transportation workers, employees at nuclear power plants, and employees at other jobs where public safety is involved. These fitness evaluations are better thought of as forensic evaluations in that there is not a primary treatment relationship with the person being evaluated and reports have to be provided to the source of referral.

Under the heading of "whistle-blowers," a number of individuals referred for these evaluations have alleged that their referrals to mental health professionals were efforts to harass and intimidate rather than being based on any concern regarding their health or safety. These referrals have achieved headlines in the press and have been the subject of several congressional hearings during the past 5 years. Of course, it is difficult for clinicians to know in advance of such an evaluation whether such an abuse is occurring. It can be helpful to screen such referrals beforehand by speaking with the referral source and/or requiring a written referral letter outlining the basis for the evaluation request. This can be especially difficult in the military, where the commanding officer has almost unlimited discretion and there are presently no practical due-process protections for review of involuntary commitment, much less for fitness evaluations.

Social Security and Worker's Compensation evaluations are more clearly forensic in nature (i.e., requests for expert opinion regarding legal questions). Generally, because of the likelihood of disruption to the treatment relationship, it is not recommended that treating psychiatrists provide this type of evaluation for their patients. In some states (e.g., New York) the treating physician's evaluation has presumptive validity in court. This may force psychiatrists to override the general admonition, especially when it may be specifically detrimental to the patient because of the legal rules.

Conclusions: Principles of Mandated Treatment and Guidelines for Its Use

The clinician must know and/or establish the conditions of treatment before beginning the therapy. A minimum list of considerations would include the following:

◆ What is being mandated, and by whom?
◆ What are the conditions, if any, of that treatment?
◆ What requirements are being made for the patient's compliance?
◆ What must the patient do to satisfactorily comply with the mandate and/or with the clinician's expectations for treatment?
◆ What behaviors will constitute a compliance failure?
◆ What are the penalties for the patient's failure? What are the reporting and monitoring requirements?

The therapist must know the answer to each of these questions and must feel comfortable doing therapy under such externally controlled and restricted conditions.

It is extremely important to deal explicitly with confidentiality issues, because reporting to a third party on the progress of the therapy will almost certainly be a component of the process. Especially with patients referred by the criminal justice system, it is important to review the statutory language and administrative regulations that govern the referral so that the legal boundaries are clear. The referral request should be obtained in writing and should spell out the basis for and conditions governing the evaluation or treatment. These limitations should be reviewed with the patient prior to beginning the evaluation.

It is useful to have an evaluation period that is distinct from treatment. Evaluation reports usually have to be provided to the referring authority with more information than is subsequently required for follow-up reports once treatment has begun. An extended evaluation will allow hidden agendas to be discovered as well as allow for time to obtain and integrate records of past treatment experience.

It is also important for the therapist to follow the conditions and, if possible, be a part of the process that sets the parameters of treatment. One cannot take on the responsibility of such treatment without enforcing the rules of the treatment. It is generally not the clinician's prerogative to bend the rules or excuse missed appointments or other noncompliance behaviors. To do so is to allow the treatment contract to erode, and, more seriously, this may place the clinician at risk of liability for the patient's future violent or destructive behavior. It is necessary, therefore, for the therapist to make the constraints and conditions of the mandated treatment contract an explicit part of the therapy.

The clinician should externalize the coercion and use it as a tool in the therapy.   Patients are not mandated into therapy by their therapists. Other external forces are the motivating factor(s). Referring to this external force can allow the patient and therapist to form an alliance to work together to satisfy this third-party requirement. The coercion can also be used to stress the issues of assuming personal responsibility, accepting the negative effects of maladaptive behaviors, and understanding the value of change and growth. With more resistant patients, the external force may simply provide the impetus to keep the patient in treatment long enough for therapy to have an effect. Thus, external coercion may make it possible to treat patients who would otherwise not be accessible to therapy because of the nature of their disorders. Character disorders and substance-use disorders are notoriously difficult to treat without constraints that limit acting out and premature withdrawal from treatment.

The effectiveness of coercion may also be dependent on personality style or traits. In reviewing data on locus of control, Strickland (1989) found that people with an external locus are more likely to conform to influence than are individuals with an internal locus.

Some of the implications of these findings are that an important part of the definition of coercion from a treatment perspective is that perceived coercion may be a significant component of someone's ability to form a therapeutic alliance. Without advocating that patients be manipulated to believe they have freely chosen something they have not, it is not unreasonable to describe how they have made a series of choices that have, in part, resulted in the current situation and that they will continue to control certain factors regarding the outcome.

Building the patient's trust is a more difficult process in mandated treatments. This difficulty in building trust is due to, in part, the patient's resistance to the therapy and, in part, the dual role that the clinician must fill as therapist and evaluator/reporter. This divided agency makes it difficult for the patient to see the clinician solely as an advocate or benefactor. Trust is further hampered by limitations on the usual patient-psychiatrist confidentiality. There are two basic tactics for the clinician to take. First, the clinician should be completely straightforward and unapologetic about the special circumstances of the therapeutic relationship. The therapist must acknowledge the various external forces in a matter-of-fact way in order to get beyond them with the clinical work. It is also very useful to acknowledge in an understanding way the patient's negative reactions to such forces. This can further enable the alliance.

The second main tactic is to enlist the support of other interested third parties. Patients, because of the divided agency, may not see the therapist as being "on their side." They may, however, see their lawyer or various supportive friends or family members as being squarely on their side. It is often effective to utilize a trusted lawyer to present information to the patient. Cooperating with the legal advice of counsel may be less threatening to the patient than cooperating with the "shrink." Gradually, it becomes possible to unite the helping services of lawyer (and/or family or friend) and clinician. This can be facilitated through joint meetings with the patient, attorney, family, friends, and clinician. In such meetings, patients can get a good deal of supportive feedback and begin to see that treatment is a means to a desired end.

Mandatory treatment is treatment; there is no need to be apologetic about it.　The purely voluntary patient is a rarity, if not a plain myth. Clinicians are trained to deal with various forms of coercion in nonmandated treatment. The coercive elements in mandated treatment are simply more explicit and perhaps more extensive. Establishing a treatment alliance can be a difficult clinical task, but here again, most clinicians have successfully treated patients who were resistant to treatment. Not only is mandated treatment not necessarily inferior to nonmandated treatment, but there may actually be some advantages to it. It may be possible to treat some patients who, without a mandate, would be untreatable. Also, because of the sociopolitical interest in mandated treatment, resources may be easier to obtain. This societal interest can be a double-edged sword, though, because it is often predicated on fear and may thus increase stigma.

Clinicians must maintain a sense of control over the treatment.
Too many times clinicians tolerate treatment noncompliance to a degree that the treatment would be viewed as below reasonable standards of care or negligent if some harm occurs. Patients may not reasonably refuse to comply with medication or blood tests such as lithium levels or antidepressant levels, or random urine screening for substance abuse. Clinicians sometimes allow unrea-

sonable periods of time to elapse before making it clear that treatment cannot continue unless certain minimum standards are being followed. Mandated psychotherapy patients who consistently refuse to discuss any meaningful issues session after session in a fashion that connotes "abuse" of the treatment should also be informed that treatment will not be allowed to continue. At the same time, the consequences of discontinued treatment should be reviewed.

Professionals in clinic settings are prone to feel trapped in a treatment relationship where no treatment alliance has developed; they incorrectly feel that treatment must continue no matter what the patient does, short of violence, just because the patient is mandated. They also do not want to feel responsible for sending someone back to prison or "causing" him or her to lose a job. This is a situation ripe for a disaster, and consultation or supervision may be helpful in reviewing such impasses.

There are good reasons to agree to provide mandated treatment. Many of the patients who are mandated are those severely and chronically ill individuals who have not responded to customary nonmandated treatments. It can thus be very rewarding for the clinician who provides a mandated therapy that results in a significant alleviation of suffering and improved quality of life for the patient.

Mandated treatment can be a humane way of dealing with individuals in difficult situations. Such treatment may provide alternatives to persons who are losing their jobs, or being incarcerated for substance abuse problems, or being punished for acts for which they are not blameworthy, or being otherwise rejected, isolated, or institutionalized in various scenarios. Thus, through the willingness of mental health professionals to provide treatment in nontraditional, mandated formats, we are able to realize important, humanistic goals of our society and health professions. The extra time and energy expended in attending to the demands of providing mandated treatment are well worth the investment—both for clinicians and patients.

References

American Medical Association Council on Mental Health: The sick physician: impairment by psychiatric disorders, including alcoholism and drug dependence. JAMA 223:684–687, 1973

American Psychiatric Association, Brief Amicus Curiae, Ford v Wainwright (No 85-5542) (U.S. January 30, 1986)

American Psychiatric Association, Task Force on Involuntary Outpatient Commitment (Starrett D, chair): Involuntary Commitment to Outpatient Treatment (Task Force Report No 26). Washington, DC, American Psychiatric Association, 1987

American Psychiatric Association/American Medical Association, Brief Amicus Curiae, Perry v. Louisiana (No 89-5120) (U.S. October Term 1989)

Appelbaum PS: Empirical assessment of innovation in the law of civil commitment: a critique. Law, Medicine & Health Care 13:304–309, 1985

Appelbaum PS: Competence to be executed: another conundrum for mental health professional. Hosp Community Psychiatry 37:682–684, 1986

Beaumont PB, Allsop SJ: An industrial alcohol policy: the characteristics of worker success. Br J Addict 79:315–318, 1984

Blankstein H: Organizational approaches to improving institutional estimations of dangerousness in forensic psychiatric hospitals: a Dutch perspective. Int J Law Psychiatry 11:341–345, 1988

Bloom JD, Williams MH, Rogers JL, et al: Evaluation and treatment of insanity acquittees in the community. Bull Am Acad Psychiatry Law 14:231–244, 1986

Bloom JD, Bradford JM, Kofoed L: An overview of psychiatric treatment approaches to three offender groups. Hosp Community Psychiatry 39:151–158, 1988

Bonnie RJ: Dilemmas in administering the death penalty: conscientious abstention, professional ethics, and the needs of the legal system. Law and Human Behavior 14:67–90, 1990

Bureau of National Affairs: Employee Assistance Programs: Benefits, Problems, and Prospects. Washington, DC, Bureau of National Affairs, 1987, p 89

Commitment following an insanity acquittal. Harvard Law Review 94:584–625, 1980–1981

Cook LF, Weinman BA, et al: Treatment alternatives in street crime, in Compulsory Treatment of Drug Abuse: Research and Clinical Practice (NIDA Monogr No 86) (DHHS Publ No (ADM)88-1578). Edited by Leukefeld CG, Tims FM. Rockville, MD, National Institute on Drug Abuse, 1988, pp 99–105

Cox M: Dynamic psychotherapy with sex offenders, in Sexual Deviation. Edited by Rosen I. Oxford, UK, Oxford University Press, 1979, pp 306–350

Eisner HR: Returning the not guilty by reason of insanity to the community: a new scale to determine readiness. Bull Am Acad Psychiatry Law 17:401–413, 1989

Ford v Wainwright, 106 S Ct 2595 (1986)

Geller JL: Rights, wrongs, and the dilemma of coerced community treatment. Am J Psychiatry 132:1259–1264, 1986

Gibbens TCN, Soothill K, Way C: Psychiatric treatment on probation. British Journal of Criminology 21:324–334, 1981

Harris GA, Watkins D: Counseling the Involuntary and Resistant Client. College Park, MD, American Correctional Association, 1987

Heilbrun KS: The assessment of competency for execution: an overview. Behavioral Sciences and the Law 5:383–396, 1987

Heilbrun KS, McClaren HA: Assessment of competency for execution? A guide for mental health professionals. Bull Am Acad Psychiatry Law 6:205–216, 1988

Ikeda R, Pelton C: Diversion programs for impaired physicians. West J Med 152:617–621, 1990

Inciardi JA: Compulsory treatment in New York: a brief narrative history of misjudgment, mismanagement, and misrepresentation. Journal of Drug Issues 18:547–560, 1988

Kurtz NR, Googins B, Howard WC: Measuring the success of occupational alcohol programs. J Stud Alcohol 45:33–35, 1984

Lamb HR: Incompetency to stand trial: appropriateness and outcome. Arch Gen Psychiatry 44:754–758, 1987

Lamb HR, Weinberger LE, Gross BH: Court-mandated outpatient treatment for insanity acquittees: clinical philosophy and implementation. Hosp Community Psychiatry 39:1080–1084, 1988

Larke J: Compulsory treatment: some practical methods of treating the mandated client. Psychotherapy 22:262–268, 1985

Lipsitt DR: The doctor as patient. Psychiatr Opinion 12:20–25, 1975

Maddux JF: Clinical experience with civil commitment, in The Compulsory Treatment of Drug Abuse: Research and Clinical Practice (DHHS No [ADM]88-1578). Rockville, MD, National Institute on Drug Abuse, 1986

Miller RD: The treating psychiatrist as forensic evaluator in release decisions. Journal of Forensic Sciences 32:481–488, 1987

Miller RD, Fiddleman PB: Outpatient commitment: treatment in the least restrictive environment. Hosp Community Psychiatry 35:147–151, 1984

Miller RD, Maher R, Fiddleman PB: The use of plea bargaining in civil commitment. Int J Law Psychiatry 7:395–406, 1984

Miller RD, Doren DM, Van Rybroek G, et al: Emerging problems for staff associated with the release of potentially dangerous forensic patients. Bull Am Acad Psychiatry Law 16:309–320, 1988

Mossman D: Assessing and restoring competency to be executed: should psychiatrists participate? Behavioral Sciences and the Law 5:397–409, 1987

Musto D: The American Disease: Origins of Narcotics Control. New Haven, CT, Yale University Press, 1973

National Medical Association, Section on Psychiatry and Behavioral Sciences (Bell CC, chair): Position statement on the role of the psychiatrist in evaluating and treating "death row" inmates [undated]

National Treasury Employees Union v von Raab, 109 S Ct 1384 (1989)

Norko MA: A developmental perspective on the treatment of insanity acquittees. Paper presented at the 21st annual meeting of the American Academy of Psychiatry and the Law, Coronado, CA, October 1990

Omnibus Budget Reconciliation Act of 1990, PL No 101-508

Perry v Louisiana, 111 S Ct 449 (1990)

Prins H: Dangerous clients: further observations on the limitation of mayhem. British Journal of Social Work 18:593–609, 1988

Prins H: Some observations on the supervision of dangerous offender patients. Br J Psychiatry 156:157–162, 1990

Radelet ML, Barnard GW: Ethics and the psychiatric determination of competency to be executed. Bull Am Acad Psychiatry Law 14:37–53, 1986

Rappeport JR: Enforced treatment—is it treatment? Bull Am Acad Psychiatry Law 2:148–158, 1974

Reuborne E: More top firms test workers for drugs, USA Today, June 21, 1990, B1

Salguero RG: Medical ethics and competency to be executed. Yale Law Journal 96:167–186, 1986

Scales CJ, Phillips RTM, Crysler D: Security aspects of clinical care. American Journal of Forensic Psychology 7:49–57, 1989

Schmidt MJ, Geller JL: Involuntary administration of medication in the community: the judicial opportunity. Bull Am Acad Psychiatry Law 7:283–292, 1989

Schottenfeld RS: Involuntary treatment of substance abuse disorders: impediments to success. Psychiatry 52:164–176, 1989

Shore J: The Oregon experience with impaired physicians on probation; an eight year follow-up. JAMA 257:2931–2934, 1987

Skinner v Railway Labor Executives Assn, 109 S Ct 1402 (1989)

Stackel L: EAPs in the work place. Employment Relations Today 14:289–294, 1987

State of Louisiana v Perry, WL 296230 (La 1992)

State of Vermont v Mace, 578 A2d 104 (Vt 1990)

Stone A: Mental Health and Law: A System in Transition. New York, Jason Aronson, 1975

Strickland BR: Internal-external control expectancies. Am Psychol 44:1–12, 1989

Ward BA: Competency for execution: problems in law and psychiatry. Florida State University Law Review 14:35–107, 1986

Weisner CM: Coercion in alcohol treatment, in Broadening the Base of Treatment for Alcohol Problems: Report of a Study by the Committee of the Institute of Medicine. Washington, DC, National Academy Press, 1990, pp 579–609

Wrich JT: Beyond testing: coping with drugs at work. Security Management 32(6):64–73, 1988

Zanni G, de Veau L: A research note on the use of outpatient commitment. Hosp Community Psychiatry 37:941–942, 1986

Chapter 10

The Psychiatrist's Use of Family Involvement

Stuart Sugarman, M.D.

F amily therapy is a skill that residents often do not learn in depth during psychiatric training. Consequently, they perceive family therapy to be in the province of other mental health professionals, especially social workers. Yet, an increasing number of family-oriented psychiatrists see this work as necessary for optimal treatment of their patients and use this approach or feel they should be using this approach (Lansky 1985). Thus, issues raised in this chapter should be helpful to the practicing clinician.

I first present a conceptual framework to orient the psychiatrist to various clinical options involving the family. This typology provides the psychiatrist with a model for using systems interventions that are consistent with psychiatric training and belief systems. Detailed examples of family work are incorporated within each conceptualization. Although this conceptual framework does not focus immediately and directly on clinical issues involving difficult patients, my view is that most psychiatrists do not have a sufficient theoretical framework for deciding when and how to use family interventions in the clinical arena. Thus, rather than focusing solely on interventions with "difficult" patients, my emphasis in this chapter is on giving the practicing psychiatrist a clinical framework for using this method. Such a framework should then make family involvement a useful tool in the therapist's armamentarium of approaches to the patient who is difficult to treat. Examples of difficult clinical situations are woven into the explication of the conceptual framework. In addition, specific types of patients are discussed at the end of the chapter.

Throughout this chapter *family* is used synonymously with *family system*. Family therapy and systems therapy have close enough connotations in the literature that I use them interchangeably. I do not separate couples therapy from family therapy because couples therapy is family therapy with one particular subsystem of the family. Although some readers will disagree on these usages, a full discussion of the nuances of definitions is beyond our scope here.

The demographics of families have changed significantly over the last 50 years. It is useful to view family therapy theory and practice from the perspective of the change in family demographics over this period. Much of the initial family therapy literature addressed the nuclear family. When the literature developed in the 1940s and 1950s, the nuclear family (consisting of mother, father, and a second generation of children) was the prototypical family available for clinical work. Grandparents were also sometimes involved. Much of the family therapy literature has discussed strategic changes with regard to these two- and three-generational systems (Nichols and Schwartz 1991).

With the rising divorce rate, the nuclear family has become less prevalent, resulting in an atypical clinical population. Psychiatrists also are seeing more severely dysfunctional families than in the past. Divorced families, low-income families, abusing families, and remarried families make up a growing, large share of the general population. Both clinical practice and the theoretical literature have evolved over the last few decades to reflect these demographic changes (Becvar and Becvar 1988).

A Conceptual Framework

One of the problems that psychiatrists have with "family" involvement is that they have been been trained to deal with the individual as the unit of assessment and intervention rather than with the family as a whole. At times, it makes sense to focus on family issues within a primary dyadic perspective, while at other times it is better to focus primarily on the family unit itself (Sugarman 1982). I will refer to the former as a *family as background* perspective and the latter as a *family as unit* perspective. An intermediate point between these two concepts is the notion of *family as context*. These concepts provide a framework for strategic thinking about applying family concepts to clinical situations. In the major part of this chapter I will deal with an exposition of this framework and give clinical examples to illustrate their usefulness.

Family as Background

The *family as background* concept considers the individual as the primary unit of assessment and intervention. The family is involved only in the assessment phase, but not as an active participant in treatment. The diagnostic interview and "permission giving" interventions described below are two examples of *family as background.*

A family diagnostic interview is a useful way of getting additional clinical information. Traditionally, there has been a reluctance in psychiatry to pursue the family approach based on the premise that the individual is the patient and that bringing anyone else into the therapy room will interfere with the therapist-patient relationship, distort transference, and/or violate confidentiality. However, recently, psychiatrists have become increasingly willing to utilize family contact, realizing that the positive benefits gained from the family diagnostic approach may outweigh the negative aspects.

For example, consider a situation in which a psychotic patient comes into the emergency room. His mother and sister are sitting in the waiting room. Should the therapist bring them into the room for a joint interview? When I presented this scenario to third-year residents 15 years ago, I found that frequently they resisted this approach, believing the social worker or psychiatrist should see the family in a separate session. Over the years it has become clear to many that the family interview is a reasonable way to get, at a minimum, additional diagnostic information on the family situation, and potentially to make effective therapeutic interventions. For instance, in the psychotic patient's situation it is possible to get the family's point of view concerning what is going on and how the psychotic episode started, and a feeling for how the family functions in regard to the patient.

We can apply the same kind of analysis to a variety of other clinical situations, some simple and some more difficult. For example, a 33-year-old man comes into the clinic for an outpatient appointment and complains of anxiety and depression with a duration of 1 year. Dysthymia and panic attacks are under consideration as possible Axis I disorders. However, during the interview the psychiatrist learns that the man's marriage of 3 years has become extremely difficult and that his wife is threatening divorce. Traditionally, this information did not deter the psychiatrist from proceeding with the individual approach for both diagnosis and treatment.

However, what if the psychiatrist suggests that the second interview with the man involve a couple's assessment? In this particular case, such an assessment occurred. Information obtained in the couple session included the fact that the man's symptoms were intimately tied to events involving the marriage, in particular, an affair that the husband had engaged in for several years but had recently terminated. The wife was able to add significant history about her husband's symptoms and the interplay between events and these symptoms.

The psychiatrist went on to treat this patient with a combination of individual therapy and psychopharmacology. However, much of what came up with the wife in that diagnostic interview was helpful in the subsequent individual interviews. In addition, when the psychiatrist reviewed the videotape of the couple's session months later, he evolved new perspectives concerning the impact of the affair on the marriage. The psychiatrist brought these ideas up in the next few sessions, which led to additional fruitful discussions concerning the patient's guilt. Thus, the diagnostic couple's interview was helpful for the ongoing individual assessment and treatment of this particular patient.

Another useful family involvement is family consultation with the purpose of "permission giving." Consider the following situation: A 26-year-old woman makes an appointment, with the encouragement of her individual therapist, to attend a partial hospital program (PHP). She tells the interviewer that she will think about the issues involved and call back if she feels that the program is suitable for her needs. Nothing is heard from her for several weeks. A call from her individual therapist encouraging us to accept her into the program is met by the PHP staff's response that they are concerned that she has not followed up on the initial interview herself and that possibly her motivation is not sufficient for a successful outcome. The therapist understands the PHP staff's concerns and plans to discuss it further in his next interview with his patient.

The PHP staff gets another call from the woman the following week and makes another appointment to interview her. She is still ambivalent and makes the appointment primarily because of pressure from her therapist. As the PHP staff explores her ambivalence, it becomes clear that her husband is very opposed to psychiatry, and the patient feels that she would be disloyal to him if she entered PHP. The staff asks her to bring her husband to the next interview. She is reluctant but says she will try. Eventually, they succeed in having a couple's interview and find out that the husband is quite suspicious about the staff's efforts to have his wife in PHP. The PHP staff explores this further with him and also explains how they feel the program will help the wife without harming the marriage. After further discussion, the husband reluctantly agrees to let his wife try the program. The staff makes it clear that if he has any problems with the program, he is to let them know immediately.

The initial couple's interview with the subsequent "permission" from the husband was necessary before the patient could start PHP. Furthermore, an additional couple's interview during the program kept her from prematurely dropping out. Thus, diagnostic and permission-giving family interventions, as examples of a *family as background* perspective, can be very useful, particularly with difficult clinical situations.

Family as Context

The *family as context* is the middle perspective, one that, until recently, has not been given enough attention in the theoretical and clinical literature as a legitimate form of family involvement. An individual is viewed as the patient, but the therapist attempts to have the family in the therapy room both for assessment *and* for help in treating the individual patient. The goal is to reduce the family's role as a stressor and/or to increase them as a resource and facilitator.

Various models have developed over recent years that have employed this *family as context* concept. One is the psychoeducational model for treating schizophrenia. In this model schizophrenia is viewed as an illness in one person. Family involvement concerns educating the family about the illness, reducing the family as a stressor (i.e., moving the family from high expressed emotion [EE] to low EE), and also enhancing the family as a resource for the patient. The appropriateness of this model is not confined simply to patients with schizophrenia, but can be used with patients who have other types of psychopathology and who are at other levels of dysfunction. For instance, the psychiatrist might see a neurotic spouse as the individual patient but will decide to see both spouses together to help in the treatment of the individual. This is entirely different from seeing the couple as the "unit" of intervention.

There are strengths and weaknesses in using the *family as context* format. A strength is that the therapist has an individual patient defined as such. Thus, there is a clear contract regarding the boundaries of the "unit of therapy," and all of the clinical knowledge base regarding individual psychopathology and treatment is easily acceptable. A weakness is that the clinician has limited ability to intervene with the whole system. If the therapist attempts to work with the whole family system, he or she may encounter substantial resistance. In the case of the psychotic patient discussed in the previous subsection, the family had come to the emergency room with their "patient" clearly and rigidly defined. The implicit (and often explicit) contract is that there is an identified patient who needs treatment. I have seen many examples in which patients and families feel confused, offended, and unsupported by this change in contract. In summary, the *family as context* format is a very useful way of retaining the definition of an individual patient while at the same time using some of the strengths of the family approach through an effective engagement of the family.

Family as Unit

The third perspective of family involvement is the *family as unit.* In this approach, the unit of intervention is a family group greater than one individual. In the case of a marital relationship, the unit of assessment and intervention is the couple. The goal is to change the pattern of the relationships within the larger group. *Family as unit* is often a difficult concept for psychiatrists to appreciate and feel comfortable with, because our training teaches us to use the template of the "individual" as the patient. As an example, many residents and young psychiatrists who have not received family/couples treatment training will say: "I feel very uncomfortable with couples and families. It takes all my knowledge and energy to assess and understand the facts associated with one individual (e.g., the mental status, past history, diagnosis, treatment). To do the same with two to four individuals within the same time frame seems overwhelming, if not impossible."

My response is that to work from a *family as unit* point of view, the therapist must give up working at the level of the individual. This is analogous to individual psychotherapy, in which there is no reason the clinician needs to know everything about what goes on in *all* of the patient's subsystems. For example, the therapist does not have to know all of the biological information that an internist must know. In the same way, the clinician does not have to know all the individual psychological information when working with the family. The frame of reference shifts to a different level of assessment and intervention: the styles and patterns of interactions among family members.

Issues in Utilizing the Three Family Concepts

In clinical practice it is often difficult to move between these concepts of *family as background, as context,* and *as unit.* It is useful to establish which concept to use at the beginning when making the treatment contract with the patient system. Changes in this contract can be effected. Doing so must involve an explicit discussion and agreement with all of the participants, acknowledgment of the difficulties involved in this transition, the consideration of therapist-patient loyalties when moving from individual to systemic therapy, and even the need for new clinicians.

As an example of "previous loyalties" in the *family as background* or *family as context* perspective, the therapist is the ally of an individual patient. Movement to *family as unit* entails the therapist becoming the ally for the whole unit. Co-therapy is useful in such a situation. For instance, in changing from *family as context* to *family as unit,* the individual therapist can continue to be loyal to the individual and thereby continue with the previously established contract. The co-therapist can "contract" with the whole family in the new *family as unit* perspective.

For example, a 25-year-old schizophrenic man has been seen by a therapist for several years individually in a *family as context* model. Both the patient and his family have seen the therapist as the *patient's* therapist. There is a therapeutic contract (that both the patient and his family have agreed upon) that the family is there to help the therapist help the patient. With many families like this one, this context is sufficient for progress. However, the patient's situation is improving only slowly, even after years of work including intensive psychoeducational protocols.

The therapist decides that the individual therapy is stalled. The parents seem to pay lip service to the procedures but sabotage them after a period of time. It appears that marital conflicts as well as complex triangulations that involve the patient and his sister contribute to the failures of the interventions in this *family as context* model. The therapist decides that it is necessary to switch to a *family as unit* perspective that would allow the therapist to do intensive, change-oriented work with the whole family.

Although the family seems to agree, after a few sessions with this new perspective, the patient feels abandoned because his previous individual therapist is supporting the women in the family (i.e., the patient's mother and sister). In addition, both parents seem to resent the therapist's "intrusive" interpretations. Part of this resentment seems to be related to the fact that they saw the therapist as being much more supportive of them when the therapist was doing *family as context* work. In that mode, the therapist did not seem to be so "therapeutic."

It is possible to make this transition from a more supportive psychoeducational relationship to a more dynamic therapeutic relationship. However, adding a co-therapist would save much time and avoid many failures.

Often, only a part or a fragment of a family is available for clinical work. This is especially common when we are using the perspective of *family as context* and have an identified patient with severe psychopathology. Not all family members are willing to come in, for various reasons. My view is that with *family as context,* it is generally best to proceed with available family members. There is little to lose, from a clinical point of view, by not moving ahead with the family members who are willing to come in. Other family members may be willing to attend sessions later, either on their own or as a result of persuasion by the therapist or participating family members.

When working with the *family as unit,* the clinician is advisably more demanding concerning this issue of attendance to sessions. The therapist can say simply that he or she is not going to work with the family unless more members are present. There are sound clinical reasons for taking this stance at certain times, particularly with difficult families.

As an example, one patient and her family had many previous treatment failures in individual as well as family therapy. The family therapy failures seemed to involve therapeutic attempts to engage a family that, from the start, was extremely ambivalent about therapeutic involvement. This ambivalence was demonstrated by an important family member simply not showing up for the interviews. Sometimes the father would not attend, and at other times one particularly significant sister would not show up. The therapist would go ahead with the work in spite of the absences. Each of three family therapy courses failed, after 2 to 7 months.

In looking back at the previous therapies, it appeared that the absent member contributed to the failure. For example, in one failure, the patient and her father were in constant conflict at home. When the father did come into the therapy, he felt that the rest of the family, as well as the therapist, were against him. He was angry that many of the family secrets were discussed "behind his back." Similar dynamics occurred with the sister.

In the current therapy, when the mother called to make an appointment for treatment, the psychiatrist told her, "Because of your past treatment failures, I feel it is not in the family's interest for me to see you unless everyone is present." The mother was very angry and said that she would seek another psychiatrist. However, after thinking about their previous therapeutic failures, the rationale made sense to her. She then persuaded her husband to come in and stay involved. This round of therapy was finally helpful.

This is not to say that the therapist should hold arbitrarily and rigidly to this attendance requirement. There are certainly times when one loses little by compromising it. However, with some difficult families, this firm boundary is a crucial precondition to clinical success. Clinical judgment must be the ultimate guidepost in this territory.

The Treatment Context

Site Considerations

Inpatient services. It is difficult to use *family as unit* interventions on an inpatient unit. In its purest form, this would only occur if the whole family were to be hospitalized. There are rare programs around the world, as well as in this country, in which an entire family is hospitalized concurrently. However, if only one individual is hospitalized, it is still possible, although much more difficult, to have a primary *family as unit* model. Some child and adolescent units succeed with this approach, and there have been attempts over the years to organize some adult units in this manner. In general, though, the organization of hospitals mitigates against the *family as unit* model when an individual patient is hospitalized.

Usually, *family as background* or *family as context* is the most effective way of involving the family in the inpatient hospitalization (Whitley and Zankowski 1986).

Over the last few years, most psychiatrists with whom I have talked around the country seem sophisticated about family issues related to a given individual's hospitalization. However, I am dismayed that in actual clinical work, covert theoretical blind spots or practical necessity mitigates against a reasonable consideration of the family dimensions during inpatient stays. Frequently, patients are discharged against medical advice because the family felt that the staff was against them or did not respond to their needs. I continue to see clinical omissions of family approaches even in specific situations involving an inpatient in which family issues are clearly primary and need immediate intervention. Family therapy is still relegated to the social worker in many sites. Such relegation reflects the view that these issues are considered less important and mitigates against using them as a crucial part of the treatment.

Comprehensive treatment must involve the family (Group for the Advancement of Psychiatry 1982), particularly as shorter inpatient stays become the standard of practice. Inpatient work is changing dramatically because of managed care. Thus, involvement of the whole staff with the patient's life context is crucial. Currently there are some managed care groups that are making family therapy of up to two to three times a week a necessity for authorization for continuation of care (Health Management Strategies International 1991). This does not seem unreasonable, for the new goals of hospitalization—stabilization and movement to a less intense level of care—require dealing with the family environment. Even employing the *family as background* perspective—that is, simply sitting in with the social worker at the first assessment interview—can be clinically useful.

One crucial question often posed on inpatient units is whether the patient should return to the family environment. This question has to be answered clinically on a case-by-case basis. While there probably is very little disagreement at the extremes about what constitutes a good or bad environment, most of the debate concerns the large gray area of appropriate family context for a given individual. My experience over the years is that a reasonable number of these living contexts that were unacceptable without family work can become acceptable when family work is added.

Family work accomplishes two goals in these ambiguous instances. First, a more comprehensive assessment can occur than is possible without the family perspective. Mental health professionals often get a skewed, distorted view of the family situation, such as villain/victim issues, from their exclusive contact with the patient. These distortions often diminish with ongoing family involvement or even merely by conducting the family assessment. Second, a marginal living environment can be changed into a more acceptable context through therapeutic work.

Outpatient services.   The outpatient arena offers the freedom for utilizing any of the three types of family involvement described above. *Family as background, as context,* and *as unit* all make sense in the outpatient arena. Because all options are available, the issues that often come up are how to choose among the three concepts. This is related to the larger issue of modality selection criteria that has received more attention over the last decade. For example, when should one choose a family approach as opposed to an individual, group, or combined approach? This is a controversial area, and a full discussion of these issues is beyond the scope of this chapter. However, some comments are pertinent in light of the issues we are discussing.

Practitioners and theorists are divided along a spectrum. At one end are those who believe that clear, definitive standards of practice can be established for every clinical situation. At the other end of the spectrum are those who believe that each clinical situation can be well handled by any number of different approaches. I believe this latter approach more accurately reflects clinical realities in the early 1990s.

If the clinician is free to take a *family as background, as context,* or *as unit* approach, which perspective for family involvement is best for a given patient? In most cases, I believe the criteria are based on the therapist's experience, not on the clinical situation. There are no good controlled studies that definitively identify when any one approach is clinically indicated. A skilled and interested therapist can make any of these perspectives work.

Although I argue for the therapist's primacy in adopting a particular perspective, I temper this view by suggesting that there are certain additional clinical variables that might favor one approach over another. The family's motivation is important to consider. *Family as unit* work demands the most motivation on the family's part. Family availability is another factor. Although availability may reflect the family's "motivation," it also may reflect independent factors, such as geography. *Family as unit* models can be attempted over long distances, using speaker phones and conference calls, or by having members travel to the therapy location. Often it is more practical to employ the other models in such situations. Furthermore, a family that conceptualizes their problems in a manner congruent with one of the three approaches that I have described favors the therapist's choosing that particular perspective. An evaluation of the family's capacity to use one approach or another is also important.

The treatment site can limit options. As stated above, inpatient treatment is much more congruent with *family as background* or *as context* interventions. Often, the nature of the inpatient hospitalization limits the therapeutic options. If the service is only for stabilization, with extremely short lengths of stay, only *family as background* interventions are possible.

The patient's diagnosis should also be considered. Patients with clear biological pathology (e.g., schizophrenia) do better in outpatient settings with *family as context* interventions. Difficult clinical situations involving Axis II pathology can often be treated starting with either *family as context* or *family as unit* interventions. If an impasse or failure occurs, the therapist should consider switching to another perspective, keeping in mind the caveats discussed previously.

Partial hospital services. A partial hospital program (PHP), as in the outpatient arena, lends itself to all three types of family involvement (Sauer 1984). The PHP therapeutic community with whom the patient "lives" day after day and becomes quite involved functions in many ways as a surrogate family. Patients can act out and process issues regarding their family lives by transferring them onto the PHP community, allowing a sort of proxy family therapy. This is not to say that therapy with the patient's actual family members is not additionally indicated.

Many PHPs provide a formalized family psychoeducational module or family support group (*family as context*) as an optional or even required part of the therapeutic package. The combination of therapeutic formats available and practiced within a PHP can be quite powerful in helping difficult patients to integrate the various dimensions of dysfunction within their lives. For example, when the therapist identifies a self-defeating role within the patient's family, it is useful to encourage the patient to work on this issue within family sessions. Furthermore, if the role is acted out in group therapy with other patients and treatment staff, this difficulty can be clarified, interpreted, and worked through.

Therapist Considerations

Combined format. Often, difficult families are seen in a *combined format.* I am using this term to describe any situation in which more than one therapist is involved with the family, and the second therapist is seeing the family, or a subsystem of the family (sometimes just an individual), at a different time (thus distinguishing this approach from conjoint co-therapy). An example of the combined format is an adolescent who is being seen in individual and family therapy in a residential treatment setting. The mother is in a PHP many miles across the state and, in addition, is involved in couples therapy with her husband at the PHP. Another therapist is involved in treating the entire, larger family network.

Another example of the combined format that occurs frequently is when a psychiatrist who has a patient in individual therapy identifies significant couple or intergenerational issues that are not likely to resolve spontaneously with his or her individual clinical interventions. The psychiatrist refers the couple to a family therapist for ongoing systems work. However, the psychiatrist and his or her individual patient continue individual therapy because they believe it is still productive.

Both these situations, which often occur when treating difficult families, are examples of the combined format. For the combined format to work, the therapist must address a variety of clinical issues. The most important consideration is that the therapists must have a partnership characterized by adequate communication among themselves and joint treatment planning. Although helpful, it is not absolutely necessary that the therapists have worked together before. Effective communication must include a mutually agreed-upon conceptualization of the problem, treatment plan, goals, and interventions. Within this broader framework, there must be agreement on how the separate interventions will work together. Therapists who have reasonably similar treatment beliefs and some goodwill, and who are not excessively competitive with each other, can do well in such situations. Initial planning and ongoing communication are essential.

The combined format can fail for a variety of reasons. Communication is perhaps the most common reason for failure. Sometimes therapists are simply too busy or do not see the necessity for consultation. Splitting, particularly with difficult families, is the most common result of a lack of communication. Competition, one-upmanship, and deliberate triangulation in the family are only a few of the reasons for failure when the therapists are poorly prepared and badly motivated.

Co-therapy.   Co-therapy is a format in which two or more therapists treat the same family at the same time. The earlier example of the treatment of a schizophrenic patient and his family illustrates the potential usefulness of co-therapy. There has been significant debate over time about the efficacy of this format. Many clinicians in the family therapy world argue that co-therapy is a superior method for treating any system. Carl Whitaker, a well-known psychiatrist, has often stated, "It takes a system to treat a system." Although data-based studies have not demonstrated Whitaker's conclusion, considering the methodological difficulties in this kind of study, it is quite plausible that co-therapy makes a difference in particular clinical areas. Some difficult families, for example, may benefit from the co-therapy arrangement. Complicated families can overwhelm an individual therapist with transference and countertransference issues. In a co-therapy situation, it is possible to have more "therapeutic power" and to have increased degrees of freedom to intervene. For example, if one of the co-therapists is "limited" by a particular transference/countertransference situation with a given family member, the other therapist, free of such entanglements, can intervene.

An example of the benefits of co-therapy is provided by a 25-year-old borderline patient who has had multiple hospitalizations over the last 5 years. Her degree of psychopathology is such that stabilization in partial hospital and/or outpatient settings has been impossible up to now. Family therapy with one therapist had been tried several times. The therapist found himself unable to keep the family in therapy; he often felt that he was coerced into doing individual therapy because of worries about issues of liability and the patient's threats of suicide. Frequently, he felt that he was not free to maneuver in a way necessary to work on the family dynamics. Furthermore, the therapist felt that it was impossible to keep an empathic connection and to stay "joined" with each member of the system.

A year ago, this therapist added a co-therapist to his patient's treatment system and things began to change very quickly. As a team, the two therapists were less frightened by the patient's suicidal threats. Together, they were able to share responsibility and make less emotional decisions about when to make no-suicide contracts, when to commit her (this happened twice over the subsequent year), and when to simply throw the responsibility back to her and the family as a way of dealing with issues.

What about combining psychopharmacology?   There has been controversy about whether the psychiatrist should prescribe psychopharmacological agents for the individual patient if, in addition, family therapy is being used. The reasons for not prescribing are in some ways similar to those for not combining family therapy with individual psychotherapy. The therapist ends up focusing on the psychological dysfunction of one family member while trying to persuade the family to address their interactional issues. This transmits a muddled message to all family members. This issue is significantly more problematic in some types of family involvement than in others. For example, it causes little difficulty when family consultations are utilized to enhance an individual therapy. However, using a *family as unit* model makes it almost impossible for one to prescribe medication without getting caught in the bind of trying to move between the systemic and individual levels of the family. This switching can be done, but only with great difficulty.

My experience has been that while utilizing the *family as unit* model, the therapist should have someone else prescribing psychotropic medications. However, with the *family as context* model, it is much easier to do both the psychotherapy and the prescribing. In this situation, there is no contradiction between theoretical constructs. In other words, because there is an "individual patient" in the *family as context* model, the psychiatrist is not working against himself or herself in prescribing psychotropic medications. Of course, to the extent that the psychiatrist is doing any psychotherapy, the same issues of concern about diluting the motivation for psychotherapy and transference/countertransference complications arise when prescribing psychotropic medications.

Family Diagnosis

There is no section on "family diagnosis" in DSM-III-R (American Psychiatric Association 1987). However, preliminary meetings of the DSM-IV study groups have considered family diagnosis proposals. Over the years there has been a strong belief among significant members of the national family therapy leadership that a diagnostic framework would limit clinical practice. This has been based on the theme that an objectification of the family as "separate" from the therapist is not consistent with the systems model (Whitaker 1976). The crucial system, the argument goes, is the "meta-system" of the therapist and family, not one or the other. In addition, another factor that has mitigated against a consensually agreed-upon typology has been the multiplicity of major perspectives in the field. The intergenerational, structural/strategic, and experiential perspectives have each had, over time, a kind of typology, with some more developed than others (Gurman and Kniskern 1981). However, each is very different from the others, and, thus, any attempts at consensus have been stalemated.

Despite the lack of an agreed-upon typology, most clinicians have at least some informal diagnostic framework (Howells and Brown 1986). I will indicate briefly those "distinctions" that I have found most useful in clinical work.

One approach is to label a family by the pathology of the identified patient: the schizophrenic or anorexic family has at least one family member with schizophrenia or an eating disorder. This is useful because there are problems that are common to all families that have a schizophrenic member, as there are problems common to families that have a member with an eating disorder. It is important not to take this separation too far, because many of these families overlap in terms of crucial characteristics. Thus, I find it useful to look at the family itself rather then separate the families by an identified-member typology.

When one looks at the family as a whole, a simple typology that is often useful is separation by demographics. For instance, nuclear families (two generations, with both parents) are very different from single-parent families or from remarried families. It is useful to have a sense of the general differences among these various kinds of families.

I find it useful also to separate families along a continuum from "normal" or functional to mildly, moderately, and severely dysfunctional. There is a clinical literature that focuses on defining functionality in terms of various family "tasks." These tasks include boundary functions, effect of stability, problem solving, and so forth.

An important categorization includes distinguishing "enmeshed" from "disengaged" families. Enmeshed families are extremely overinvolved with each other. Object-relations theorists might say that there is an overuse of part objects for self representations. On the other hand, disengaged families are those in which members have little contact with one another.

Another continuum I find clinically useful is that of motivation for change of the family as a whole. On one end are those families that believe (either initially or with a little education from the therapist) that family work can be very helpful for a particular goal. These families are very different from families at the other end of the continuum who are unmotivated to change and/or are so anxious that they will not come to sessions or will allow crucial family members to miss sessions (the "absent member maneuver"). In between are families who are persuaded to come for reasons other than a belief in the efficacy of family work but are severely resistant or even oppositional in sessions. In general, the more a family is motivated, the greater the likelihood that *family as unit* work will succeed. *Family as context* and *family as background* fit best with families in the middle of this continuum. My experience has been that significant mistaken placement in terms of where the family fits on this continuum can result in profound clinical difficulties.

Specific "Difficult" Patients

I will highlight only a few "difficult" patient types that deserve particular comment. There are many other difficult clinical situations involving "difficult" patients, as illustrated throughout the chapter.

The Suicidal Patient

The advantage of any of the family therapy approaches with a suicidal patient is that one is in a better position to make an assessment and intervention than in an individual situation. Within a *family as background* perspective, the assessment involves getting other family members' views of the difficulties. This has been described in detail in the literature of suicidality and emergency psychiatry. A principle of emergency psychiatry is that a discharge to a supportive family context is much safer than a discharge to either no family or to a conflictual, unsupportive situation.

It is possible to create a support system within the family and to use it to cope with the suicidality. The *family as context* perspective supports doing this in an overt manner, maintaining a focus on the identified patient while also directly attempting to decrease the "friction" in familial relationships. The *family as unit* perspective presupposes that such therapeutic work will evolve within the context of deeper, insight-oriented therapeutic work. Co-therapy, as discussed above in the case of the borderline patient, is often an important therapeutic maneuver useful in these situations. Not only is the family supported in their burden of concern for the suicidal patient, but each co-therapist likewise is supported by the other therapist and by family members. A full team is at hand to manage the severe situation.

The Schizophrenic Patient

The formulation of the *family as unit* was tried for several decades (during the 1950s and 1960s) as a way of treating schizophrenic patients (Wynne et al. 1958). However, the results were equivocal at best and tended to alienate the family, who felt blamed for the illness of the identified patient. During the 1970s and 1980s, a psychoeducational model was developed for family intervention of schizophrenic patients (Hahlweg and Goldstein 1987). This model is essentially a *family as context* model in which the schizophrenic patient is seen as the unit of assessment and intervention. The family sometimes constitute a significant stressor to the patient (i.e., a high EE family), so a primary clinical goal is to change them into a support system for the patient over time. Ian Falloon, Robert Lieberman, and Carol Anderson are among those who have developed the best protocols for a psychoeducational approach (Falloon et al. 1984).

Essentially, behavioral family therapy protocols are used that focus on education, problem solving, and communication training. Large-scale studies by the National Institute of Mental Health (NIMH) are currently in progress that may shed some light on the question of how to best use these protocols. For example, whether to use home visits versus clinic visits, whether to have 12 sessions or 24 sessions, and how much follow-up is needed are among the questions these studies are striving to answer.

Important support groups have developed over the past two

decades for these families. Many of them are related to the National Alliance for the Mentally Ill (NAMI). Many states have developed their own chapters. My experience has been that these groups provide significant support for the schizophrenic patient as well as for his or her family. Although they are not for everyone, it is worth encouraging families to try out these groups.

Patients With Other Axis I Disorders

Patients with Axis I disorders have not been studied in as much detail as have schizophrenic patients. However, there is evidence that the same concepts are applicable to them. An ongoing NIMH study is using a psychoeducational protocol to study *family as context* work with bipolar patients. Also, diagnosis-specific support groups exist in many cities for patients and their families struggling with bipolar disorder, eating disorders, substance-use disorders, etc. Interventions for patients with obsessive-compulsive disorder and other anxiety disorders are the least developed, but are fertile grounds for development of similar models in the near future.

Patients With Borderline Personality Disorder

This is a very important group of patients, but a definitive, elaborate clarification of family involvement has not yet evolved. A significant body of literature in the 1970s and 1980s suggested *family as unit* involvement as the intervention of choice. As with schizophrenia, controlled studies have not documented the usefulness of such an approach. Gunderson has suggested a primary focus on individual or *family as background* approaches at the start of psychotherapeutic treatment with most borderline patients, with the understanding that this will evolve into *family as context* or *as unit* work with some families. Protocols for psychoeducational approaches (i.e., *family as context*) have yet to be elaborated with this group.

Conclusions

In this chapter I have presented concepts intended to assist the practicing psychiatrist in involving patients' families in clinical work. Delineating family involvement into three separate perspectives or degrees of involvement has been most useful in my practice and that of the residents I have trained with over the last 14 years at the University of Connecticut. It enables the clinician to involve the family in a legitimized, coherent, and helpful manner without having to know, in depth, many of the technical strategies of systemic family therapy. However, there are times when full family systems intervention is appropriate. Ideally, clinicians will, with the benefit of experience from family consultations, be able to identify these situations, develop more in-depth skills themselves if they are so inclined, and/or refer these patients to colleagues or specialists who have such training.

References

American Psychiatric Association: Diagnostic and Statistical Manual of Mental Disorders, 3rd Edition, Revised. Washington, DC, American Psychiatric Association, 1987

Becvar DS, Becvar RJ: Family Therapy: A Systemic Integration. Boston, MA, Allyn and Bacon, 1988

Falloon IRH, Boyd JL, McGill CW: Family Care of Schizophrenia. New York, Guilford, 1984

Group for the Advancement of Psychiatry, Committee on Family: The Family, the Patient, and the Psychiatric Hospital: Toward a New Model (GAP Rept No 117). New York, Brunner/Mazel, 1982

Gurman AS, Kniskern DP: Handbook of Family Therapy. New York, Brunner/Mazel, 1981

Hahlweg K, Goldstein MJ: Understanding Major Mental Disorder: The Contribution of Family Interaction Research. New York, Family Process Press, 1987

Health Management Strategies International: Mental Health Review Guidelines—HMS Criteria Manual. Gaithersburg, MD, Instruction Writers, 1991

Howells JG, Brown AWM: Family Diagnosis. Madison, CT, International Universities Press, 1986

Lansky MR: Family Approaches to Major Psychiatric Disorders. Washington, DC, American Psychiatric Press, 1985

Nichols MP, Schwartz RC: Family Therapy: Concepts and Methods. Boston, MA, Allyn and Bacon, 1991

Sauer RJ: Family therapy in a partial hospitalization setting. Family Therapy 11:211–215, 1984

Sugarman S: Combining family therapy with other clinical interventions, in Questions and Answers in the Practice of Family Therapy, Vol 2. Edited by Gurman AS. New York, Brunner/Mazel, 1982, pp 135–143

Whitaker CA: The hindrance of theory in clinical work, in Family Therapy: Theory and Practice. Edited by Guerin PJ. New York, Gardner Press, 1976, pp 154–164

Whitley MJ, Zankowski GL: Family therapy in a hospital setting: a model for time-limited treatment. J Psychoactive Drugs 18(1):61–64, 1986

Wynne LC, Ryckoff IM, Day J, et al: Pseudo-mutuality in the family relations of schizophrenics. Psychiatry 21:205–220, 1958

Chapter 11

Working With Sued Physicians

Sara C. Charles, M.D.

It might be suspected that physicians who seek psychiatric consultation as a result of having been sued offer therapists the opportunity to work with ideal patients who are bright, verbal, and well motivated. Although eager to return to their former state of psychological equilibrium, these doctors are often impeded in their ability to do so by a host of problems inherent both to their own usual mode of functioning and to the litigation experience itself.

In addition to dealing in a straightforward manner with any psychiatric disturbances identified in a sued physician-patient, the psychiatrist needs to have some understanding of the unique dimensions of this event. This includes an appreciation of the personality traits of physician patients, of the elements of the litigation experience that may be unfamiliar to the therapist but impinge on the therapeutic work, and of a variety of therapist transference and countertransference reactions. The following case vignette will illustrate many of these issues:

> Dr. A. is a 48-year-old obstetrician-gynecologist who has been in a solo private practice in the southeastern United States since completing his residency training 18 years ago. He sought psychiatric consultation after he read an article that described the effects of litigation on doctors. He had done well until he was sued for malpractice in his 10th year of practice. The case involved a

fetal death subsequent to complications of an amniocentesis that he had correctly diagnosed and for which he correctly initiated a caesarean section. He described having penetrated an aberrant vessel that caused the complication, the first such instance since his residency training. Following initiation of the suit he briefly experienced symptoms of depression, fleeting suicidal ideation, insomnia, and difficulty in concentration, but was generally able to function adequately throughout the process. Experts testified that the doctor was not negligent and the case was settled within the year. He continued to perform amniocenteses regularly with no undue anxiety or subsequent complications.

Seven years after the initiation of that first suit, he was again named in a suit for an incident that had also occurred in his 10th year in practice. He had delivered a fellow physician's child who had suffered minor neurological deficits, first noted when the child entered school. Shortly after being served with the summons, he became distraught and experienced depressed mood, increased appetite, anxiety, insomnia, periodic suicidal ideation, self-doubts, irritability, lack of concentration, preoccupations, and lack of sexual interest. He began to avoid performing amniocenteses. He discussed his problems with his wife, who suggested he give up the practice of obstetrics. He felt that she was emotionally unavailable and did not understand his concerns. She became increasingly dissatisfied with his lack of interest in family activities and in the couple's sexual relationship. Within 8 months, the doctor had developed a relationship with a nurse who he felt understood his distress, and, shortly thereafter, separated from his wife. His symptomatology has diminished and his malpractice case is still pending, although legal counsel has advised him that there is no evidence of negligence.

Dr. A. is an attractive man, elegantly attired, comfortable with his accomplishments but anxious about his current situation. He has always denied himself time for outside interests but has been generous and caring of his family. He feels guilty about leaving his wife and children. He is also ashamed of the changes he has introduced into his practice, especially because patients now have to obtain amniocentesis from a physician in a neighboring town. Dr. A. denies any current symptoms except for periodic crying spells. His most prominent symptom during the interview was intermittent overwhelming anxiety when certain subjects were broached. He would then say, "I'm confused . . .," and would lose the train of thought, recover gradually, and change the subject. He ruminates continuously about the events that led to his first malpractice suit, admitting that it is a distraction and affecting his concentration. He also states that his lack of availability to perform certain high-risk procedures has affected his practice base. He has considered leaving the practice of medicine but currently finds that solution untenable.

Elements in the Physician-Patient

Personality Characteristics of Physicians

Obsessive-compulsive personality traits are probably the most widely used adaptive approach by modern men and women as they attempt to achieve some illusion of safety and security in an otherwise uncertain world (Salzman 1980). Doctors are especially vulnerable to the development and nurturance of this mode of adaptation in the face of their limited control over the forces of nature, their awareness of both what they do and do not know, and their feeling that they are being pressured to possess both knowledge and control over illness and death. A central motivating dynamic derives not only from physicians' own need to control their environment but also from their patients' needs and expectations that they do so as well.

In a survey of 100 randomly selected physicians, Krakowski (1982) reported that 100% described themselves as having compulsive personalities. Gabbard has highlighted the normal doctor's vulnerability to feelings of self-doubt, guilt, and an exaggerated sense of responsibility. Such doctors tend to possess an inappropriate sense of responsibility for things beyond their control, experience chronic feelings of "not doing enough," have difficulty in setting limits, and have excessive feelings of guilt as well as confused ideas about selfishness and what constitutes healthy self-interest (Gabbard 1985). Such traits may characterize the individual drawn to a medical career. Medical training, however, reinforces these traits in an attempt to consolidate a professional identity that values not only personal competence and responsibility but also a commitment to placing the patient's welfare above self-interest. Although doctors may find their work absorbing, and therefore satisfying, these very traits may also be maladaptive, vulnerable to defensive excesses, and detrimental to physicians' psychological health (Gabbard 1985).

Malpractice litigation impels into the psychiatrist's office many physicians who function in this compulsive manner and who otherwise would not need or seek therapy. Dr. A., in the example above, has been successful, has raised a family, and has been well regarded in his community. He has a stable family of origin, and, although he has maintained good relationships with them, he has not needed them for many years. Nor has he required much affection or sensitivity from his own spouse, his children, or his peers. He managed his solo practice and his first malpractice case relatively well. Only when he received his second summons did he feel the full brunt of the accusation that he had failed. Given his basic personality, Dr. A. has developed excessive anxieties about the degree of control he had over the events in question, feels ambivalent and guilty, and questions his decision-making capacities. His compulsivity reinforced, he devotes more time to work, worries constantly, and is less available emotionally.

The Work of the Physician

The nature and ongoing transformation of medical practice are further complicating factors of the litigation experience. Rene Fox has described medical practice as morally and existentially serious work from which doctors derive pressure to "define their work as limitless in time and potential urgency" as well as encounter the "uncertainties that stem from how much and how little they know." She maintains that no matter how much training or experience doctors may have, the "basic, human-associated stresses and dilemmas . . . cannot be eliminated" (Fox 1979). Added to these intrinsic pressures are a range of economic and legal intrusions associated with medical practice (Charles et al. 1987). Many of these intrusions have contributed to the breakdown of the accepted role of the physician as a trusted and competent authority in the community. The fabric of support afforded to physicians, both from society as a whole and from within the medical community, has deteriorated, leaving these individuals increasingly vulnerable to feelings of isolation. How individual doctors react to and manage these stressors is important in assessing the stressfulness of their litigation experience.

Doctors cope with the ordinary stressors of practice in a variety of ways (Linn et al. 1985). Vaillant et al. (1972) noted that doctors tend to use characteristic defense mechanisms such as reaction formation, hypochondriasis, and altruism; those with the least stable childhoods were more vulnerable to the occupational hazards of medicine and were, therefore, more likely to develop problems requiring psychiatric intervention. McCue (1982) suggested that doctors suppress their emotions, withdraw from the nonmedical world, and use denial and irony. We have found that most doctors tend to deal relatively effectively with ordinary practice stressors by identifying the source of stress and by actively addressing the problem (Charles et al. 1988b). When physicians are sued for malpractice, however, their usual pattern of coping temporarily fails, which results in the development of symptoms and the use of maladaptive strategies (Charles et al. 1985).

The Doctor as Mistake-Maker

Much attention has been paid in recent years to the potential for physicians to make mistakes. In early 1991, results of the Harvard Medical Practice Study suggested that adverse events occurred in almost 4% of hospitalizations, a goodly portion due to what was defined as substandard care (Brennan et al. 1991). Concomitant with this is the growing literature about the humanity and fallibility of the physician (Skelly 1990). David Hilfiker's (1985) writing on his own capacity for error in the context of a medical practice that prized care and competency enunciated for many practitioners their own deep and hidden concerns about their vulnerabilities.

When a bad outcome, misjudgment, or mistake occurs, the doctor is often the first to sense it. It may involve the permanent disability or death of a patient, which generates feelings of anger, guilt, shame, and a loss of self-esteem. In order to continue working in the face of these strong emotions, the doctor must often use massive denial and/or suppression (which might be expressed as "It wasn't my fault") or projection (e.g., "If that resident had checked on that blood level . . ."). Underlying these statements, however, is the knowledge, or at least suspicion, of failure. Much as doctors may wish to talk about and acknowledge such failures openly, the threat of litigation often limits their freedom to do so. If, after all, a doctor acknowledges a mistake to a patient, there is little defense if future litigation should occur. In addition, most physicians are well schooled by risk managers, whose advice to anyone involved in a potential "incident" is, "Don't talk to anyone about it." This powerful dynamic in the current climate of medical practice inhibits most doctors from freely acknowledging their "mistake-making" capacity.

The Doctor as Defendant

When the doctor is sued, the normal, useful adaptive obsessional personality traits that serve doctors and their patients well in ordinary times are the source of many of the problems associated with malpractice litigation.

A malpractice complaint almost invariably alleges a failure on the part of the physician to control the events that precipitated a negative outcome. For sued doctors, the central psychological event is the accusation that they have, in some manner, failed. This represents a narcissistic injury and an assault on their sense of personal integrity. It also dislodges the delicate equilibrium maintained by most doctors between their feelings of fallibility and vulnerability on the one hand, and the internal and external pressure to be infallible and omnipotent on the other. The resulting disequilibrium complicates their ability to continue the decision making that is integral to their work.

Unless an individual can be absolutely certain about the choices and decisions made, there exists the risk of making mistakes. For sued physicians, this prospect generates increased anxiety, especially in instances surrounding certain procedures or types of conditions that are high risk and/or are the focus of an already pending malpractice complaint.

The process of litigation is designed to determine who was in control in a given situation and who, therefore, was responsible for the outcome. The doctor's defense against the allegation almost always counters with evidence that the events could not be fully controlled. The nature of litigation is to weigh the one side against the other throughout the lengthy process, playing on the degree of personal responsibility to be borne by the accused physician. Given their compulsive adaptive style, and irrespective of litigation, doctors are constantly struggling to moderate their mildly neurotic demands to be ever more competent, knowledgeable, and conscientious within the context and awareness of their humanity against their pressure to devote more time to their personal lives. A lawsuit, which is an accusation in the public sector, externalizes the conflict and exacerbates physicians' vulnerability to self-doubt, guilt feelings, and an exaggerated sense of responsibility. The doctor's response often is, "It really is true. If I make a mistake or oversee a serious complication, I can be held legally liable. Therefore, I must try even harder to be perfect."

For many doctors, the conflicting demands in an environment so filled with risk are no longer psychologically tenable. Their compulsivity renders them unable to adapt effectively to both elements of the conflict. Overwhelmed and immobilized by anxiety, they in many instances withdraw from the source of their conflict. In Dr. A.'s case (see beginning of this chapter), the anxiety surrounding amniocentesis became intolerable and thus led to his decision to limit his practice in an effort to reduce his exposure to further litigation. The increasingly common reaction to refuse to perform procedures often generates more guilty feelings as doctors judge themselves harshly for acting out of self-interest. This cycle renders the affected doctor less able to seek the help so desperately needed to interrupt the process. Symptoms are minimized and anxiety increases; self-initiated behaviors designed to dampen the anxiety only serve to complicate it, and the fear of dependency and of loss of control leads the suffering physician to reject offers of help so that he can "work it out himself."

The Doctor as Patient

Doctors tend to adapt to the role of patient poorly largely because of their obsessive personality features. In order to become a patient, or, at minimum, to request help from another professional, the doctor needs to acknowledge a degree of vulnerability and dependency and give up some degree of control. Because many doctors perceive dependency as being out of control, becoming ill represents a personal failure (Marzuk 1987). As a result, they often minimize their symptomatology by using denial, which serves to defend against their feelings of lack of complete control over their body and emotions (Vaillant et al. 1972). They also tend to delay seeking help until they can diagnose themselves, which allows them to anticipate the nature of the potential workup and treatment plan. Armed with this knowledge and psychological advantage, they can approach the specialist with some measure of "self-control." When they are unable to accomplish this, doctors often feel anxious and become more compulsive, and, therefore, are even less able to seek help.

Dr. A. initially managed the effects of his first malpractice suit. He kept "control" over his feelings and maintained his practice. The case was settled, which meant he bore no legal guilt. His vulnerability to mistake-making and potential failure that was underscored by his first litigation experience, however, remained a nidus for self-doubt. His feelings of responsibility for the event were clearly unresolved, so that the first incident reemerged as *the* accusation upon being served with the second complaint. As his practice base declined and his family became increasingly alienated, Dr. A. finally decided to seek psychiatric consultation in a manner that assured him of being "in control," miles away from home in a "safe" environment.

Elements in the Litigation Experience

The Epidemiology of Malpractice Litigation

In the early research on physicians who had been sued, striking features of their experience were the feelings of social isolation and the loss of self-esteem associated with being singled out as a "bad doctor." Acquiescing to legal advice, doctors did not talk to anyone about their litigation, making them feel even further isolated. When data on the incidence and prevalence of litigation became more available, doctors became aware not only that, indeed, they were not alone but also that litigation is not an uncommon experience in medical practice. Such knowledge is the cornerstone of primary interventions aimed at diminishing the lack of social support so keenly felt. Psychiatrists engaged in work with these doctors will do well to keep abreast of trends in medical malpractice litigation in order to appreciate the feelings of the affected physician within the context of the litigation climate.

In the first half of the 1980s it was estimated that one of every four physicians was sued for medical malpractice at least once (American Medical Association 1989). Although the incidence of litigation decreased sharply after 1985, largely because of tort reform initiatives, there has once again been a gradual ascendance in the incidence of claims. In Cook County, Illinois, for example, the year 1990 saw the highest incidence of claims since 1985 (Cook County Jury Verdict Reporter 1991). Closely allied to incidence of malpractice claims is their prevalence in the physician population. A 1990 survey of Illinois physicians found that 54% of respondents were currently involved in litigation (Illinois State Medical Insurance Exchange 1990). However, this high prevalence may be due, in part, to the length of time it takes to process a claim. Many of the cases that went to trial in Cook County in 1990, for example, were filed in 1979 and 1980.

Certain specialties are particularly vulnerable to claims. The average obstetrician/gynecologist has been sued three times (eight times for New York State doctors), and approximately 78% of them have been sued at least once (American College of Obstetricians and Gynecologists 1990). The responses to this experience by this segment of the physician population, which includes distancing themselves from high-risk work, are beginning to raise public policy questions. Psychiatrists who treat these doctors need to appreciate the profound personal reverberations of litigation not only on physicians but on their patients as well.

The Outcome of Litigation

If outcome is any measure of the appropriateness of these allegations, then it is clear that most physicians accused are found to be not guilty of negligence. Nationally, a 1984 study revealed that an estimated 57% of malpractice claims resulted in no payment to the plaintiff (U.S. Department of Health and Human Services 1987). The physician-owned insurer in Illinois has closed approximately 21,000 claims in its 16-year existence, 83% of which resulted in no payment to the plaintiff (Illinois State Medical Insurance Exchange 1990). This provides a curious counterpoint to the widely publicized studies that suggest that far more medical injury occurs than is reflected by the number of malpractice claims filed (Brennan et al. 1991). Nonetheless, the fact that an average of four out of every five claims are determined to have no legal basis underscores the serious repercussions that flow from the *allegation* of medical malpractice. It is usually the allegation of negligence, not the specific outcome of the case, that generates the symptomatic and behavioral changes that ensue and that prompts the physician to obtain psychiatric consultation (Charles et al. 1988a).

No matter how diligently physicians try, because of the nature of their work, they are vulnerable to error and poor outcomes and, therefore, to legal liability under the current tort system. The commonly accepted rationale that the current medical malpractice system exists to assure the public of the highest quality of care does not, in fact, achieve that goal. Rather than ensuring competence, the current malpractice system addresses the issue of compensation, albeit ineffectively (Danzon 1985). What is clear, irrespective of the arguments for and against, is that, under a cloud of the accusation of incompetence, many well-functioning, highly competent, albeit excessively compulsive, doctors are exposed to a major life event that ultimately compromises their ability to function optimally, alters the climate of mutual trust between doctor and patient, achieves little gain for most plaintiff-patients, and may, in the long run, compromise access to care for certain segments of the patient population.

Psychological Implications of the Process of Litigation

An allegation of malpractice cannot be factored into the average doctor's practice just as the "cost of doing business." It plunges the doctor into an alien environment, a legal system that proceeds according to its own rules and time frame and confers on the doctor a new and unfamiliar identification, that of a defendant. Because most doctors possess little semblance of control within the legal environment, they often feel impotent and anxious. They become largely dependent on the process itself for resolution and on their attorneys for guidance and direction. No matter how they might wish to influence, interrupt, or terminate the process, doctors are generally frustrated in their attempts to do so.

As shown in Table 11–1, the process of litigation is a series of events, each imbued with its own degree of stress. The chronicity of the process, the feeling that the charge of incompetence is used primarily to determine compensatory damages, and the lack of predictability of outcome all contribute to its stressfulness. If the case is not dropped or terminated for technical reasons, it is often settled. In this instance, the issue of control again becomes a central psychological factor. When a doctor settles a case, there is no assessment of legal guilt, but neither is there a statement of vindication. When settlement is forced by the insurer, without consultation or the acquiescence of the involved physician, the psychological repercussions may be quite different than if the doctor, in consultation with the involved parties, chooses to settle.

When a judgment of negligence is assessed at trial, the defendant physician often experiences feelings of low self-esteem, isolation, and depression. This is particularly evident in those doctors who are confronted with a negative judgment associated with an untoward occurrence or misjudgment in an otherwise competent and well-regarded practice. It is not uncommon for psychotherapy to be indicated for these physicians in order for them to regain emotional equilibrium and deal with such issues as suicidality, retirement, or specialty and practice changes.

Two developments related to outcome are beginning to increase the stressfulness of litigation for physicians. Settlements of any amount, even the most negligible sum, are now reported to and held permanently in a federal data base, the National Practitioner Data Bank. It is too early to determine what, if any, long-term repercussions this will have on an individual physician's

---

Table 11–1.　The litigation process

The summons　The summons, a formal legal document issued by the clerk of the court and usually served by the sheriff, is notification that a suit has been filed.

The complaint　This document accompanies the summons and tells in legal terms the nature of the complaint. It may be preceded or followed by a notice in the local newspaper.

The pleading stage　Shortly after the complaint is filed, the attorney begins to communicate with the court by filing *motions,* a request addressed to the court to do something.

The discovery stage　A process designed to discover information relevant to the case. This includes *interrogatories* (i.e., written questions) and *depositions* (i.e., oral questions and verbal responses taken before a person empowered to take testimony under oath). The discovery may also request *inspection of documents* and/or *physical and mental examinations.* For the psychiatrist, this stage often raises conflicts about confidentiality issues.

Expert witnesses　A case proceeds only if each side presents experts who will give an opinion about whether the facts relevant to the case represent a deviation from the accepted standard of medical care.

Summary judgment　The summary judgment is a decision entered by the judge when it is clear that all the facts indicate that one or other side of the case should win. If a judgment is issued, the case is resolved.

The trial　This phase may be preceded by a series of pretrial maneuvers that may or may not contribute to a resolution of the case by settlement or some other method. If these fail, the case goes to trial before a judge or a judge and jury as determined by laws in a given location.

The verdict　The verdict is the decision reached by the deciding body.

Posttrial activities　If a participant fails to receive a favorable verdict, the law permits a number of procedures to appeal the outcome. A *posttrial motion* must be submitted within a prescribed period of time and is a request to the court to void the verdict usually on technical grounds. A formal *appeal* may also be initiated to overturn the verdict on legal grounds.

career. It represents, nonetheless, an added source of anxiety for physicians who wish to settle. A second development relates to the fact that, previously, a trial verdict rarely assessed damages beyond the physician's insurance coverage. An increasing number of recent judgments, however, have exceeded insurance coverage and threaten the safety of the physician's personal assets. The threat of financial ruin exacerbates to a frightening degree the physician's already stressful experience of having been judged as negligent.

A useful paradigm for understanding doctors' reactions is the one utilized by Folkman and Lazarus (1980). They describe two factors—the context of the event and how it is appraised—as critical influences on the complex process of how an individual copes with a life event. The context of an event is "what it is about" in terms of the person's health, work, family, or other dimensions of life. Appraisal involves concomitant cognitive processes that evaluate the meaning or significance of an event as well as what can and might be done about it. When an event such as an illness is appraised as having few possibilities for change or influence, the individual's coping response tends to be more emotion-focused—that is, geared to regulate uncomfortable emotions. When an event occurs, such as in the work environment, that is appraised as alterable by taking specific action, problem-focused coping responses predominate. Folkman and Lazarus note that while both styles are used in most events, the proportion of their use varies as a function of the individual's appraisal of the event.

The context of litigation is primarily the work environment that the doctor theoretically "controls." The meaning of the event is usually assessed in both personal and professional terms related to issues of control, integrity, and competence. The accusation is experienced as "I am not only a bad doctor but a bad person." These feelings are further influenced by the nuisance value of the suit, by the amount of publicity that accompanies it, and by the nature and intensity of the relationship that the physician had with the accusing patient.

We found that the appraisal of litigation as the most stressful event in one's life may be a useful predictor of coping response (Charles et al. 1988a). Doctors who reported this as their most stressful life event had significantly more symptoms, especially of depression, and used emotion-focused coping more often than did doctors who mentioned some other previous life event as being most stressful. In this instance, no doctor who rated litigation as his or her most stressful life event had been divorced or had suffered the death of a spouse or child, events acknowledged as more stressful by the other doctors. Physicians in this latter group were more likely to use problem-focused coping styles in response to both ordinary stressors and their most stressful life event.

Evaluation and Treatment of Sued Physicians

Evaluation

In addition to conducting a thorough psychiatric evaluation, the psychiatrist needs to be mindful of elements of the litigation experience and personal history that are particularly relevant to the physician population (see Table 11–2). In many instances, the evaluation process serves also as a therapeutic intervention and therefore must be thorough, empathic, and, perhaps, more active than

---

Table 11–2.   Psychiatric evaluation of the sued physician

Specific areas of inquiry in addition to the routine assessment include
- ◆ A short history of the litigation experience
- ◆ Current stage of litigation
- ◆ Expert opinion offered regarding the case
- ◆ Advice of insurance and legal counsel
- ◆ Past and present medical history
- ◆ Past psychiatric consultation and/or treatment
- ◆ Child and adolescent adjustment history
- ◆ Past and present prescribed medications
- ◆ Family history of psychiatric illness
- ◆ Recreational drugs and/or alcohol use
- ◆ Changes in practice behavior secondary to litigation
- ◆ Suicidal ideation

---

might otherwise occur. Some interpretive work may be not only appropriate but welcomed depending on the degree of receptivity of the patient.

Many doctors who in the past have questioned their mode of psychological functioning use the occasion as an entrée for seeking psychiatric consultation. In these cases, it is not the litigation itself that is the central issue, but a marital problem, misuse of drugs or alcohol, conflicts about career and/or retirement, or a long-term psychiatric problem. There are also many doctors for whom the litigation experience activates latent conflicts and/or pathology so that the resulting symptomatology necessitates some kind of consultation.

Irrespective of their motivation for seeking psychiatric consultation, these doctors recognize that their current state of disequilibrium has become untenable. This awareness enables them to break through their compulsive need to "be in control." For the majority, an evaluation alone gives them sufficient relief and some increased understanding of their feelings and reactions. For another group, although psychotherapy is recommended, there is a "flight into health," so that after one or two sessions they say, "Now I understand, and therefore I can handle it myself." The return of equilibrium may represent realignment of either healthy ego defenses or, in some cases, more maladaptive defenses. The psychiatrist may recommend treatment to doctors from this latter group that may be accepted. It is not uncommon, however, for such patients to fail to follow through, because their own sense of self-esteem and their compulsive style prevent them from doing so. In addition, there are many doctors who clearly recognize some of their shortcomings and the fact that psychotherapy would enable them to gain better control, but they fear the potential changes required for a successful resolution of their conflicts.

Transference and Countertransference Issues

Psychiatrists, because of the nature of their work and their patients, often evoke ambivalent feelings within the medical community. Psychiatrists' own strivings for omnipotence and grandiosity are enhanced when patients, often quite prominent in the community, seek consultation about their litigation experience. A psychiatrist who is singled out as one who could possibly understand and help in such instances may develop feelings that could influence treatment. Most common is the psychiatrist's attempt to secure physician-patients' trust by offering them evidence of their own trustworthiness as physicians. The psychiatrist thereby assumes that the physician-patient is knowledgeable about the psychiatric examination and therefore deviates from his or her usual routine of inquiry by allowing the doctor to offer spontaneously any relevant information. Striving not to offend or discomfort the physician-patient, the psychiatrist may conduct a limited, nonproductive, and ultimately harmful evaluation. A clear drug and alcohol history, mental status assessment, suicide potential, sexual history, medical history, and/or other pertinent elements of the evaluation might therefore be minimized, overlooked, or avoided. Related to these transference feelings are Marzuk's (1987) reminders of how doctors manage the issues of privacy, control, and support with their physician-patients.

One of the complications involved in the care of doctors is that the treating physician often has the same personality characteristics as the patient (Galloway 1981). Doctors' compulsive personality style renders them prone not only to self-criticism but to ready criticism of their peers. Psychiatrists are no exception to this rule. They do, however, possess specific skills that enable them to be cognizant of these psychological interferences that inhibit successful work. Especially important is the objective assessment of a doctor's relative guilt related to the event at issue. Many psychiatrists working with sued physicians, because of the threat that litigation poses to them as practitioners and their own need to disavow it as a potential threat, automatically presume that an allegation is most likely a sign of guilt. Psychiatrists, however, can only be helpful if they are relatively free of their own transference distortions. It is important to carefully listen to the sued physician about the assessments of negligence and the advice offered by defense counsel, insurance personnel, and experts as the case progresses. The degree of real versus neurotic guilt that the sued doctor experiences is a central issue in his or her ability to successfully cooperate in the defense of the case.

Countertransference feelings, defined as transference reactions to the patient's transference feelings, are particularly relevant when psychiatrists treating physician-patients have themselves had a previous or current malpractice suit filed against them. This situation may easily lead to overt identification with the accused and interfere with the objective evaluation and/or therapy of the doctor. Physicians' struggles to balance their professional and personal life, and their obsessive struggles relative to control over their work, as well as the conflicts inherent to the litigation process, all can stimulate reactions in the psychiatrist that can compromise the patient's freedom to proceed without interference.

A significant source of countertransference distortion occurs when the psychiatrist judges the sued doctor to be impaired and, therefore, presumably guilty or harmful to patients. No empirical research has established a relationship between malpractice litigation and physician impairment. Anecdotal evidence suggests that impaired physicians are proportionately less likely to be sued than the general physician population because they tend to see fewer patients and engage in less high-risk work. The role of the psychiatrist in these instances, therefore, is to maintain neutrality, recognize and deal with his or her own countertransference feelings, and treat the psychopathology of the patient directly. The fact that these patients often use denial vis-á-vis their degree of disability and their level of professional performance complicates this task.

A physician-patient accused of undue familiarity provides another source of countertransference feelings. Countertransference rage is not uncommon, and these feelings are complicated by the knowledge that some of these doctors use denial regarding their culpability and engage in "stonewalling" maneuvers, often for lengthy periods during the process. At issue for the patient is the potential for earning a livelihood if a final judgment is rendered. Aware of this, the treating psychiatrist should nonetheless proceed cautiously regarding the patient's relative guilt. Related issues that complicate this stance include conflicts about the potential harm done to the patient, the psychiatrist's professional ethical obligations, and the potential for involvement in subsequent related litigation and disciplinary proceedings. On occasion, personal consultation is indicated to separate out the psychiatrist's personal reactions from the professional duty to the physician-patient and the latter's ethical obligation to patients.

Treatment

Any diagnosable psychiatric illness can be precipitated by the stress of litigation and should be treated accordingly, although psychotic illnesses are infrequent. Alcohol and drug abuse may emerge or may represent the exacerbation of a previous illness. When indicated, the doctor should be referred to a substance abuse program. This may require the participation of the local impaired physicians' committee, especially when a referral is rejected or felt to be inappropriate.

The most common diagnoses necessitating treatment include an adjustment reaction, posttraumatic stress disorder, and a personality disorder, especially of an obsessive-compulsive nature. Major depressive disorder is not uncommon, but relatively few doctors actually seek treatment for it.

Psychiatric evaluation often reveals evidence of a newly developed physical illness or the exacerbation of a previously diagnosed one. The opportunity to enumerate physical symptoms and express concerns about them often enables the doctor to break through the denial previously in place and accept the referral for medical evaluation. The most common illnesses are those associated with stress, such as coronary artery disease, hypertension, and gastrointestinal disorders.

Adjustment reactions.   For most doctors, after being named in a claim, especially the first time, there is a temporary period of emotional disequilibrium in which insomnia, anger, lowered self-esteem, anxiety, irritability, depression, and/or diminished interest in work and pleasure are prominent. Given their commonly shared compulsive personality characteristics, doctors are more comfortable in control and feel vulnerable if perceived as out of control. Consequently, insurers and medical societies who work with these doctors have initiated programs aimed at quickly providing "buffers" against the impact of litigation. These programs are designed to provide the physician with information utilizing print literature and audio- and videotapes that doctors can use in privacy. This allows doctors the opportunity to regain control on their own, which is an enormous aid to their damaged self-esteem.

Other more public programs aimed at providing education and support are also useful. The primary goal of these and the previously described interventions is to support the doctor's healthy defenses so that he or she can return to optimal functioning as soon as possible.

The majority of doctors will respond well to a self-initiated and/or organized program of intervention that provides social support, some feeling of mastery over their environment, and increased self-esteem, and enables them to change the meaning of the event. Because the litigation has already occurred, these interventions only serve to buffer the impact of the event itself.

The single most important intervention in any major life event is social support (Cobb 1976). This is no less true in the case of sued doctors. The common myths associated with medical malpractice litigation theoretically mitigate against the provision of social support because sued doctors are assumed to be "bad doctors" and, therefore, undeserving of support. Associated with being named in a suit is rejection and isolation not only from society as a whole but from within the medical community as well. Many doctors also impose an isolation on themselves by withdrawing from peers in a variety of ways. As noted previously, when a doctor is notified of pending litigation, defense counsel immediately cautions against discussing the case with anyone, which results in further isolation. In more recent years, in recognition of the detrimental psychological effects of the prohibition against physician-patients sharing their personal anguish about the litigation, not only have doctors begun to talk about its effects on them personally, but many medical societies have taken bold steps to provide social support for their affected members during this critical time.

Active suggestions for enhancing feelings of mastery and increased self-esteem (Pearlin and Lieberman 1979) include doctors' taking the initiative to educate themselves about the legal process, seeking more input from their attorneys and insurers, reevaluating priorities in their personal and professional life, and reassessing risk-management strategies in their practice and among their office personnel (Charles 1989). These suggestions are especially useful when the psychiatrist has assessed the doctor to be basically healthy but symptomatic because of an inability to control the events associated with litigation. By offering strategies that enhance self-esteem and give the doctor some feeling of control over those areas of practice that lend themselves to change and mastery, the psychiatrist can be of enormous help. It is also useful to encourage doctors to enhance their feelings of competence by taking more time for continuing education, special courses, writing articles, and/or participating as an expert witness.

The common meaning attributed to litigation is that the doctor is bad, incompetent, and deserving of sanction. As long as doctors accept this, they will remain symptomatic and their work will be sorely compromised. A range of psychological maneuvering is immediately and instinctively set into motion by most people experiencing a major life event in order to change the meaning of the event (Pearlin and Schoolar 1978; Pearlin et al. 1981). Doctors express this as, "I'm not a bad doctor. This was a bad outcome, but . . ." The psychiatrist can contribute to this effort by helping the doctor review the relative defensiveness of the case, by actively recommending relevant literature, and by supporting the doctor's healthy defenses, including denial. These doctors need to change the "meaning" of the event, that is, to find a way to think about themselves as both "good" and competent in order not only to continue their work but also to function as a good defendant throughout the process of litigation.

Some authors have suggested that the most effective intervention in terminating the symptomatic effects of the litigation experience is to settle quickly and, ideally, to deal with the issue in psychotherapy (Horowitz 1989). A legal settlement does not assess guilt, nor does it vindicate the accused. It does terminate the process so that further associated stressors are prevented. The drawback for many doctors, however, is that a settlement is not vindication, so lingering doubts may persist, much as they did in Dr. A's first case (see beginning of chapter). Many doctors, especially the more compulsive ones, have great difficulty forgiving themselves without some objective vindication but, having settled, have no remaining legal redress. Dr. A. was unable to settle many of the psychological issues associated with his first case until he was sued again. Psychiatrists treating patients in such a situation should review not only the short-term pros and cons of settlement with the defendant physician but the potential long-term effects as well. Each individual must review an agreement to settle in the light of its meaning for him or her individually. For many doctors, vindication is the only healing solution. The recent requirement that all settlements are to be reported to the National Practitioner Data Bank further complicates these considerations.

The majority of doctors respond well to the suggestions offered above. When symptoms linger, brief dynamic psychotherapy (most often time-limited) is useful. Techniques utilized include some elements of support and interpretation as well as cognitive restructuring. Periodic sessions during the critical periods of the litigation process are often also useful.

Posttraumatic stress disorder. Although many doctors experience a moderately severe stress response syndrome, the frequency of posttraumatic stress disorder subsequent to litigation is estimated to be low. When it does occur, it is not the litigation event that most often stimulates the response, but rather the event that precipitated the litigation in the first place. In Dr. A.'s case, it was the perforation of the aberrant vessel that led to exsanguination, which led to a fetal death. This was the "violent" act that Dr. A. not only witnessed but oversaw. The literature that reviews the relationship between the development of symptomatology associated with life events underscores the importance of events that not only are undesirable but also are to some extent within the person's control (Fairbank and Hough 1979). Dr. A.'s conflict over the degree of control he could acknowledge relative to this event was at the core of his symptoms. If he assessed himself as fully responsible, he deserved to feel guilty. Despite his capacity to continue to work effectively when initially sued, he continued to struggle with how much control he did or could have exerted over the event. Settlement may have been a practical solution at the time, but it did not vindicate him or erase its impact. Subsequent litigation uncovered the unresolved issues surrounding the event.

For doctors with this diagnosis, time-limited psychotherapy, such as outlined by Horowitz (1989), can be helpful. The use of anxiolytics and/or antidepressants is not generally recommended in this population, nor are these agents often accepted when recommended. Doctors, however, are often amenable to the short-term use of hypnotics as an aid to sleep. These, of course, should not be self-prescribed but used under medical supervision.

In Dr. A.'s case, psychotherapy was recommended. He was concerned that a short-term psychotherapy aimed at relieving his symptomatology would reveal his need for a longer-term therapy related to his compulsive adaptation. This, he felt, could be potentially disruptive. He did, however, agree to a few sessions in which he and the therapist could further explore the possibility of committing himself to a course of psychotherapy.

Obsessive-compulsive personality disorder.   Doctors with obsessive-compulsive personality disorder tend to seek therapy when the stress of litigation compromises their defensive posture and leads to symptoms of dysphoria and other symptoms of depression. As Salzman has noted, the problems implicit in therapy with this group derive from their defensive structure, which is antithetical to the therapeutic task (Salzman 1980). They tend to be controlling, perfectionistic, grandiose, and indecisive, and can easily draw the therapist into a "tug of war." Of central importance is the reminder noted earlier, that psychiatrists are themselves more similar than dissimilar to these patients in terms of their personality characteristics (Galloway 1981). Unless the therapist is careful about his or her own feelings of control and omnipotence, the therapy can be unduly prolonged, poorly focused, and ultimately unsuccessful.

Conclusions

The goal of the evaluation and treatment of sued physicians is to quickly assess and correctly diagnose the degree of disequilibrium experienced so that they can be restored as closely as possible to their premorbid level of functioning. An additional goal is to prevent the development of long-term disability and/or impairment.

Almost irrespective of their final diagnosis, sued physicians who seek psychiatric consultation have one commonly shared characteristic: they want immediate relief. Most did not have significant symptomatology prior to the litigation. They feel they have been unjustly accused, and they find the disruption afforded by litigation unnerving and untenable. They tend to pressure the psychiatrist for a "short-cut" or "quick cure" and have unrealistic expectations about the nature of psychiatric treatment, and they will often express frustration with and rejection of the therapist's efforts. Acquainting physicians with this dimension of their personality functioning is often helpful in preparing them for treatment recommendations.

Most doctors develop at least a temporary period of emotional symptomatology. Despite this, they are not and should not be viewed as impaired. Just as the military has learned to reassure soldiers suffering from battle fatigue and to quickly restore them to their units, so should psychiatrists who work with sued physicians reassure them that the latter's responses to litigation are not signs of major mental illness but normal and expected reactions to a major life event.

A basic philosophical premise underlying this work is that the majority of these doctors are fairly healthy, competent, and well functioning, and that litigation is a major life stressor. The stressor is not easily dismissed; sometimes lasting for many years, it initiates a whole series of events that will cause further stress. Doctors, therefore, often need help in their efforts to diminish symptoms, to deal as effectively as possible with the event, to exercise a degree of control over their reactions, and to continue to deliver high-quality and competent care to their patients. In large measure, physicians' ability to maintain some level of self-esteem and self-

confidence during the process is highly dependent on their ability
to continue to work effectively.

References

American Medical Association, Specialty Society Medical Liability Project
(AMA/SSMLP): Trends in Medical Liability. Chicago, IL, American
Medical Association, 1989, pp 4–5

American College of Obstetricians and Gynecologists: Professional liability and its effects: report of a 1990 survey of ACOG's membership.
Washington, DC, American College of Obstetricians and Gynecologists, 1990

Brennan TA, Leape LL, Laird NM, et al: Incidence of adverse events and
negligence in hospitalized patients. N Engl J Med 324:370–376, 1991

Charles SC: Stress associated with malpractice litigation, in American Psychiatric Press Review of Psychiatry, Vol 8. Edited by Tasman A, Hales
RE, Frances AJ. Washington, DC, American Psychiatric Press, 1989,
pp 531–548

Charles SC, Wilbert JR, Franke KJ: Sued and nonsued physicians' self-reported reactions to malpractice litigation. Am J Psychiatry 142:437–
440, 1985

Charles SC, Warnecke RB, Wilbert JR, et al: Sued and nonsued physicians:
satisfactions, dissatisfactions, and sources of stress. Psychosomatics
28:462–466, 468, 1987

Charles SC, Pyskoty CE, Nelson A: Physicians on trial: self-reported reactions to malpractice trials with a comparison to previous studies. West
J Med 148:358–360, 1988a

Charles SC, Warnecke RB, Nelson A, et al: Appraisal as a factor in coping
with malpractice litigation. Behav Med 14:148–155, 1988b

Cobb S: Social support as a moderator of life stress. Psychosom Med
38:300–313, 1976

Cook County Jury Verdict Reporter (CCJVR): 1990 Medical Malpractice
Suit Index. Chicago, IL, Max Sonderby, January 1991

Danzon PM: Medical Malpractice: Theory, Evidence and Public Policy.
Cambridge, MA, Harvard University Press, 1985

Fairbank DT, Hough RL: Life event classification and event-illness relationship. Journal of Human Stress 5:41–47, 1979

Folkman S, Lazarus RS: An analysis of coping in a middle-aged community sample. J Health Soc Behav 21:219–239, 1980

Fox RC: The human condition of health professionals. Lecture given at University of New Hampshire, Durham, NH, November 19, 1979

Gabbard GO: The role of compulsiveness in the normal physician. JAMA 254:2926–2929, 1985

Galloway G: Are doctors different? Reflections on the psychodynamics of physicians. J Fla Med Assoc 88:281–284, 1981

Hilfiker D: Healing the Wounds. New York, Pantheon, 1985

Horowitz MJ: Post-traumatic stress disorder, in Treatments of Psychiatric Disorders, Vol 3: A Task Force Report of the American Psychiatric Association. Washington, DC, American Psychiatric Association, 1989, pp 2065–2082, 1989

Illinois State Medical Insurance Exchange: Loss analysis and report. Chicago, IL, Illinois State Medical Insurance Exchange, January 1992

Illinois State Medical Society, Membership survey. Chicago, IL, Illinois State Medical Society, 1990

Krakowski AJ: Stress and the practice of medicine, II: stressors, stresses, and strains. Psychother Psychosom 38:11–33, 1982

Linn LS, Yager J, Cope D, et al: Health status, job satisfaction, job stress, and life satisfaction among academic and clinical faculty. JAMA 254:2775–2782, 1985

Marzuk PM: When the patient is a physician. N Engl J Med 317:1409–1411, 1987

McCue JD: The effects of stress on physicians and their medical practice. N Engl J Med 306:458–463, 1982

Pearlin LI, Schoolar C: The struggle of coping. J Health Soc Behav 19:2–21, 1978

Pearlin LI, Lieberman MA: Social sources of emotional distress, in Research in Community and Mental Health, Vol 1. Edited by Simmons R. Greenwich, CT, JAI Press, 1979, pp 217–248

Pearlin LI, Lieberman MA, Meneghan EG, et al: The stress process. J Health Soc Behav 22:337–356, 1981

Salzman L: Treatment of the Obsessive Personality. New York, Jason Aronson, 1980, p xii

Skelly FJ: When doctors aren't perfect. AM News, November 23–30, 1990, p 25

U.S. Department of Health and Human Services: Report of the Task Force on Medical Liability and Malpractice. Washington, DC, Department of Health and Human Services, 1987, p 57

Vaillant GE, Sobowale NC, McArthur C: Some psychological vulnerabilities of physicians. N Engl J Med 287:372–375, 1972

Section III:

Therapist Factors

Introduction to Section III

The authors in the three chapters of this final section deal with countertransference problems as well as therapist behaviors. Victor Altshul, and Michael Selzer and John Grimaldi, in Chapters 12 and 13, respectively, give us two different views on countertransference issues, one with patients who present certain characteristic resistances and one with psychotic patients. Dianna Hartley, in Chapter 14, provides us with a particularly useful account of psychotherapeutic mistakes and demonstrates a way of thinking about these difficulties that is especially valuable to the clinician. Hartley makes the point that mistakes are ubiquitous and must be dealt with forthrightly by the therapist.

Chapter 12

Some Characteristic Initial Resistances in Psychotherapy

Victor A. Altshul, M.D.

Patients entering therapy tend to have ideas about it that are very different from those of the therapist. They may think the point of therapy is to be understood by the therapist rather than to engage in a difficult process that aims to overcome resistance and promote self-understanding. They may think the point is to evoke the therapist's sympathy and thus may experience a neutral or detached response as a hostile attack. Patients' conception of words themselves may be different from the therapist's. They may view words as not having any importance in and of themselves—as not being connected to anything real. They may see words not as vehicles for communicating significant ideas or feelings, but rather as devices for evoking and manipulating affect in the therapist.

Ordinarily, as therapists, we view these differences as signs of *initial resistance*. This usage seems problematic, because before the patient arrives there has been no agreement about what he or she is supposed to be doing there. What, therefore, can the patient be said to be resisting, when he or she may have no idea what the purpose of the enterprise is supposed to be? Nevertheless, I propose to retain the term, partly because the usage is conventional and partly because these characteristic ideas, styles, and expectations soon become used in the service of opposing insight.

The resistances I will describe tend to be massive. They do not

347

present themselves as discrete, articulated wishes not to engage in a process of self-understanding, but rather involve the entire character structure of the patient. In other words, the resistance itself consists in the very character patterns evinced by the patient in the first two or three interviews. Because the therapist is initially unfamiliar with the patient's character style, the therapist often may not conceptualize the patient's presentation of himself or herself as a resistance. Instead, the therapist may be aware of discomfort and incongruities within himself or herself, for which he or she cannot easily account.

The therapist may, for example, find himself talking at cross purposes with the patient and be unable to find the reason for it (Altshul 1977). The therapist may experience a disruption of his empathy with the patient, or, more severely, a failure to experience empathy from the beginning. He may even find himself frankly disliking the patient without knowing why (Altshul 1980; Maltsberger and Buie 1974). In trying to account for these feelings he may have fantasies that he and the patient are "not on the same wavelength" or that the patient seems to espouse value systems that are not congruent with his own (Giovacchini 1975).

I believe that such inner experiences can be examined more fruitfully as manifestations of character resistances of the patient than as manifestations of value discordances or of problematic countertransference (Altshul and Sledge 1989). It is my aim to help the therapist translate his or her initial feelings of discomfort and incongruity into conceptualizations of resistance. In the service of providing a "road map" for the therapist, I offer a typology of resistances as well as some illustrative case material.

We may divide the resistances into five types: 1) ethical, 2) erotic, 3) aesthetic, 4) cognitive, and 5) ideological. This typology is offered as a conceptual convenience to the therapist. It is not intended to allow psychodynamic inferences, which would vary widely from patient to patient within each group. This typology does, however, offer two other advantages. One is that it might provide diagnostic clues that may not be clearly apparent from external signs. For example, an ethical type of resistance might alert the therapist to the presence of a narcissistic or sociopathic disorder;

an erotic resistance might indicate hysterical or borderline pathology; and the cognitive type might point to psychotic or obsessional disturbance, depending on the subtype.

The second advantage the typology offers is that it helps the therapist identify the kind of "countertransference trap" he or she is facing and needs to avoid. Each resistance to be described exerts a "countertransference pull" on the therapist; it puts psychological pressure on him or her to respond impulsively and untherapeutically, in either an overidentified or an adversarial way. This then interferes with the capacity for empathy, in my view the cornerstone for any effective therapeutic strategy. The therapist needs to be better able to contain the patient's offerings and the therapist's own initial reactions to them, so that he or she may "metabolize" them into a less intense, more neutral, and more therapeutic verbal response (Giovacchini 1975). Because each resistance tends to mobilize more or less characteristic countertransference reactions, it may be helpful for the therapist to have a conceptual framework within which to locate his or her own reaction.

Initial Resistances

Ethical Resistance

A resistance falls within the ethical category when the patient relates to the therapist in such a way as to cause the therapist to feel that a major value discordance exists between the patient and himself. The patient talks as if an ordinarily shared assumption about the way in which people ought to behave in our culture is absent from the patient's thinking. The patient appears not to notice that the therapist may feel disturbed about what he is hearing and may want to raise questions about it. Feeling that he cannot ask necessary questions for which the patient would not be ready, the therapist may feel stymied, impatient, and possibly even judgmental. The therapeutic task then becomes to restore or create an empathic bond with the patient through a fuller understanding of the resistance.

Case 1

Mr. A. presents for therapy after leaving his wife. He tells me he left the day before the birth of their first child. He says "stresses within the relationship" had made it impossible for him to stay, but does not say what they were. Mr. A. calls attention to his pain and loneliness and acts as if he expects me to sympathize with him. He shows no curiosity about the possible role of the baby in his decision to leave; he appears to be so caught up in his "pain" that the idea has probably not occurred to him. It also does not seem to have occurred to Mr. A. that he has hurt his wife and that others may criticize him for it; he does not attempt to justify his behavior to me. I feel so distracted by his apparent callousness that I think it would be a waste of time to raise questions about his feelings toward the baby; he would not be interested.

I wonder if I am dealing with a sociopathic personality. Combating the rush to premature judgment, I reflect that he is probably engaged in a massive effort not to think about the role of the baby and about the real nature of what he glibly calls his "pain." The blindness to his wife's pain and the bid for my sympathy may then be seen not as sociopathic maneuvers but as defensive shifts in emphasis. What had begun to appear as an ethical value discordance now looks more like a defensive constriction of the psychological field. I remind myself that the patient is not obligated, as I am, to interest himself in issues of dynamic relevance.

Immediately I feel less anxious and more attuned to the patient's psychological state. It is as if I have analyzed my own resistance in the act of analyzing his. I say, "You must indeed have been feeling a great deal of pain, or you would not have taken so drastic a step at such a critical time in the life of your family. Nevertheless, I am still quite unclear about the nature of this pain, and I am sure you are too. We need to work very hard together to understand it fully, to understand the connections between what you have been feeling and everything that has been going on in your life." I look at him and see that I have held his attention throughout my speech. The therapeutic alliance has begun.

Erotic Resistance

In erotic resistance the patient is preoccupied chiefly by fantasies of a romantic and sexual character, which come to center on the person of the therapist. In extreme cases these fantasies take the form of a concrete intent to seduce the therapist.[1]

For the patient with this resistance the medium of therapeutic exchange revolves around the wish to be loved by the therapist. This wish, and only this wish, is regarded as curative and preemptive. The patient is unmoved by, unmindful of, or scornful of the therapist's conviction that therapeutic progress involves not the gratification of feeling loved, but rather the psychological mastery that comes from renunciation, reflection, and understanding.

The wish to feel loved may be overshadowed by fantasies of a more sadistic nature, so that the seductive assault may become a frankly hostile attack. The patient may be motivated by an urge to demonstrate that the whole enterprise is corrupt and thus to destroy the therapist entirely, at least as a therapist.

Whatever the patient's motivation and fantasies, the situation presents grave clinical risks. For example, a patient's commitment to his or her own set of values may be stronger than the therapist's commitment to his own set of values. This may be particularly so at times in the therapist's life when his narcissistic vulnerabilities are at their highest, as for example when he is going through a divorce. At such times the therapist may find it easier to provide rationalizations and excuses for some slippage of his normal therapeutic frame of reference, which may then begin to move imperceptibly toward that of the patient (Langs 1982). The therapist may compound the difficulty by sending subliminal signals, outside his awareness, of his own neediness, which may then encourage the patient to redouble the intensity of the seductive behavior. As the therapist becomes more guiltily aware of his enmeshment in the process, he may lose sight of where the seductive impulse originated. At this point personal therapy for the therapist may be the only practical means of averting disaster (Altshul and Sledge 1989).

If the therapist has been able to withstand the assault and to refrain from compromising his therapeutic stance, a vigorous con-

---

[1]Despite my use of gender-specific pronouns, this kind of erotic assault may be mounted on a therapist of either sex by a patient of either sex.

frontation is often necessary. However, even the most gentle and empathic confrontation at this point is likely to humiliate the patient. Yet not to confront the patient in some measure would be to collude with the erotic resistance. The task of identifying the resistance without arousing undue shame will try the resources of the most inventive therapist. If one can, one should try to address the shame and deep sense of unlovability that almost always underlie this manner of presentation.

Case 2

A young general medical officer seeing psychotherapy patients in an army hospital under my supervision anxiously sought on-the-spot consultation. Ms. B., a young woman complaining of marital problems, voluptuously shaped and revealingly clad, had ended the first hour by offering her hand. With her thumb she slowly and circularly massaged the therapist's anatomical snuff-box (i.e., an area between the tendons of the proximal phalanx of the thumb, just beyond the wrist) while running the tip of her tongue slowly across her lips. At the end of the second hour he again allowed his hand to be taken. She repeated the maneuver, standing so close to him that her breast touched his hand; pursing her lips, she asked him to kiss her.

"My third-year psychiatry clerkship didn't prepare me for this," he said. "I didn't know what to do."

"So what did you do?" I asked.

"I improvised," he said. "I said, 'No, I don't think it is a good idea.' She asked, 'Why isn't it a good idea?' My mind went blank, but I remembered a resident telling me it doesn't hurt to be honest. So I said, 'I don't know why it isn't a good idea, I'm not thinking too clearly at the moment, but I've read somewhere it isn't a good idea, and if you'll just wait a week, I'll look it up and let you know, or maybe I'll discuss it with Captain Altshul and see what he has to say about it.' She was indignant about me telling you, but I said, 'Don't you think a chaperon wouldn't be such a bad idea?' She laughed at that, so I was able to get out of the session without kissing her, but God, did I want to. It was a close call."

"I think you did well to drag me into it," I said. "But next week you're going to have to face her alone again, and you'd better use this time to figure out the answer to her question."

He used the time well, as was evidenced by his review of the next session: "I began the next session by saying, 'I'd better deal with the problem between us right now, so the tension doesn't mount during the session. I'm not going to let you touch me any more, even to shake my hand. You're scared to tell me how bad things are with you, so you want to turn this into a sexual encounter. But this is therapy, not sex. It's therapy you badly need and therapy I want to provide. The last thing you need is another disastrous romantic encounter; I suspect you've been injured enough by those already.'"

"She was scornful. 'Captain Altshul has given you some pretty good lines,' she said. But I was ready for her reaction. 'I see that I embarrassed you by bringing him into it, and you're upset and sore about it. I don't blame you. But I needed to do that to cool us both down. And these are *my* words, not Captain Altshul's. I stand behind every one of them. Now let's get to work.' And by God, she did."

The young doctor recounted his surprise as she tearfully told him of her alcoholic father and of her long-standing inability to feel real love for any man.

Cognitive Resistance

The term *cognitive resistance* refers to the style in which some patients approach questions of thinking and knowing. It also refers to the differences between the patient's style and the therapist's. Of course, to the extent to which they deal quizzically or contemptuously with the therapist's psychological-mindedness and interest in exploration, all patients can be viewed as resisting in this fashion. I am referring, however, to a larger character style that seems to predominate above all others.

This category of patients is subdivided into two classes. The first describes the patient whose basic view of cognition is, from the therapist's point of view, *hyporational*. Diagnostically this group includes patients with a psychotic condition with disordered thought, with or without paranoia. The basic feature of this condition is the deterioration or absence of syllogistic reasoning.

There is a characteristic response on the part of many therapists to a florid display of psychotic verbalizations from the patient.

Often the therapist will feel confused, anxious, agitated, and incapable of framing a reply. Sometimes these affects are the result of a projective identification of the patient's state of mind. These affects may also be understood, however, as an anxious response to what may feel like an aggressive assault on the therapist's assumptions about cognition, which rely on empirical evidence and intact syllogistic logic. The patient may be unmindful of the therapist's presumptions about rationality, just as the therapist is distrustful of the patient's presumptions about rationality, and the patient may intensify his efforts to get his point of view across, thus exacerbating the sense of assault. My impression is that much of the dread commonly experienced by therapists in the presence of psychotic patients has as its basis this terror of a massive attack on the syllogistic structure of the therapist's thinking.

Case 3

> Mr. C., who was receiving outpatient treatment for schizophrenia, complained that he was unable to develop relationships beyond the most superficial level. He would go to dances by himself, strike up conversations with women, and, after some initial pleasantries, find that he was utterly unable to think of anything to say. The paralysis of thought and speech was accompanied by debilitating anxiety. Feeling that he was not interested in the woman anyway, he would turn away from her in an apparent effort not to recognize that she had already begun to turn away from him.
>
> It was clear that in the face of a threat of human closeness the patient would become disorganized and disoriented, unable to locate within himself a structured feeling or perception from which to generate a response. He was terrified of exposing the extent of his debility and nonachievement, of which he was deeply ashamed. Moreover, he knew that if he opened up to the woman, he would show her his looseness and disorientation, which would seem crazy to her.
>
> The therapist realized that the patient was expressing a displaced fear of opening up to him, of engaging with him on any but the most superficial level. However, he had an unforeseen personal response to the patient's behavior. In the face of the

looseness, the quick changes of subject, the repeated denigrations of therapy, and the derisive and inappropriate hoots of laughter, the therapist had a sense of having lost his place, of feeling anxious and confused, and of not knowing just how to respond.

The therapist could identify many possible reasons for his reaction. One was that the patient's contempt and rage were so palpable. Another was that through projective identification the patient was causing the therapist to feel the same kind of tongue-tied debility and disorientation of which the patient himself had been complaining [Ogden 1979]. But even more interesting were the bizarreness and incongruity of the patient's behavior, which appeared to amount to an assault on the possibility of meaning itself, an assertion that the very notions of logic and sequential meaning were absurdities. What could the therapist say in the face of such a savage attack on the premises of his thinking?

In time the therapist did find something to say, and it was really quite simple: "I feel anxious and confused right now, and I can't think of anything to say. Is this what you feel like at dances, and here with me?"

"Sort of," said the patient with a dismissive shrug, but it was the first time he appeared to recognize that there was another human being in the room with him.

The other subdivision within the category of cognitive resistance describes the patient whose basic view of cognition is, from the therapist's point of view, *hyperrational*. This group includes the "intellectualizer," particularly one who uses intellectualization in the service of competitiveness and aggression. He so values intelligence over all other human attributes that the therapist is evaluated solely in terms of how smart he is, and an interpretation is measured only by its cleverness and originality. Therapy thus becomes a competitive game in which the patient expects both participants to display their brilliance, for the purpose either of stimulating or defeating each other. Therapists who practice in university towns often see this kind of patient, whose solely intellectual engagement in the therapy is merely a continuation of the kind of relationship the patient has with his or her faculty peers (and often, one may imagine, spouses). Unbeknownst to the patient, of course, the therapist is operating on an entirely different set of assumptions about the expected nature of activity. For the therapist, brilliance may be a pleasant enough attribute if one has it, but it is utterly irrelevant to the conduct of or participation in therapy. What matters infinitely more is emotional engagement and psychological-mindedness. It may take the therapist a while before he has figured out that he and the patient are talking at cross purposes (Altshul 1977).

Case 4

Mr. D., a graduate student, complains of chronic despair and intense suicidal urges. A previous psychotherapy had been a failure; the patient tells me that he had repeatedly tried to shake his therapist out of his silence and into some more helpful behavior, but that the therapist remained silent to the end. Finally, partly to get his increasing desperation through to the therapist, he made a serious suicide attempt. He says he is again suicidal, but hopes for better things from me.

I suggest that he is wondering whether he will have to go that far with me or whether I will be able to show some understanding of how terrible he feels earlier than his previous therapist did. I expect him to look relieved. He does not. He looks scornful and disappointed and silently leaves the office when the time is up.

I begin the next hour by saying that he seemed to have an intense and unpleasant reaction to my observation and asking him to tell me about it. He replies that if that is the best I can do, then clearly hoping for better things was a self-induced mirage. I wonder aloud what he can possibly be so frightened of, that he would need to spurn my effort to help him with such withering contempt. He tells me that that question is no better than my earlier comment, that it is "formulaic," trotted glibly out to fend him off, "unsubstantive," and generally without intellectual merit.

And so it goes for a few sessions: he, ever more haughty and disdainful; I, feeling increasingly chastened, inept, and querulous. I have no idea what this young man with an IQ of 150 is trying to tell me, other than that he is smarter than I am, which should have been obvious to both of us from the start.

Suddenly an inspiration hits me. Reasoning that as a graduate student he must be used to lectures, I figure that if I give him a good one, I may get his attention and at least get him to stop beating on me for a while. Throwing my training in brevity to the winds, I say: "I perceive that you have the notion that you can be treated only by someone who is as smart as you. I don't know why you think that, but it isn't so. Ordinary competence will do just fine. If you like, I'll concede from the outset that you're lots smarter than I am. But you are also frightened, desperately frightened of letting me know what you feel about yourself. Perhaps you're terrified of getting suicidal again. Perhaps you're afraid that if you tell me about yourself in a serious way, you will be put down, mocked. Maybe that has happened to you a lot in the past, which is why you put me down, mock me, to turn the tables."

I am surprised by what I say. I had not realized I had been thinking all these things. I am also surprised by the rising heat in my voice, but even more surprised by the patient's response. He looks stunned, blank. After a long while he says in a small voice, "Okay."

Aesthetic Resistance

A fourth general category of resistance is what I term *aesthetic resistance*. This category applies to the patient who offends the therapist through his physical presentation of himself. The patient may do so through a visual modality (i.e., through physical appearance alone), an auditory modality (i.e., by emitting unappealing or disgusting sounds, often nonverbal in nature), and/or an olfactory modality (i.e., by being inattentive to issues of personal hygiene). This type of assault is often particularly difficult to deal with. One gets the impression that a major part of the patient's aggression may be energetically deployed in this fashion. The patient, however, may be entirely unaware of the offensive way he is presenting himself; and if he were to be made aware of it, he would remain unaware that it had any psychological significance. The therapist, for his part, schooled as he is in genteel, liberal values, is often loath to make even the most gentle confrontation for fear of hurting the patient. An ensuing standoff may then threaten the entire therapy.

Case 5

Ms. E., age 38, begins her first hour by telling me she needs "treatment" for her "depression." She does not define either term. She says that a previous psychiatrist told her it was a biological depression and that she needed only medication, not therapy. She didn't like him because he hadn't listened or talked to her. On the advice of a friend she is now going to try psychotherapy, even though she knows it isn't going to work. She tells me she expects me, like her husband and father and all other men she has ever known, to let her down. She demands that I contact my predecessor. Even though she knows he is no good, at least he knows something about drugs, as she is sure I don't. She says all this with a surprising lack of overtly aggressive affect; it is as if she has no idea she is being demanding and petulant.

I comment that she seems to be working very hard to assure both of us that no good can come of our contact, and ask if she may have any ideas about why. She sighs rather theatrically and tells me that no one has ever really understood her—that no one has ever wanted to. Why should she expect anything different from me? "Okay," I say, "but why work so hard to make that point?" I ask her if she is afraid of getting her feelings hurt? Tearfully, bitterly, she says that everything hurts her feelings; there isn't a thing that anyone can say to her that soothes and supports her. She hears everything as a put-down. This has the ring of truth to it, but it still sounds contrived, and I pick up the hint of a challenge to me in it.

At this point my attention is drawn to her appearance and mannerisms. She is moderately obese. Her hair has thinned to the point of partial baldness. The skin of her face is marred with numerous unsightly raised red lesions, some of which are weeping. The unaffected areas of skin are sallow and visibly oily. Between sentences she emits a complex smacking sound, half click and half chew, which has no discernible rhetorical purpose but serves only to unsettle and annoy me. Whatever she says, she says it with an incongruous and purposeless grin, of which she is evidently unaware. I feel disoriented and anxious.

I reflect that the paralysis of thought and feeling I am experiencing is precisely what she has had in mind for me. I find myself idly wondering if she beats her children, and this leads to musings about her sadism. It is too early to deal with this, however, and I have another thought. I am fascinated by her skin and its disfigurement and think that no one could possibly want to touch her. Suddenly it strikes me that she is working to ensure that she will remain untouched by me. At this point I ask her to tell me more about how things are going with her husband.

She replies that he is very kind to her, but that he is not sexually interested in her and repels her advances. She says she cannot understand why. She associates to a former therapist whom she occasionally visits. When she tells him how bad she feels, he takes her in his arms and holds her. She says she finds this enormously comforting. She grins incongruously and makes a smacking noise, which I now understand to be signs of embarrassment.

Ignoring the transference implications, I say that I can understand why that might feel particularly comforting to her. Looking interested, she asks why I say this. I answer, "Because I have the idea that, in spite of what you say about your husband, you don't truly believe that anyone could really want to touch you." She begins to weep softly, this time not in a theatrical manner.

Ideological Resistance

The fifth and final type of resistance I wish to describe is *ideological resistance*. This type of resistance refers to patients who operate in major ways in accordance with ideologies that are antithetical to those of dynamically oriented psychotherapy. When one initially sees such patients, their commitment to these ideologies often seems grossly exaggerated.

There are a number of such ideologies. For instance, the patient in the preceding example at first showed an implacable determination to view her encounter with her new therapist as yet another opportunity for a biological intervention. This value conflict—the biological-psychological split—is, of course, a very common ideological discrepancy and often serves as a significant source of resistance early in the therapy.

Nowadays an interesting type of ideological resistance has emerged from the springing up of numerous self-help groups, such as Adult Children of Alcoholics (ACOA), which offer simplified conceptions of human psychology. These groups may offer considerable support for suffering people and provide them with a new way of understanding the nature of their suffering. The groups may also help to prepare their members for future use of psychotherapy.

There may be, however, a difficulty in the transition from group membership to therapy. The group's ideology usually seeks to establish that there are broad commonalities that characterize all persons who fall within its purview and that the commonalities have far more significance than the differences that might distinguish people from one another. The actual events of the past, then, have greater significance than any individual's inner fantastic elaborations of them; for example, for the purposes of the group's processes, all people are believed to react to the stresses of growing up in an alcoholic family in much the same way. Therefore, the experience of any one member of the group can be shared and validated by any other. Because the road to the "truth" is already known, it becomes unnecessary for the member to embark on any voyage of individual self-discovery. Such a belief may present a knotty resistance early in the psychotherapy, as is illustrated in the following case.

Case 6

Ms. F., age 46, entered therapy for a rapidly worsening depression, apparently secondary to a badly deteriorating family situation. Her son was destroying himself with drugs and alcohol, and her third husband was on the verge of divorcing her. For support and relief she had turned to a local Adult Children of Alcoholics (ACOA) group—both her parents had been severely alcoholic— but her degree of distress had been so pronounced that she had been told she would need a more intense type of help than the group could provide.

In spite of her obvious frenzy and desperation, she approached therapy extremely warily. She said she had been warned by ACOA not to trust most psychiatrists. They were schooled, she thought, in irrelevant Freudian dynamics but knew nothing of the particular problems faced by children of alcoholic persons, of the terrible injuries they have sustained to their self-esteem, of the way in which they all repeat destructive early patterns in their contemporary lives. She had heard that I was better than most, and because she was so needy right now, she would give it a try. She hoped I already knew something about ACOA and its tenets so that she would not have to explain it all.

I replied that I did not know very much about it—that I had read about it in the newspaper but had never read any of its more basic literature. I understood that it might be tedious for her to go through it all again, but would she do so anyway, so that I could better understand the nature of her pain. In spite of her clear impatience, something about the ingenuousness and directness of my reply seemed to move her, and with a sigh of resignation she began a lengthy lecture about the history and theory of ACOA. Instead of confronting her and interpreting the resistance I listened sympathetically and at length. Finally, I commented that I could understand how she had come to feel that nobody in the world could help her and that, indeed, nobody seemed to want to. The patient burst into tears and said that she had not been able to tell anyone how she had been feeling; even the participants at ACOA had been put off when she had tried.

Thus began a productive year-long therapy, during which the patient was able to stop thinking of herself as poisonous to anyone who came into contact with her. She reconciled with her husband, and her son, with the help of a substance-abuse program, was able to stop taking drugs. Periodically she would lecture me on the tenets of ACOA, but with my help she came to see that she did so only when anxious, in particular about the possibility of not being understood sympathetically by me. Thus, what had begun as a fixed ideological divergence shrank in size and became interpretable as a symptom of anxiety.

Discussion

Taken as a whole, the resistances I have described tend to give the therapist the impression that a major value discrepancy exists between the patient and himself or herself. The first indication a therapist may have that such a resistance is in process is a sense of mounting irritation within himself or herself, accompanied by a sense of frustration that genuine communication is not taking place. Whatever efforts the therapist may make to break through the impasse and get his or her point across only meet with greater resistance and mutual incomprehension. Soon the therapist is forced to recognize that an adversarial character has developed around the still nascent relationship.

In order to forestall the disintegration of the therapy and to retain its therapeutic character, the therapist must act decisively. Once the therapist recognizes the existence of a major resistance, he or she should try to identify its type and begin to speculate about the nature of the anxiety that is giving rise to it. Because of the sense of confusion and irritation with which the therapist is struggling, he or she will often not find it easy to think clearly about these issues. Fortunately for those therapists who are able to trust their inner processes, such "thinking" often takes place preconsciously, as was illustrated by the confrontation of Mr. D., the graduate student, in Case 4.

The therapist's options range from persisting empathy to tactful confrontation. In the cases of Ms. E., the repellent woman in Case 5, and of Ms. F., the woman who believed in ACOA in Case 6, no confrontation was necessary at all; continued empathy sufficed to provide a sufficient therapeutic alliance. In the case of Ms. B., the disdainfully seductive patient bent on destroying the therapy at any cost (see Case 2), however, a clear and vigorous statement of the therapist's aims and procedures was required from the outset, because any failure to provide it would have been understood as a tacit compliance with the patient's aims. As was seen in the cases of Mr. A., the separated man in Case 1, and of Mr. D., the graduate student in Case 4, most situations fall between these extremes, and a combination of empathy and gentle confrontation will work toward a resolution of the difficulty.

Lest these recommendations about technique sound too facile, we must remember that both empathy and confrontation are being offered in the midst of significant countertransference turbulence. While these pressures do in fact complicate the therapist's technical tasks, the clinical material presented here does offer some further generalizations about what is necessary for an effective response.

First, the content of the resistance itself can be used as a tool for helping the therapist generate effective responses (Altshul and Sledge 1989). In the cases of Mr. D. and Ms. E., the therapist used his feelings of victimization and of repugnance to make dynamic inferences that were then incorporated into the response. In both cases these processes took place outside the therapist's awareness. Perhaps the therapist's responses had a particular poignancy for the patients precisely because they were so spontaneous. Undoubtedly, patients will tend to feel more addressed if they sense that what they have offered the therapist is coming back to them in recognizable, if transmuted, form.

Second, the therapist must clearly avoid the countertransference trap that is being laid for him by the particular resistance. He does this partly by becoming as clear as he can about the type of resistance he is dealing with. The therapist may often be unable to do so at the beginning, however, and some degree of "gritting of psychological teeth" may be necessary before his feelings settle and his clinical judgment returns. These processes are part of what is meant by the "metabolizing" that takes place within the therapist, whereby raw affect propelled by countertransference becomes transmuted into a clinically useful response (Giovacchini 1975; Ogden 1979).

Third, the effective interventions come after a period of stress and strain both within the therapist and between the therapist and the patient. Without this kind of pain there tends to be insufficient engagement on the part of the therapist and inadequate contact between therapist and patient; the latter is likely to feel that his or her concerns are being insufficiently addressed.

Fourth, the most effective interventions come from the therapist's heart. Products as they are of his turmoil, these interventions have a certain degree of conviction and passion behind them. Without these attributes the therapist would probably not succeed in getting the patient's attention, in breaking through the resistance, and in making the patient understand, to his or her surprise, that he or she is capable of making any real impression on the therapist at all. In other words, the metabolizing process should never be so complete as to render the interventions bloodless. This is not to say that there is no place in therapy for more purely intellectual observations; but in the case of these massive initial resistances something more affectively engaged is required.

It should be noted, however, that the strength of the confrontation does not and must not depend on the intensity of the therapist's anger or sexual arousal or on the strength of whatever projective identifications have taken place. If these parameters are used as guides, the confrontation is certain to be too harsh and destructive. The presence of a significant degree of anger or signs of projective identification should be an indication for pause and further reflection. If reflection and introspection alone are insufficient to reduce the intensity of the anger, frustration, and other strong affects, immediate consultation with a colleague should be undertaken, whatever the level of the therapist's experience. This is particularly critical in the case of the sexually seductive patient, whose activities represent a terrible danger not only to his or her own therapy and life, but also to the career and self-respect of the therapist as well.

Finally, however experienced we may be and however much therapy we may already have had, we must never be too proud to recognize that in extreme cases, when countertransference affects become unmanageable by ordinary means, it may be not only wise but necessary to undertake personal therapy for ourselves.

References

Altshul VA: The so-called boring patient. Am J Psychother 31:533–545, 1977

Altshul VA: The hateful therapist and the countertransference psychosis. Journal of the National Association of Private Psychiatric Hospitals 11:15–23, 1980

Altshul VA, Sledge WH: Countertransference problems, in American Psychiatric Press Review of Psychiatry, Vol 8. Edited by Tasman A, Hales RE, Frances AJ. Washington, DC, American Psychiatric Press, 1989, pp 518–530

Giovacchini PL: Psychoanalysis of Character Disorders, New York, Jason Aronson, 1975

Langs R: Psychotherapy: A Basic Text. New York, Jason Aronson, 1982

Maltsberger JT, Buie DH: Countertransference hate in the treatment of suicidal patients. Arch Gen Psychiatry 30:625–633, 1974

Ogden TH: On projective identification. Int J Psychoanal 60:357–373, 1979

Chapter 13

The Use of Countertransference in Intensive Psychotherapy With Patients With Schizophrenia

Michael A. Selzer, M.D.
John A. Grimaldi, M.D.

The term *countertransference*, which historically referred to the therapist's unconscious transference to the patient's transference (Brenner 1985; Reich 1960), has evolved in contemporary psychoanalytic writing to encompass any reaction the therapist has to the patient (Kernberg 1976; Loewald 1986). This broader definition is an outgrowth of interest in applying psychoanalytic technique to more severely disturbed patients, and a response to the challenge these patients present to psychotherapeutic intervention. Although countertransference as originally defined tells us little or nothing about the patient, the broader definition provides an essential element in understanding him or her. For that reason, we employ the broader definition in this chapter.

In general, the more regressed the patient and the more exploratory the work, the more difficult it is for the therapist to determine the principal source of countertransference phenomena. At times, the therapist's sorting out his or her needs from the patient's contribution requires access to either supervision or a personal analysis.

Countertransference reactions may take the form of feelings, fantasies, thoughts, shifts in levels of alertness, and somatic sensations. We will discuss ways in which the nature of the therapist's countertransference may inform a deeper understanding of the patient's subjective experience, afford a better grasp of the patient's central problem, and lead to the formulation of specific treatment interventions. Although our comments are directed primarily to therapists conducting psychoanalytically oriented individual psychotherapy, we hope clinicians working with severely disturbed patients in less traditional settings will also benefit from a better understanding of commonly experienced countertransference attitudes arising in their work.

While it is not our intention to present an in-depth review of the writings on countertransference (see Altshul and Sledge 1989), two clinicians whose seminal work has provided the foundation for all subsequent investigation regarding countertransference and schizophrenia bear mentioning. Harry Stack Sullivan (1940/1953), in asserting that schizophrenic individuals are more human than otherwise, implicitly focused attention on the (countertransference) barriers therapists erect to keep out of awareness how much they have in common with their patients. Yet for therapists to achieve personal safety, Sullivan warned they may shatter the possibility of an empathic bond with their patients. Searles (1979) showed the variety of ways in which schizophrenic patients and therapists impact on each other, including the mutual growth that can ensue if therapists allow for true emotional involvement. Searles, certainly no sentimentalist, noted that sadism was often a prominent feature in schizophrenic individuals and was likely to elicit powerful counterforces within the therapist, including the wish to drive the patient crazy. What follows, to a considerable degree, derives from these fundamental insights.

Identifying the Problem

Often the therapist's initial reaction to schizophrenic patients is uncertainty, and there is confusion about one's own feelings, what the patient might be experiencing, and how to proceed. Therapists also commonly question the appropriateness of their reactions to patients. Their questioning often carries with it some prohibition, self-judgment, or fantasied punishment or reward. The therapist momentarily loses access to the store of experiences he has acquired that would otherwise allow him to freely and openly react without expectation of some unwanted and irrational consequence.[1] Given that the primitive nature of the schizophrenic patient's experience easily fosters a return to archaic ways of thinking in therapist as well as patient, it is not surprising that clinicians may revert to magical beliefs and rudimentary systems of reward and punishment.

As a general rule, when the therapist is confused and uncertain about his reaction, he can better understand the situation by asking himself, "How would the average individual be expected to react in a similar situation?" Regardless of level of experience, every therapist comes equipped with a body of information that he can apply to that question. Rarely, the therapist finds himself so confused about the nature of the situation or so frightened about what he fears may be happening that he is unable to define it sufficiently to imagine what form a normative reaction might take. In this event, the therapist must wait to get his bearings before he can pose the question to himself. Eventually, the therapist can describe what he thinks both he and the patient are doing, and then ask himself whether his reaction falls within a normative range.

If the therapist had been critical of himself and, upon reflection, concludes that his reaction falls within the normal range of response, he can use his prior distorted self-evaluation as a clue to the patient's impact on him. Why had he held himself to such an exaggerated standard, and, more importantly, what role did the patient play in the therapist's setting it up?

The following vignette illustrates the use of the normative response as a source of information regarding a confusing patient:

---

[1] In this chapter the therapist will be referred to as "he," though it is understood that the reference applies to both men and women; the exception will be when the therapist in a given clinical vignette is female.

Case 1

A beginning psychiatric resident was assigned a patient, Mr. A., whose previous therapist had been a resident now entering his second year. The patient spent the entire first meeting angrily denouncing his new therapist for knowing less about the particulars of his diagnosis and treatment than did his previous therapist. The new therapist, in turn, felt confused about how to respond to the patient's angry and devaluing observation and, at the same time, experienced a strong inhibition against asking the patient to provide him with any information. It was as if the therapist believed that in some mysterious fashion he already should have been as familiar with his patient as his predecessor had been after 1 year of working together. Moreover, the therapist came to believe that other staff members shared his belief—that is, the staff would be critical of him if he were to openly discuss how little he knew about his patient relative to what the previous therapist knew. [At this point, the therapist might have asked himself whether meeting someone for the first time should result in the same degree of familiarity as he would obtain after 12 months of sessions. Had he been able to imagine a normative response as a guideline, the therapist could have appreciated from the outset that Mr. A. had stimulated in him a need to be omniscient, and the therapist might then have wondered what this indicated about the patient.]

After several more sessions in which the patient reproached the therapist for having failed to know "all about me" from the outset, the therapist was able to question what a normative response might be. However, despite being able to recognize that no one should expect to be fully informed about someone else prior to meeting them, the therapist nonetheless remained critical of himself and continued to feel that the staff would censure him. The fact that he persisted in feeling guilty and fearful eventually led him to appreciate that the patient was the stimulus for his sadistic and punishing attitude toward himself.

Finally, in reviewing the session, the psychiatrist asked why he had prevented himself in the first place from asking what a normative response might be. He came to understand that once he had accepted Mr. A.'s requirement for omniscience he no longer could allow himself the luxury of inquiry, because that would have implied uncertainty.

Another countertransference problem exists when a therapist concludes that it is inappropriate to compare his response to the patient with a normative one. For example, the therapist might feel the need to treat the patient in a manner that goes beyond ordinary therapeutic convention and, consistent with that belief, to reject the notion that the usual rules should apply. If so, his assuming of this burden should alert him to question the source of this demand. Is the patient creating in the therapist the need to be excessively tolerant?

Case 2

A patient, Ms. B., made a dramatic suicide attempt after experiencing a series of tragic losses, and was hospitalized. Shortly after starting work with her inpatient therapist, Ms. B. threatened to cut her wrists in front of him. She cited her recent losses as justifying her right to act destructively. "You never came close to going through what I've been through, so what gives you the right to judge me?" The therapist felt paralyzed to respond to the patient's threats. When he tried to ask himself what a normative response might be, a competing internal voice admonished him for being unfair. The therapist, thus, had accepted Ms. B.'s assertion that her unfortunate circumstances were so unique that any self-destructive action was justified.

Treatment Frame

The *treatment frame* refers to those constant aspects of the therapeutic relationship "within whose bounds the process [of treatment] takes place" (Bleger 1967, p. 511). The role and responsibilities assigned to the therapist and patient, the length and location of sessions, the consideration of fees, the time of session, and so forth are all elements of the treatment frame. The clinician working with severely disturbed individuals frequently finds himself challenged by clinical situations in which the patient threatens the integrity of the treatment frame, either through overt destructive behavior or by more subtle efforts to undermine it. In this section we will take up a particular feature of this phenomenon, the therapist's impulse to abandon his responsibility to maintain adherence to the frame and/or his collusion with the patient to violate it. In this regard, the existence of the frame allows the therapist to recognize his wish to deviate from the treatment frame. This recognition is often the single most powerful and reliable indicator of countertransference.

A major reason the therapist deviates from the frame is that, on a preconscious or unconscious level, he believes that the alliance is weak, and so he tries to manipulate the frame to strengthen it. Paradoxically, precisely the opposite behavior is required at such a moment, namely, to adhere to the frame and within its context examine with the patient the problems in their relationship. For example, a therapist working with a very disturbed individual may feel that unless he yields to the patient's wish to extend the session, the patient will experience the therapist's refusal as sadistic and withholding, and in turn reject the therapist. Unfortunately, by acceding to the patient's request, the therapist is inadvertently supporting the patient's belief that nothing should be expected of him or her and that time does not constitute a boundary. The therapist also may abandon the frame in a misguided effort to find a way into the patient's world, to befriend him or her, or to demonstrate that he is different from all the previous therapists who have been uncaring and aloof in playing by the rules. In the latter instance the therapist believes he must compensate for the patient's earlier deprivations by suspending the rules to "prove" the uniqueness of their relationship.

The crucial point is that a therapist working in an area so dominated by unneutralized aggression and primitive modes of defense can expect to experience intense reactions in relationship to the treatment frame. By keeping the frame as a standard against which to monitor his impulses, the therapist enhances his ability to use his responses to inform his understanding of the patient's internal world and to formulate appropriate treatment interventions.

The Wish to Violate the Frame

Case 3

The patient, Mr. C., had been a medical intern when he experienced his first psychotic break, some 5 years previously. Since that time, despite multiple short-term hospitalizations, treatment with antipsychotic medication, and several failed attempts to resume medical training, Mr. C. denied that he was ill or that his illness was associated with any vocational disability. There was one exception. During a previous brief period of transient acute psychosis he had developed a painfully experienced delusion that he had killed a patient during his internship year.

In the individual therapy hours Mr. C. boasted of his exemplary performance in medical school and during his internship, attributing his difficulties in the intervening years to the malevolence of others. For several consecutive sessions the patient's denial that he was ill intensified and took on new and irritating dimensions. He wore hospital whites to sessions, quizzed the therapist about medical trivia, and demanded that the therapist use whatever influence he had to secure Mr. C.'s readmission to a training program in internal medicine. When the patient's demand that he be "permitted" to practice medicine became particularly insistent, the therapist was tempted to terminate the session, believing that no further work could be accomplished on that day.

The therapist began to despair about Mr. C.'s capacity to benefit from treatment altogether and entertained the idea of terminating treatment and referring the patient to a clinic for monthly medication maintenance. He rationalized termination as the only effective means of confronting the patient's denial. While discussing the treatment with a colleague, the therapist began to recognize that his impulse to end "unproductive" sessions early or terminate the treatment altogether stemmed more from his own frustration than from a reasoned understanding of the patient's predicament.

Because each session, by prescription, lasted for 30 minutes (regardless of whether or not the session was productive), ending early would have been a clear violation of the frame and would have signified to the therapist his own incompetence and negligence. Further, for the therapist to end treatment altogether would have been consistent with being a bad doctor who brought harm to his patient. The wish to act in a manner consistent with being a bad doctor was a result of Mr. C.'s having projected his feeling about himself onto the therapist. Had the therapist acted on his impulses he would have lost the opportunity to help Mr. C. become aware of his belief that he, rather than the therapist, was the bad doctor, an idea he had dramatically expressed in his delusion of having killed a medical patient during his internship.

In contrast to deviating from the treatment frame, the therapist may adopt a position of stultifying rigidity with regard to creating and maintaining the frame. In this situation, the therapist only superficially preserves the frame while violating its underlying intent. Just as permissive disregard of the treatment frame may reflect the therapist's fear of setting limits and/or his own wish to regress, too strict adherence generally signals that the therapist feels overwhelmed and is trying to exert control, or that he feels angry and is using the frame to attack the patient. Attitudes of rigid adherence and permissive disregard, unfortunately, are further strengthened by the misguided clinical notion that severely regressed patients are beyond psychodynamic understanding.

Case 4

Mr. D., a schizophrenic patient on a long-term inpatient unit, developed tardive dyskinesia midway through what had been a successful treatment. In response to the developing tardive dyskinesia, the psychiatrist reduced the antipsychotic medication while keeping all other aspects of the treatment constant. On reduced medication the patient became more anxious and impulsive and experienced difficulty tolerating the full 45-minute psychotherapy sessions. Despite the patient's frequent insistence that he needed to leave sessions for a drink of water or a cigarette, the psychiatrist insisted on scrupulously maintaining the full length of sessions. In supervision, the supervisor asked the psychiatrist whether he had considered that Mr. D.'s behavior might signal that he was feeling overwhelmed and that a change in their arrangement might be indicated. The psychiatrist responded by saying, "I never gave it a thought. I felt that since we set it up that way, it should stay that way."

The psychiatrist's rigid refusal to consider the possible usefulness of altering the time and/or place of sessions was in the service of avoiding facing that the patient's clinical state had worsened and was overwhelming both him and the patient.

It is common for patients, once they begin to improve, to deny the possibility of future regression. In the example above, by not allowing the frame to accommodate for the setback, the psychiatrist colluded with Mr. D.'s wish to believe that progress, once it begins, follows an exclusively uphill course. If the psychiatrist had suggested a change in the frame—that is, having shorter, more frequent sessions in the patient's room on the unit, rather than in the office—the patient would have been faced with his feelings about having a chronic disease that will require him at times to alter his life circumstances.

Countertransference With Neurotic Patients and Schizophrenic Patients: Problems in Alliance Formation

Patients with schizophrenia provoke intense and perplexing reactions in anyone trying to work closely with them, in part because they often lack the social conventions that serve to ease human interactions. As a consequence, the therapist, unable to rely on his patient to utilize the usual forms of politeness and civility, feels especially vulnerable and exposed. The therapist, because the schizophrenic patient may attack him if he attempts to use social conventions, may find it difficult to conceal his vulnerability.

Sharing social customs can also provide the basis for imagining that collaboration is possible. Some fundamental code of behavior that is assumed by both patient and therapist provides at least the illusion of relatedness. A neurotic person is able to present himself as a reasonable person interested in and able to engage in a collaborative process. Whether this is the case or not, his capacity to appear *as if* he can and will collaborate permits the therapist to feel as though a working relationship is likely to take place. However, with schizophrenic patients, no such shared assumption about civil behavior exists, making it difficult for the therapist to consider that an alliance will ever be possible.

In addition, the neurotic patient is more likely to acknowledge the ego-dystonic aspects of his symptomatology than is the schizophrenic patient, who frequently regards his symptoms as favorable. Even when he does not view them as ego-syntonic, the schizophrenic person will resist identifying his symptoms as the product of inner conflict. This blanket resistance leads to powerful countertransference reactions that may take the form of the therapist blaming the patient, as the following example indicates:

Case 5

A patient, Ms. E., created a delusional world in which she claimed to need no one because she belonged to a "master race." At the same time, her behavior in the therapy hours indicated that she was extremely dependent on her therapist. Ms. E. implored the therapist to intervene on her behalf in a variety of situations and had trouble leaving the office at the end of the sessions. Ms. E. attributed her dependent behavior to the devil, who was forcing her to act this way to humiliate her. The patient insisted, "I'd be fine on my own except I hear his [the devil's] voice commanding me to come to session." The therapist, after repeatedly trying to make the patient aware of the contradiction between her claim of needing no one and her behavior, began to challenge her: "If you're so independent, why can't you leave my office?"

As the example indicates, the schizophrenic person's tendency to externalize conflict can create problems in alliance formation. From the viewpoint of the therapist's countertransference, the alliance is most likely to suffer when the therapist limits his empathic involvement with his patient so as to protect himself from making contact with aspects of himself that are ego-alien. Unfortunately, the more primitive the patient, the more the patient threatens to make the therapist aware of forbidden aspects of his own self. To prevent this from happening, the therapist may choose to view the patient as incomprehensible so as to put a barrier both between himself and the patient, and between the reasonable and primitive aspects within himself.

Case 6

The patient, Mr. F., refused to eat because he was afraid that the world's food supply had become contaminated. As a consequence, Mr. F. was admitted to the hospital and force-fed. The patient insisted that the staff would kill him by making him eat "these toxins." The therapist told his supervisor that he found it hard to understand how Mr. F. believed what he did. "He must know somewhere inside himself that the food is not really contaminated." Consistent with his statement to the supervisor, the therapist tried to cajole Mr. F. into eating, hoping he might be able to "tease him out of it." The patient's condition worsened, yet the therapist, as part of his treatment regimen, continued to make light of Mr. F.'s efforts at self-starvation.

As the patient's medical condition deteriorated, an internist was called for consultation. The consultant, witnessing the way the therapist approached Mr. F., took him aside and angrily asked, "How can you keep this banter up when your patient may be dead soon?" At that moment the therapist began to understand the similarity between the patient and himself. Both had wished the patient dead. Once the therapist could admit his own destructive wishes, he was able to recognize them in the patient.

In the above example, the therapist shielded himself from his own destructive impulses by refusing to recognize the similarity between himself and his patient. The therapist also may create a barrier in the opposite fashion, seeing himself as more similar to the patient than he actually is, as in the following example:

Case 7

The patient, Ms. G., believed that she spent her life alone in a spaceship orbiting earth. The ship was light-years from earth, which was visible only through an extraordinarily powerful telescope. Because Ms. G. knew herself to be alone in outer space, she interpreted other people's, including her therapist's, belief that they were interacting with her as their folly. Despite Ms. G.'s vehement protest that she and the therapist existed on different planets and therefore could not possibly have contact with each other, the therapist persisted in his interpretation that Ms. G. was

defending against her wish to be connected to him. In exasperation, the therapist insisted that Ms. G.'s experience was similar to
what many people felt in their day-to-day life. After repeatedly
failing to persuade the patient of this interpretation, the therapist finally appreciated that he was trying to force his interpretation on her out of his need to protect himself from experiencing
Ms. G.'s sense of profound disconnectedness. The therapist recognized that he was misidentifying Ms. G.'s experience as ordinary social anxiety, while, in fact, the patient's isolation was a
reflection of her belief that she was not human. Although it also
may have been true that underlying her isolation the patient experienced a wish to be connected, this need for connection
could only have been reached by first appreciating Ms. G.'s sense
of discontinuity. Paradoxically, the therapist's insistence that the
patient immediately acknowledge a wish for connectedness left
the patient feeling more alone.

Sustaining the Work

Work with both neurotic and psychotic patients is sustained by the
therapist imagining a new and higher level of maturity (Loewald
1960) that the patient is capable of achieving. Yet, for each of the
two groups, maturity may suggest very different meanings. With
the neurotic patient, good treatment outcome is described by
metaphors that emphasize growth, healing, awareness, and development; with psychotic individuals, however, a good outcome is
often described as acceptance of chronic illness and its attendant
despair. At the same time, the therapist working with schizophrenic patients must also contend with society's mandate to heal, as
well as his own intrapsychically determined strivings to cure. To
accommodate these pressures and sustain his investment in the
work, the therapist often creates the illusion that more can come
of treatment than is realistically possible. Ironically, if he could acknowledge the realistic limitations and his feelings about not being
able to remedy everything, he would be in a better position to help
his patient.

How does a therapist working with psychotic patients sustain
himself in the face of such limited possibilities, keep his sense of

hopefulness alive, and not succumb to the seductive promise that unrealistic hope engenders? This aspect of the work is too subtle and complex to yield any general prescription. Perhaps some brief clinical examples will serve to illuminate a few of the commonly encountered countertransference reactions related to the difficulty defining and maintaining realistic goals.

In the case of Ms. G., who believed herself to be traveling in a spaceship, the therapist began making contact with her only after he permitted himself to acknowledge the patient's profound sense of alienation from everyone, including him. Although he now felt closer to the patient, he also had to be able to appreciate that he and Ms. G. might never bridge the gap between them. Certainly, the therapist could realistically expect for a long time the patient to make only occasional forays onto earth. Should the therapist desire more from Ms. G., he might easily translate his expectation into a demand, which would send her farther away. Another example further illustrates this dilemma:

Case 8

In her work with Mr. H., a schizophrenic patient hospitalized on a long-term unit and approaching discharge, the therapist became aware of feeling distracted and bored in team meetings, particularly when details of her patient's discharge plans were being discussed. In contrast, other members of the team were anxious about Mr. H.'s upcoming discharge. In spite of Mr. H.'s history of homelessness, including an incident in which he nearly froze to death while sleeping in a park the previous winter, the therapist rationalized her indifference by telling herself that disposition planning was the social worker's job. The therapist examined what she was doing only after another team member angrily questioned her directly about what she and Mr. H. talked about regarding his life after hospitalization. Caught off guard by the intensity of the staff member's challenge, she began to review what she and the patient were discussing, namely Mr. H.'s fantasy that they would coauthor a book about the patient's treatment that would become a bestseller and ultimately be made into a movie. Rather than treating this fantasy as a resistance against the painful work of examining how meager the patient's life might actually be, the therapist, in discussing the book, was colluding with the patient's denial. A detailed examination of Mr. II.'s functional capacities would have demonstrated how pervasive and disabling an effect his illness continued to have on his life.

Splitting

Splitting, a predominant defense in patients with primitive mental states, has been described by Bion (1955) as ministering to the patient's greed: "Splitting-action is the outcome of the determination which can be expressed verbally as an intention to be as many people as possible, so as to be in as many places as possible, so as to get as much as possible, for as long as possible, in fact timelessly" (p. 223). It is precisely this refusal to be pinned down, to accept finiteness, that makes the schizophrenic patient so hard to engage. The moment the therapist feels he has discovered an important issue, the patient turns it into its opposite. The therapist can become so frustrated by the patient's elusiveness that he challenges the patient to become more reasonable—"Surely you can see what you're saying makes no sense . . ."—as if he might exhort the patient to act more rationally.

More regressed patients are likely to deal with objects by splitting, whereas better organized patients are far more likely to experience objects ambivalently. In parallel fashion, the therapist working with a less disturbed patient can be aware of liking his patient while at the same time remembering how annoyed he had been just moments before, whereas the therapist working with a schizophrenic individual has difficulty remembering the side of the patient that conflicts with his current experience. The therapist who now wishes to prematurely end the session with his schizophrenic patient will have trouble remembering that this is the same person who yesterday inspired in him the wish to extend the hour.

Splitting can be used by the patient to abolish time. Because the patient refuses to hold to any fixed position, anything is possible, and therefore the limitation that time imposes is no longer recognized. One by-product of splitting is that the patient will not have a continuous sense of his or her relationship with the therapist. The patient's discontinuity may be similarly experienced by the therapist so that the experience of the history of the relationship is either shattered or never established.

Recall, for example, Mr. C. (see Case 3), the patient who had been a medical intern at the time of his first psychotic break. Five years later he was still unable to resume his medical training, yet he stubbornly maintained that if only his therapist would help him with the application process, he could successfully resume his training. The therapist reacted by agreeing to review the application forms with the patient. In so doing, the therapist acted in accord with Mr. C.'s wish to be treated as someone who had not been episodically psychotic for 5 years, but rather as someone requiring help securing a residency position. The therapist had subscribed to the timelessness of Mr. C.'s position.

Problem of Interpretation and Use of Projective Identification

The interrelationship between projective identification and countertransference is well known. Several contributors in the field (Ogden 1989, 1990; Racker 1968) have described the pivotal role that projective identification plays in the therapist's understanding of more regressed patients, and how the therapist's countertransference reactions provide the major link in understanding the particular projective identification. The more regressed the patient is, the more the therapist relies on his countertransference as the primary, if not the exclusive, window through which to view the patient. It is essential that the therapist recognize that his countertransference is in response to the patient. However, as the recipient of the patient's projections, the therapist can have difficulty maintaining a boundary between himself and the patient. If the therapist fails to do so, he will inaccurately view his reactions as one-sided and may miss the patient's contribution. The following clinical example illustrates this process:

Case 9

Mr. I., a patient hospitalized on a long-term inpatient unit, jumped out of a window and sustained severe physical injuries. Because Mr. I. believed himself to be omnipotent, he had expected to be unharmed. Prior to his jump, Mr. I. had taunted the therapist, declaring that she was a mere mortal, while he was the ruler of a "master race." After his jump, Mr. I. became convinced that the therapist had stolen his powers out of envy. The patient now saw himself as totally weak and dependent on her. Mr. I. experienced the damage to his body as greater than it actually was, and remained in a wheelchair well after he was able to walk. Similarly, on a psychological level, Mr. I.'s sense of impotence extended to all spheres of his life— past, present, and future. This included his inability to comprehend that he had actively tried to take his life—he was not able to imagine himself capable of engaging in such forceful activity—or that he would be able to consider doing so in the future.

At the same time that Mr. I. was proclaiming his ineffectuality, the therapist began to disagree with the ward staff over whether the patient remained a suicide risk. The ward staff wished to keep him on a severely restricted status, whereas the therapist insisted on giving the patient full privileges, arguing that she would somehow "know" if he were again suicidal. She went so far as to insist that she could guarantee that the patient would not harm himself. She was unable to appreciate the legitimacy of the staff's concerns or Mr. I.'s potential for self-destructiveness, or that her ability to protect him was limited, because she had accepted the patient's projection of omnipotence. She would have been able to help Mr. I. accept responsibility for his suicide attempt and the attendant damage he had done to himself if she had identified, rather than acted out, her countertransference. Similarly, had she removed the blinders resulting from having "accepted" the projective identification, she also could have appreciated Mr. I.'s internal resources and thereby helped him take responsibility for lifting his ward restrictions.

Language

Various theoreticians (Bion 1959; Klein 1930/1968) have provided useful concepts for understanding the schizophrenic person's verbal communication. These explanatory concepts also provide a means by which the therapist can better understand his countertransference.

Bion (1959) posits that the patient defensively attacks the psychological processes by which meaning is attached to experience. Further, we have observed that when the patient engages in such an attack, typically the therapist experiences one of two countertransference reactions: either he agrees with the patient that he has destroyed meaning, or he insists that he has not. To prove his case, the therapist will identify a particular meaning before there are enough data to support it.

Case 10

A supervisor asked a therapist to present an audiotape or process notes of an individual psychotherapy session. The therapist repeatedly failed to bring either to his supervisory hours. He explained that he felt unable to ask the patient, Ms. J., if she would agree to tape sessions, and could not write process notes because he could not reconstruct a picture of what transpired in the session. Rather than reflecting on how his confusion might be a clue to understanding Ms. J., the therapist instead ascribed to the notion that nothing was happening.

In the supervisory hours, the therapist became aware that he was afraid the audiotape or notes would reveal that his work with Ms. J. was meaningless and that she would be better off without him. Gradually, the therapist began to discuss in supervision the ways in which Ms. J. had convinced him to abandon the search for meaning. The patient would sneer at any attempt the therapist offered to attribute significance to what she was saying, insisting that the therapist was not "man enough" to face up to the truth—that it was all "just words." Repeatedly, Ms. J. would use the meaninglessness of their experience together as proof of her contention: "You think words change anything?" the patient mockingly challenged, and then reminded the therapist of how long she had been in the hospital.

What proved most difficult for the therapist was that whenever he thought he was developing a rudimentary grasp of how to talk with Ms. J., she would subvert his efforts by using nonsense syllables, which she expressed in a sing-song cadence. Rather than confronting the patient about how she was using language in a defensive attempt to depict all life as absurd, the therapist had come to agree with Ms. J. that in fact there was no meaning. In the supervisory hours, the therapist was acting out his agreement by not bringing in the tapes or notes, and in the therapy sessions by not interpreting the way in which Ms. J. used words.

The alternate countertransference reaction—that of insisting upon meaning before it has emerged—is illustrated by the following example:

Case 11

A therapist presented for supervision his work with an articulate, hospitalized chronically schizophrenic young man, Mr. K. The patient was well read, and in a droning voice filled the hours reciting from whatever book he was currently reading. The therapist, in turn, skillfully pointed out the similarities between the characters in the novels and Mr. K.'s own dynamics. After listening to several hours of process notes, the supervisor remarked that the material made him think of lullabies. The supervisor's association caused the therapist to recall that during several therapy sessions he had found himself fighting the urge to fall asleep. His drowsiness had made him uncomfortable, and he had reacted by searching ever more diligently for meaning in Mr. K.'s words. Rather than interpreting the patient's behavior as Mr. K.'s effort to devitalize him, the therapist insisted that the content of the patient's statements conveyed symbolic meaning. By interpreting only the content, the therapist avoided examining the dynamic meaning of the patient's behavior. Mr. K. had drained all meaning from his speech by reciting from the book in a mechanical voice. This understanding was evident once the therapist became aware of his wish to remove himself by sleeping.

According to Klein (1930/1968), symbol formation and language acquisition require the child to progress from the paranoid-schizoid to the depressive position. Words stand for something else, fixed and separate from the essence they represent. By definition, they imply the loss of actual experience. In addition, giving an object a name defines it in a static way, thereby limiting what it can and cannot be. Accepting the symbolic function of language means relinquishing the omnipotent fantasy that even though an object is defined as X, it also can be magically defined as Y. To the extent that persons with schizophrenia have difficulty acknowledging loss, they will limit the application of language as a symbolic communication, frustrating the therapist's efforts to engage in secondary process discourse.

On the other hand, when the therapist feels confused by the patient's idiosyncratic use of words, he may fail to appreciate the patient's embryonic efforts to use language symbolically. The therapist may then insist on his own sense of what the patient is saying rather than assisting the patient in utilizing language in a more symbolic form. The therapist may even convince himself that he is more expert than the patient at reading the patient's signs.

Case 12

One patient, Ms. L., when preoccupied about her poor sense of identity, would speak of her previous therapist, Dr. Denton. Each time, the therapist felt bewildered by the irrelevant mention of Dr. Denton's name and responded by asking the patient to identify Dr. Denton. Ms. L. would look puzzled and repeat what she had said. The therapist grew increasingly frustrated and retaliated by tuning out. It took several months before the therapist recognized that Ms. L. used Dr. Denton's name as a shorthand way of alluding to her confused sense of identity—that is, that the name "Dr. Denton" contained four letters in the same sequence as the word "identity." Had the therapist considered that the name "Dr. Denton" might have had some meaning other than that of a previously known actual person, the therapist might have been able to discover Ms. L.'s early effort to use language to voice her concern about her own identity.

Words as Actions

Discovering the "meaning" of the patient's communication is often difficult, painstaking, and frustrating. Therapists naively assume that, although there may be disagreement between themselves and their patients about any particular meaning, therapist and patient agree that words function linguistically, rather than as a vehicle for action. The patient's use of words as action can produce intense countertransference reactions. When the therapist begins to appreciate that the patient is using words as things unto themselves, he often feels confused and betrayed, and may retaliate by refusing to recognize what the patient is communicating.

Case 13

A patient, Mr. M., was describing the New England countryside on a lovely spring day. Though Mr. M. used conventional words to refer to a pleasant bucolic setting, the therapist found herself tensing up each time the patient spoke. Eventually she noticed that she was not responding to the content but rather to the aggressive and forceful manner with which Mr. M. spoke his words. The content was at odds with the patient's inner state, which Mr. M. revealed through his delivery.

Not uncommonly, patients with schizophrenia believe, as in the following example, that by naming something they can control or destroy it:

Case 14

One patient, Mr. N., believed that the world would end on Monday. To prevent cosmic destruction, Mr. N. decreed that no one was to mention the word "Monday." His therapist consequently felt he could not discuss "Monday" nor bring up any topic related to it. The therapist felt sadistically controlled because he could not make any efforts at interpretation or even study the process further.

When words are used as an expression of omnipotent thought, they are experienced countertransferentially as tools of control. Words also may be used by the schizophrenic patient to split off parts of the self, as in the following example:

Case 15

One patient, Ms. O., bitterly implored her therapist to treat her as special. However, whenever the therapist asked Ms. O. to describe herself, the patient instead read in a monotone from her dog-eared copy of Kraepelin's criteria for schizophrenia. Consistent with this behavior, Ms. O. also refused psychological testing, haughtily telling her therapist that the test results were already in Kraepelin's text. Ms. O. refused to complete an application for disability insurance, explaining that a description of her mental disability was covered in Kraepelin and, if necessary, the pertinent sections could be copied and sent with the form. These recitations and protests contained within them the split-off, devalued part of the patient and in turn induced in the therapist the wish to see Ms. O. as belonging to a category, Kraepelinian schizophrenia, rather than having any unique properties.

Dynamics as Resistance

Our entire discussion thus far has treated language as a capacity that is subject to the patient's motivational states. In fact, research evidence (Maher 1972) suggests that the majority of language problems in persons with schizophrenia reflect an incapacity to apply the computational strategies of linguistics to intentionality. As Sledge has suggested, "the episodic disturbances of language production in people with schizophrenia are more like aphasia than they are like verbal parapraxes" (W. H. Sledge, personal communication, 1992).

Attributing dynamic meaning to all aspects of schizophrenic pathology is as much a resistance to recognizing the totality of the schizophrenic patient's experience as is treating the patient as if he or she were completely devoid of intentionality.

Because we depend on what our patients tell us to develop our insights, we are vulnerable to succumbing to the sometimes erroneous belief that patients are always able to inform us. We like to think that the only thing standing in our way is the patient's resistance to communication, itself amenable to change through language, rather than a deficit requiring compensatory methods and skills acquisition. In our example, although we focus exclusively on the dynamic aspects of the patient's use of language, we acknowledge that underlying deficits in linguistic functioning contribute significantly to a patient's disordered communication.

Countertransference in Nontraditional Settings

Team meetings and staff meetings commonly provide a setting for expressing countertransference feelings experienced in work with schizophrenic patients. It is particularly important to recognize the different forms these countertransference reactions may take, because in the patient's absence his contribution is easily overlooked. Instead, conflict among team members may be erroneously attributed to personality differences or discrepancies in level of skill. By the same token, staff attitudes about the meeting's agenda may more accurately reflect the patient's influence rather than the group's inherent ability to work together.

For example, various staff may hold contradictory views of the patient, or they may be sharply divided regarding a particular clinical decision. This situation commonly occurs in work with regressed patients. Unfortunately, the staff's behavior is then generally explained away as a manifestation of the patient's primitive use of splitting mechanisms. Whereas the staff members' opposing views may indeed be emblematic of the patient's internal world, the relevant countertransference issues are contained in the staff members' attitudes toward each other. Individual staff members may act as if they alone have "the true picture" of the patient, or they may be unable to listen to each other's view of the patient and/or may act contemptuously of formulations other than their own. In all these instances, a parallel process is being enacted on several levels. For example, the staff's insistence that they do not need each other to understand the patient may reflect the patient's disowned contempt, a product of his burgeoning awareness of his need for others. The essential point here is that staff must focus on how they are treating each other as a countertransference clue, rather than exclusively focus on speculations about the patient's actions.

Staff reactions to the agenda reveal clues about important countertransference feelings. For example, the usual agenda may be superceded by a particular patient's personal item, without any staff member protesting. Similarly, a particular patient may consistently be a priority item on the agenda, week after week, without any staff member registering a complaint. Conversely, the team may act as if everything is going so well for a particular patient that he need not be discussed at all. The former situation usually indicates staff's difficulty dealing with feelings stimulated by the patient's narcissism, especially his contempt for time or the needs of others, his sense of entitlement, or his exploitativeness. The patient who is frequently on the agenda often is one whom the staff wishes to keep in a dependent position, whereas keeping a patient off can indicate the treatment team's unwillingness to grapple with the individual and/or the problems he represents.

Another indication of countertransference in meetings concerns the withholding and sharing of information. A staff member may experience the impulse to withhold information while consciously recognizing the importance and appropriateness of disclosing what he knows. More overtly, a staff member may "make a deal" with a patient, guaranteeing absolute secrecy in exchange for information. These countertransference reactions involve the wish to protect the patient *and* the fear of betraying the patient or having him be misunderstood by other team members. Appreciating that these reactions are expressions of countertransference is essential. They provide important clues to significant underlying paranoid and psychopathic transferences that may otherwise go unnoticed. For example, a staff member may feel that information the patient has given him will be misunderstood by the staff, and thereby withhold the data to "protect" the patient. Becoming aware of his suspicions about how his colleagues might treat the information permits him to recognize that it is the patient who feels himself to be in an unsafe environment.

Just as violation of the treatment frame signals countertransference problems in individual psychotherapy, attacks on the patient's treatment plan may indicate unrecognized countertransference feelings occurring in team or staff meetings. These attacks may be subtle, such as consistently permitting a patient a small extension of the time he has requested for a pass. Bending of the treatment plan by certain staff is often accompanied by other staff withholding their protest of the infraction, reflecting their sense that their opinions would not be taken into account, or that they are alone in their objection. These countertransference reactions indicate staff's difficulty in dealing with the patient's contempt for shared conventions and the need for collaboration.

A variety of common countertransference reactions arise in counselors working with schizophrenic patients in settings such as case management, vocational counseling, skills learning instruction, and supervised residences, which may not rely on psychodynamic understanding. Even though it may be inappropriate for the counselor to utilize psychodynamic techniques in his interventions with the patient, it is nevertheless necessary that he accurately identify his reactions as reflections of the patient's psychopathology, or else collaborative work will suffer. For example, when a case manager regularly finds himself unable to imagine *any* task for which he might ask the patient to assume responsibility, he should ask himself how the patient has managed to convince him that he, the patient, is without any areas of competence. The therapist should challenge the patient's presentation of himself as totally incompetent. In the same vein, failure to imagine that the patient has any desire or wishes is a way of avoiding the painful task of helping the patient identify and assume responsibility for his areas of competence. Calling a patient by his first name or by a nickname, or fashioning an agenda that does not take into account the patient's goals or wishes, signals the presence of this type of countertransference reaction.

A number of countertransference reactions occur when a counselor feels inappropriately gratified by the patient's intense but unacknowledged dependency longings or his wish for an omnipotent savior. The counselor may believe he cannot go on vacation because he cannot convey all the necessary information about the patient to the person covering for him in his absence. The counselor also may be unable to conceive of ever terminating with his patient, or he may step out of role by advising the patient about medication or making psychodynamic interpretations.

Conclusions

If the therapist working with severely disturbed individuals seeks conventional signs of progress as motivation for his continuing participation, his efforts will be thwarted. Rather, it is the therapist's ability to recognize and apply what appear to be his vexing, strongly charged, and personally felt reactions to the patient that sustains his interest and hope. Historically, therapists have used their reactions as justification for abandoning hope of engagement with this group of difficult patients. Paradoxically, the therapist must first face his own reactions to the patient. Having recognized and accepted his own fantasies, feelings, and prejudices, the therapist can then begin to understand the connection between his reactions and the patient's subjective experience. As the work progresses, the therapist develops and maintains a sense of who the patient is, which he can eventually share with the patient, thus relieving the patient of his sense of isolation and need for withdrawal.

References

Altshul VA, Sledge WH: Countertransference problems, in American Psychiatric Press Review of Psychiatry, Vol 8. Edited by Tasman A, Hales RE, Frances AJ. Washington, DC, American Psychiatric Press, 1989, pp 518–530

Bion WR: Language and the schizophrenic, in Klein M: New Directions in Psychoanalysis. Edited by Klein M. London, Tavistock, 1955, pp 220–239

Bion WR: Attack on linking. Int J Psychoanal 40:308–315, 1959

Bleger J: Psycho-analysis of the psycho-analytic frame. Int J Psychoanal 48:511–519, 1967

Brenner C: Countertransference as compromise formation. Psychoanal Q 54:155–163, 1985

Kernberg OF: Transference and countertransference in the treatment of borderline patients, in Objects-Relations Theory and Clinical Psychoanalysis. New York, Jason Aronson, 1976, pp 161–184

Klein M: The importance of symbol-formation in the development of the ego (1930), in Contribution to Psycho-Analysis, 1921–1945. London, Hogarth Press, 1968, pp 236–250

Loewald HW: On the therapeutic action of psycho-analysis. Int J Psychoanal 41:16–33, 1960

Loewald HW: Transference-countertransference. J Am Psychoanal Assoc 34:275–287, 1986

Maher B: The language of schizophrenia: a review and interpretation. Br J Psychiatry 120:3–17, 1972

Ogden TH: The Primitive Edge of Experience. Northvale, NJ, Jason Aronson, 1989

Ogden TH: The Matrix of the Mind. Northvale, NJ, Jason Aronson, 1990

Racker H: Transference and Countertransference. New York, International Universities Press, 1968

Reich A: Further remarks on counter-transference. Int J Psychoanal 41:389–395, 1960

Searles HF: Countertransference and Related Subjects: Selected Papers. New York, International Universities Press, 1979

Sullivan HS: Conceptions of Modern Psychiatry: The First William Alanson White Memorial Lectures (1940). New York, WW Norton, 1953

Chapter 14

Therapists' Contribution to Negative Therapeutic Reactions

Dianna E. Hartley, Ph.D.

S ince the beginning of the practice of psychotherapy, negative
therapeutic reactions in the forms of treatment impasses, stalemates, premature terminations, or poor outcomes have been significant clinical and theoretical problems. Lambert et al. (1986)
concluded after an exhaustive review of the research literature that
psychotherapy "can and does cause harm to a portion of those it is
intended to help" (p. 183). Such outcomes may include exacerbated depression, increased confusion, lower self-esteem, increased
guilt and inhibition, diminished impulse control, erosion of valued
relationships, excessive dependence on the therapist for advice or
gratification, and disillusionment with the therapy process that pre-
cludes the person's seeking help elsewhere (Strupp et al. 1977).
While negative effects have long been acknowledged by clinicians,
and were first brought to the attention of the psychotherapy research community by Bergin in 1966, little has been specifically established about the process by which such outcomes are produced
and how they can be prevented. However, what has been learned
has important implications for diagnosis and selection of patients
for treatment, for choosing interventions, for focusing attention on
the person of the therapist and the therapeutic relationship, and
for the selection, training, and monitoring of therapists.

History of the Concept

Freud (1918[1914]/1955) first used the term "negative reaction" in his discussion of the case of the Wolf Man. It seemed to him that every time something was cleared up, the patient contradicted the new insight by an aggravation of his symptoms, like a child violating a prohibition one last time before giving up the forbidden behavior. Later, Freud wrote about "negative therapeutic reactions," saying that "something in these people" opposes recovery and dreads its approach (Freud 1923/1961). Freud viewed this phenomenon as the result, in part, of defiant attitudes toward the analyst, secondary gain of the symptoms, or narcissistic inaccessibility to a relationship with the analyst; but he attributed it primarily to a "moral factor," in that the illness seemed to be a way to atone for unconscious guilt.

Abraham (1919/1948) attributed some treatment failures to the inability of some narcissistic patients to tolerate the humiliation and diminished self-love involved in facing ego-dystonic facts. Writing from a Kleinian perspective, Riviere (1936) saw some patients as using hypomanic denial and infantile omnipotence to defend against depression, with its accompanying sense of dependent vulnerability and helplessness. Sullivan (1953) wrote of negative reactions in sadomasochistic patients who, when they are stressed and most in need of tenderness, act in defensive, malevolent ways that bring malevolence back onto themselves.

A number of theorists and clinicians have recently dissented from the idea that the problem lies within the patient. Stolorow, Brandchaft, and Atwood (1983) argue that there is no such person as an untreatable patient. They contend that therapeutic stalemates arise from the interaction between patient and therapist and cannot be understood apart from the intersubjective context in which these stalemates develop. They usually are the product of prolonged transference-countertransference disjunctions in which the therapist assimilates the material expressed by the patient into configurations that distort its actual subjective meaning for the patient. This results in chronic misunderstandings and countertherapeutic spirals that intensify, rather than relieve, the patient's suffering and fail to correct the underlying pathology. A second source of impasses from this perspective is intersubjective conjunctions in which the patient's experiences are assimilated into very similar central configurations in the mind of the therapist. Such a conjunction reflects a mutually acceptable defensive posture and strengthens resistance and counterresistance.

Reich (1933) was among the first analysts to take a more interactive perspective and to link treatment impasses with inadequate technique for dealing with latent negative transference. Recent conceptualizations of stalemates and treatment failures in the clinical and research literatures emphasize understanding the developmental level of the patient reflected in transference manifestations (Blanck and Blanck 1986; Gedo 1979, 1986; Hartley, in press), adopting a more dynamic family-systemic perspective (Lerner and Lerner 1983), and closely examining the therapist's contribution to the interactional field (Gorney 1979; Langs 1982). A recent issue of *Psychoanalytic Inquiry* (Vol. 7, No. 2, 1987), in which analysts representing different theoretical positions commented on the same case material, gives some idea of the vast differences of opinion on the subject of negative therapeutic events that exist even among a relatively homogeneous group of therapists.

Considering impasses, premature terminations, and poor outcomes from an interactional perspective raises questions about the therapist's contribution and about the treatment situation or therapeutic framework. In this chapter, we will consider the therapist's contribution in terms of both technical and personal factors, apart from countertransference (which is detailed in Chapters 12 and 13). The expert clinicians polled by Strupp and his associates (1977) in their study of the origins of negative outcomes cited such technical factors as poor clinical judgment and deficiencies in training and skills, and also inappropriate personality traits such as exploitativeness, sadistic or masochistic trends, narcissism, obsessionalism, or lack of authenticity. Robertiello and Schoenewolf (1987) discuss two types of "therapeutic blunders":

1. Technical errors include misapplying theories recently learned, selecting interventions poorly, making inadequate diagnostic

formulations, not extracting latent from manifest content, and not maintaining therapeutic attitudes and boundaries suitable for each patient.

2. Countertransference and counterresistance include instances in which therapists behave toward patients in ways that are rooted in unresolved characterological or cultural conflicts or biases, whether or not they are induced by corresponding feelings or behaviors of the patients.

We will look first at those factors that may be considered technical errors and then at those factors that are more based in personal characteristics.

Technical Errors and Mistakes

Kottler and Blau (1989) define *errors* as the failure to employ the right method in the solution of a problem, and *mistakes* as the failure to apply a certain accepted method carefully. Both errors and mistakes can occur in the practice of psychotherapy, where both problems and methods are often vaguely or ambiguously described. It is important to keep in mind at the same time that trying a strategy that does not work is not the same thing as failure. Stone (1985), in a candid discussion of his own negative outcomes with borderline patients, puts it succinctly: "To the extent that my native sense of omnipotence had suggested to me that I could treat anyone for anything, the successes I may have had along the way would only have served to perpetuate this illusion. Success is seductive in this regard; failure is instructive" (p. 145).

Adequate Diagnosis

In a major study in which experts talked about negative effects in psychotherapy, several participants stressed that a thorough diagnostic assessment in the initial phase of therapy was the best safeguard against antitherapeutic processes and the negative outcomes that usually result (Strupp et al. 1977). This assessment should include 1) full information about the presenting problem, including the decision to seek professional help and the referral process; 2) a comprehensive understanding of the patient's strengths and weaknesses, general level of ego functioning, or personality organization; and 3) the role the patient's symptoms play in maintaining a personal and a family-systems equilibrium.

Symptom diagnosis.   While symptom diagnosis of the type represented by Axis I of DSM-III (American Psychiatric Association 1980) has not been specifically correlated with negative processes in therapy or with poor outcome, Mays and Franks (1985) listed five characteristics of high-risk patients: 1) impaired or conflicted social support; 2) disturbances in the ability to communicate with others; 3) disturbances in mood or affect; 4) disturbances in identity and sense of self; and 5) disturbances in impulse control. Of course, most patients will have at least one of these problems, but significant deviation on any of these dimensions beyond what is usual in a given clinician's practice should alert the clinician to potential hazards ahead. Although there is still disagreement about the relative importance of therapist and patient factors in the etiology of negative events, a consistent finding is that the more disturbed the patient is, the more therapist skill appears to be critical to the avoidance of such events (Lambert et al. 1986).

Diagnosis of personality organization.   A survey of leading clinicians across the country revealed that certain patients are considered inherently more difficult to treat than others. The therapists surveyed included in the category of difficult patients those with paranoid, borderline, narcissistic, and antisocial personality disorders (Wong 1983). Using a framework in which borderline pathology is viewed in terms of personality organization (Kernberg 1984; Meissner 1984), and not just as a cluster of traits, most, if not all, of these patients would probably be subsumed.

The present consensus seems to be that borderline patients, by whatever criteria, are more prone than the patient population in general to negative experiences during psychotherapy, to premature terminations, and to poorer outcomes. Mays and Franks

(1985), in a major review of negative effects in psychotherapy, concluded that borderline patients seem to do worse than other patients, especially in psychoanalysis or insight-oriented psychotherapy. Their conclusion may be biased by the fact that psychoanalytically oriented clinicians tend to look at their data in terms of personality variables that often are ignored by practitioners of other types of therapy. Linehan (1989) points out the paucity of attention to borderline patients among behavioral and cognitive therapists and confirms the difficulty of treating these patients in this framework. Her own successful approach to treating borderline patients includes careful attention to the treatment contract and the therapeutic relationship as well as behavior contingency analysis. The extremely maladaptive interpersonal patterns of these patients are likely to be equally disruptive in all approaches to therapy. Because patients with borderline personality organization (using Kernberg's criteria) constitute approximately 10% to 14% of the total population (Stone 1985), it is especially important to find ways to help them use therapy productively.

Weiner (1982) concluded that the most common diagnostic error leading to negative outcomes in therapy is the overestimation of ego strength.

Wallerstein (1986), in his comprehensive and clinically rich overview of the Menninger Psychotherapy Research Project, illustrates the course of several "treatment failures." Colson et al. (1985) examined 11 of these cases who were rated as treatment failures and compared them with the 10 most successful cases. Finding, paradoxically, that the patients with poorer outcomes had higher levels of educational and occupational achievement, the authors concluded from a careful reading of the clinical write-ups that misdiagnoses in the direction of overestimating ego strength had consistently been made. The negative outcome group included primarily patients with borderline personality organization, particularly those marked by a desperate, angry search for satisfaction of chronically thwarted needs for nurturance. These persons had enormous difficulty establishing mature relationships, and most resorted to substance abuse. Because they had achieved relatively high social status despite significant psychopathology, they "tended to receive treatments which, at least at the outset, were mismatched in terms of the amount of support, containment, and structure required for a successful outcome" (Colson et al. 1985, p. 67).

Psychological testing and structured clinical interviews increase diagnostic accuracy among high-risk patients. Testing has been shown to be more accurate than other single or combined sources of information in the diagnosis of borderline disorders (Appelbaum 1977; Maltas 1978). In addition, interviews for diagnosing borderline disorders have been developed by Gunderson (1977), using a trait-oriented approach, and by Kernberg (1984), using an intrapsychic object-relations approach. Currently available structured interviews and self-report measures have been reviewed by Widiger and Frances (1989). Berg (1983) has succinctly summarized the literature on traditionally used projective measures. In the absence of such an understanding, the therapist may probe too deeply too soon and provoke negative reactions, or he or she may not challenge the patient to change for the better to the fullest extent possible.

Family-systems diagnosis.   In the national survey by Wong (1983), most therapists believed that not only the patient, but a severely pathological family system made some treatments difficult or impossible. While it is often easy to see the source of problematic behavior in the family dynamics, Colson (1982) shows the value of considering the adaptive or reparative meanings of symptoms or objectionable personality characteristics. Some patients, usually on the basis of early family dynamics, seem to feel deeply that they do not deserve a better life and that any gains they make result in suffering for others. Thus they either sacrifice their own development or punish themselves whenever they do something to enhance their lives. This kind of understanding of the interpersonal and intrapsychic meaning of the patient's problem can help the therapist anticipate and avoid pitfalls in treatment.

Lerner and Lerner (1983) emphasize that failures to change during individual therapy often can be understood by considering the adaptive functions served by the patient's symptoms and developmental failures in the context of the family system. The authors see the patient as caught between the competing pulls of *change,* represented by the treatment contract and the therapeutic relationship, and *homeostasis,* represented by loyalty to the family's overt or covert injunctions to remain the same or "change back." Behavior toward the therapist that appears to be oppositional or devaluing may take on different meanings when the systemic vantage point is adopted. Once these meanings are formulated by the therapist, they can be interpreted to the patient in a neutral way that frees the therapist from the position of urging the patient to change and allows the patient to decide whether or not to change. The systemic approach can be used not only for addressing current family activity, but also with patients who are geographically distant or emotionally disengaged from family or whose key family members are deceased. The essential aspects are a conceptual framework and techniques that allow gathering of information about how the family system works and how the patient's symptoms and resistances are embedded in it.

Considering the fact that therapy rarely occupies more than a few hours a week, it is surprising how little attention has been paid to events occurring outside the consulting room. Lerner and Lerner (1983) have stressed the importance of the patient's family system with regard to the dynamic stresses and reactions that are set off by change in the individual. The explicit and implicit messages the patient gets from family members could potentially undermine strides toward autonomy or higher levels of functioning. For example, changes for the worse often have a significant impact on a patient's family members. Their reactions may at times undermine the patient's self-confidence as well as his or her confidence in the therapist, or may reinforce the idea that the patient is bad or uncooperative. On the other hand, when there is no detectable family reaction to a patient's failure to change, increased acting out, or harsh criticism of the therapist, we wonder about the importance of the patient's symptoms or weaknesses in maintaining some particular balance in family dynamics.

Colson et al. (1985) concluded that among negative outcome cases, "significant people in the patient's life colluded to an extraordinary degree, either to sabotage treatment or to undermine opportunities for health" (p. 67). The usual pattern was one of overindulgence and encouragement of self-destructive behavior and hostile dependence on family members, alternating with periods of harsh control and rejection. Voth and Orth (1973), in their book about these cases, were struck by the parallel between the impasses in the therapies of these patients and the impasses of development in the separation-individuation phases that are, in theory, associated with borderline pathology. Gurman and Kniskern (1978) suggested that in some cases the development of alliances with key family members may reduce both deliberate and unwitting sabotage of therapy.

Therapeutic Alliance and Misalliances

In his work on therapeutic alliance, Bordin (1979) pointed out that different forms of therapy make different demands on both the therapist and the patient in terms of their personal qualities and their working contract. Langs (1982) has been particularly active in exploring the effects of violations of the basic framework of the therapeutic relationship on the therapeutic process and on the patient's level of functioning. Many therapeutic stalemates and negative outcomes are precipitated by failure to deal with issues of the framework (Langs 1982) or of the therapeutic alliance (Greenson 1967; Hartley 1985). A major component of the therapeutic alliance is the explicit or implicit understanding between the therapist and the patient about the nature of the problem, the goals they will work toward, and the means they will use in pursuit of these goals, including the responsibilities each is to undertake in accomplishing the work of the therapy. The therapist as well as the patient must be willing and able to engage genuinely in the relationship and to accomplish the tasks required for the particular kind of therapy undertaken.

Langs (1982) points out the need to consider the therapeutic interaction and the contribution of the therapist and therapist-patient collusion to disturbances of the alliance. Impairments of alliance may take the form of acute disruptions, repeated difficulties, or mutual efforts to maintain an antitherapeutic misalliance. The therapist may play a part through inappropriate attitudes, incorrect interventions, blind spots, or by necessary disruptions that are nonetheless disturbing to the patient. Even when the misalliance is initiated by the patient, the therapist's reaction—which should be first to refuse to participate and then to interpret the offered interaction—often determines the extent of harm done to the treatment process. The resolution of disruptions in the therapeutic alliance takes precedence over other therapeutic tasks. The therapist's capacity to maintain the framework and offer valid interpretations under these circumstances almost always strengthens the patient's ego and capacity for trust and enhances or renews the alliance itself.

The process of establishing and maintaining an alliance may go awry at many points and in many ways. Some psychotherapies are marked from the beginning by negative interactions between the therapist and the patient. The process of conducting the assessment interviews, and of negotiating basic contractual issues of time for meeting, fees and fee collection, and the boundaries of the treatment relationship, can either establish the foundation for a positive alliance or provide hints of forthcoming struggles.

Colson et al. (1985) found that the therapy process for patients with negative outcomes in the Menninger study was notable for the absence of cooperative and collaborative activity by the patient, based in part on the attitude that the therapist should cause the patient to feel better without the patient's active work. Therapy proceeded as though the patient had to extract solutions from a harsh, ungiving therapist. The authors also noted that therapists were remarkably inconsistent in addressing blatant violations of basic aspects of the therapeutic contract, unwittingly tolerating behavior that undermined the therapy's chances of success:

> Frequently the treatments were marked by inconsistent attendance, lateness, delinquent payment of the bill, interminable contacts with the therapists at odd hours outside the treatment sessions, persistent verbal assaults on the treater, inconsistent use of medication, and a variety of other forms of "acting out" within

and outside the treatment hours. In far too many instances the therapists patiently tolerated the continuation of such behavior, perhaps expecting that such behavior would yield to the "right" interpretations. In not one case did the treater insist that continuation of treatment would depend on an alteration in such behaviors. From our current perspective it would have been quite appropriate, and in some instances necessary, for the therapist to support treatment structures by putting the treatment itself on the line. (Colson et al. 1985, pp. 72–73)

In fact, the results of this study, which was conducted 30 to 40 years ago, taught us much that we now take for granted about the importance of the therapeutic alliance (Horwitz 1974) and of firm insistence on the patient adhering to the basic treatment structure (Kernberg 1984). It is clear from Wallerstein's (1986) review that the therapists' tolerance of maladaptive behavior in the context of the therapy perpetuated their patients' problems, whereas insisting that the patients follow the more mature, adult aspects of the contract might have led to further development in patients' other relationships as well. Such neglect of the basic framework of the treatment often feeds into the patient's poor sense of personal responsibility, poor reality testing, and poor impulse control, and ultimately creates a chronic impasse in the treatment that is exceedingly difficult for the patient and therapist to resolve or dilute.

Aside from these more blatant instances of "breaking the rules" of the therapeutic contract or allowing them to be broken by the patient, therapists need to be alert to more subtle indicators of disturbances in the alliance throughout the course of therapy. Bordin (1979) has gone so far as to assert that the process of disruption and repair of the alliance is itself one of the most important therapeutic events.

More recently, Safran and his associates (1990) proposed a framework for empirical investigation of such ruptures in the alliance. Based on intensive observation of videotaped therapy sessions in which both patient and therapist indicated problems in the alliance, the authors developed a list of seven process markers: 1) overt expression of negative feelings, 2) indirect communication of hostility, 3) disagreement about the goals or tasks of therapy, 4) begrudging or thoughtless compliance, 5) avoidance maneuvers, 6) defensive operations to preserve self-esteem, and 7) nonresponsiveness to an intervention. They note that such ruptures usually follow an empathic failure (Kohut 1984) or some behavior on the part of the therapist that enacts a dysfunctional interpersonal schema (Horowitz 1988), or failure of the therapist to "pass a test" disconfirming a pathogenic belief (Weiss et al. 1987).

At such junctures in therapy—which may vary in intensity from yelling accusations and threats to quit, to withdrawing in a barely noticeable manner—it is essential that the therapist notice and talk with the patient about the relationship problem. Foreman and Marmar (1985), in a promising pilot study of patients who showed low scores on a measure of therapeutic alliance early in treatment, found that in each case in which the alliance became better in later sessions, the therapist had explicitly addressed the issue of the poor working relationship and explored with the patient what changes were necessary. In cases with unimproved alliances and poor outcomes, the therapist avoided, ignored, or tried to seal over the problematic feelings. In one of a series of exemplary studies of success and failure in psychotherapy, Strupp (1980) noted that he did not locate in the taped sessions "a single instance in which a difficult client's hostility and negativism were successfully confronted or resolved," and that the major deterrent to the resolution was "the therapist's personal reaction" (pp. 953–954).

Even though we all have been taught that it is generally important to address negative feelings in therapy, it is probably the thing we do least well because it is an uncomfortable experience that activates concerns about our professional competence and about personal qualities we value and want to see in ourselves.

Personal Characteristics of the Therapist

In beginning this section, perhaps more than the one about technical errors, it is important to acknowledge that countertransference, counterresistance, and personality characteristics that are impediments in certain kinds of treatments are universal phenomena. The question is not do I have hindering characteristics, but rather what kind and when are they evident in my work with patients. Fortunately, extreme exploitation or mistreatment of patients is relatively rare, but we make mistakes every day, not because of severe personal problems or lack of integrity, but because we work with delicate instruments: our patients' and our own psyches (Robertiello and Schoenewolf 1987). This fusion of the personal and professional identity is unique to psychotherapy. Each of us is to some extent inconsistent and fallible, even provided with the best education, supervision, and self-analysis.

Racker (1968), a Kleinian analyst, portrayed psychotherapy as a two-sided transaction in which both persons must resolve transferences and overcome resistances. He characterized the therapist's counterresistance as coinciding with resistance in the patient concerning the same situation in such a way that both participants develop a tacit agreement to keep quiet about it. The result is a standstill in which both know they are not finished with the therapy, but neither goes ahead with it either. Such resistance could originate in the personality or the neurosis of the therapist, not just as a reaction to the patient. For example, a narcissistic therapist may not confront grandiosity and rage in the patient and instead may encourage undue idealization and reinforce a false self. A hysterical therapist may avoid erotic feelings; a sadomasochistic one avert tenderness; and a passive one foil attempts at criticism and hostility.

Cultural biases—those grounded in gender, religious affiliation, political beliefs, or other social dichotomies—may also lead to blind spots and harmful behavior. To the extent that they lead the therapist to group people as good and bad, these biases are likely to detract from the therapist's ability to work with some people (Robertiello and Schoenewolf 1987).

Therapist characteristics that increase the likelihood of stalemates and negative reactions can be separated into two categories (Buckley et al. 1979; Tourney et al. 1966). First are the "sins of commission"—that is, those that are perceived as threatening to the patient's integrity or autonomy (e.g., high levels of confrontation, inappropriate or ill-timed interpretations, overidentification with the patient, unnecessary advice or controlling behavior). Then there are the "sins of omission"—that is, those that are perceived to provide low levels of support (e.g., excessive interpersonal distance; lack of warmth; passivity in the form of failures to ask appropriate questions, to interpret when relevant, or to set clear and appropriate limits). Therapists, like all people, have their own tendencies to make one or the other of these errors in situations of ambiguity, based on preferred levels of stimulation or homeostasis and the theoretical orientation of their training programs.

Once an impasse is developing, therapists may perpetuate or exacerbate it either by neglecting to deal with the feelings involved, for fear of losing control of the process, or by responding defensively to justify their own behavior, rather than helping patients examine the realistic and unrealistic sources of their perceptions and feelings (Mays and Franks 1985). Therapists usually feel angry, guilty, and impotent at times of impasse. These feelings may be enacted in the forms of lateness, cancellations, sarcasm, or coldness; of allowing dependency; or of giving up on attainable goals—all of which exacerbate the situation and may lead to premature termination or poor outcome of the therapy.

Reluctance to deal with early signs of resistance or disruptions of alliance stems from many sources, the major one being narcissistic investment in the identity of psychotherapist. Many people who choose this profession, as do many people in the general public, idealize therapists as more intelligent, compassionate, and perceptive than others. The danger of this sense of superiority in the therapist lies in not allowing oneself the same passions, frailties, and defenses as most people, and thereby not acknowledging them to oneself, to supervisors, and to patients when appropriate. Unfortunately, this individual trend is reflected in and supported by a pejorative attitude toward countertransference manifestations. Rather than learn to use reactions for their own and patients' benefit, therapists often feel guilty and inhibit their receptivity and responsiveness.

Colson et al. (1985) found that therapists in their negative-outcome group were often slow to recognize the lack of progress in treatment and to shift to more appropriate therapeutic strategies. Particularly in psychoanalysis or psychoanalytic psychotherapies that are intended to be long term, inertia may be seen as less undesirable than impatience; however, much evidence suggests that inactivity can be just as harmful to the treatment.

It is easy to say that high-risk patients should be treated only by therapists who are able to offer high levels of empathy, warmth, and genuineness and who have the greatest knowledge of personality dynamics, interpersonal styles, and the potential pitfalls of treatment. However, studies of therapists' contribution to the therapy process and common lore among therapy researchers suggest that "high functioning" therapists are rare (Mitchell et al. 1977; Strupp 1989). To provide high levels of empathy, warmth, and genuineness in the face of powerful resistance and extreme emotion is not as easy as it might sound. Strupp (1989) refers to "the great paradox of therapy": that offering a benign and empathic relationship leaves one open to becoming the target of the patient's accumulated frustrations, conflicts, and fears. The course and outcome of therapy are determined in meeting these challenges.

Rigidity is probably the therapist's most serious obstacle. For various reasons, the practice of psychoanalysis and psychotherapy has become more ritualized and orthodox over the years. We sometimes overlook that Freud and other early analysts were rather fearless innovators. Freud (1919[1918]/1955) recounted that he evolved his rules for treatment out of his own experience after other methods cost him dearly. These rules proved suited to his personality, but he did not deny that someone differently constituted would feel impelled to adopt a different attitude to his or her patients and to the task before him or her.

Resolving Stalemates

Obviously, it is better to anticipate and deal with an impending stalemate than to come to a complete impasse, to have the treatment end prematurely, or to have the patient leave treatment in worse condition than at the beginning. Several clues may point to imminent difficulties. If the therapist makes a therapeutic contract that differs dramatically from the usual, such as setting an extremely low fee or allowing extensive outside contact, problems often ensue. Recognition of early stages of an impasse requires that the therapist have in mind a goal for treatment and the means by which to reach the goal, that is, a sound therapeutic alliance. During extended periods when no change occurs or when interactions are consistently empty or negative, reexamination of the contract may reveal that neither therapist nor patient is working toward the original goal.

At a point of suspected impasse of uncertain etiology, the therapist needs, first, to observe the therapeutic process closely and to assess honestly his or her reactions to the patient and the therapeutic process. Stolorow and his colleagues (1983) recommend that therapists be sufficiently aware of themselves that they are able to "decenter," in the Piagetian sense, from their own subjective worlds in order to grasp the meaning of their patients' experience of difficulties in the treatment relationship. Then perhaps obtaining consultation or supervision, transferring the patient to another therapist, or suggesting a vacation from therapy might be considered (Weiner 1982). The patient should be involved in the process of observation and reflection on the process of therapy in order to diagnose and decide what to do about the problem. By asking the patient to participate in the process, the therapist indicates that both are responsible for understanding the process and for the outcome of the therapy.

Obtaining consultations from other clinicians. Consultation may take the form of scheduling independent interviews with another therapist; having another person (i.e., a supervisor or a colleague) observe a video- or audiotape; or referring the patient for psychological testing. Cognitive and intellectual testing can be useful in detecting patients whose capacity for abstract thinking is impaired, or for whom other deficits make it difficult or impossible for them to attain the conceptual integration necessary for verbal therapies. Projective testing can identify problems with impulse control, impaired reality testing, or other aspects of personality organization that may alert the therapist to the need for more ego-building approaches to the treatment (Blanck and Blanck 1986). In addition to these more formal or structural aspects of cognitive functioning and personality organization, testing may alert the therapist to psychological themes that have been missed because of inexperience, countertransference problems, or other sources of empathic failure.

The process of deciding whether to obtain a consultation can itself give clues about the nature of the difficulty. A patient's hesitation to see a consultant when suggested by the therapist may indicate unwillingness to engage significantly with the therapist, a lack of motivation for the therapy, or a fear that this is the first step toward abandonment by the therapist. When a patient requests a consultation, the therapist may either suggest a consultant or allow the patient to select one. While a therapist has an obligation to state clearly his or her own professional opinion and advice, therapists who feel strongly about whom the patient sees or even whether the patient should ask for another opinion should examine their wish to control the patient or other antitherapeutic attitudes.

For nonmedical therapists or physicians who prefer not to use medications with their own psychotherapy patients, multiple treatment is an alternative to transferring patients who require pharmacological interventions. A separate physician manages medications, and the psychotherapist continues psychological treatment. This practice is most feasible within an institutional setting or in a situation where frequent communication between treaters is possible.

Transferring the patient.   When it becomes clear through exploration and observation or through consultation that the therapist does not offer the kind of treatment the patient needs or that something in the patient-therapist interaction blocks effective collaborative work together, transfer of the patient should be considered. When this occurs, both the transferring and the receiving therapists share the responsibility to help in working through the loss, resolving the problematic dynamics as much as possible, and facilitating the patient's attachment to the new therapist.

Termination or vacation from therapy.   Raising the question of stopping treatment has long been used to deal with impasses (Freud 1937/1964). When temporary or permanent termination of treatment is a realistic alternative, and not a manipulation, the therapist's mentioning it may motivate the patient to examine all the possibilities for resolving the impasse. Some patients may find that the therapist's nondefensive willingness to discuss stopping the treatment makes them feel freer to air their own feelings and ideas about the problems in the relationship. The dangers of raising this possibility are the same as those of raising the more general issue of negative aspects of the therapeutic relationship: the patient may act impulsively, or he or she may feel demoralized or abandoned.

Positive Aspects of Negative Events

Because both patients and therapists have strong emotional reactions to therapeutic stalemates and poor outcomes, it is important to work with these feelings as a problem in the therapist-patient relationship, not just as intrapsychic phenomena. Clear discussion of a stalemate itself can be a valuable experience for a patient whose previous relationships have been based on mutual blame instead of mutual responsibility. Anger, guilt, helplessness, and frustration can be turned to therapeutic advantage by direct expression. Weiner (1982) stresses that mutual exploration must take place in the context of an adequate therapeutic alliance, and not be used to seduce a patient into remaining in therapy or as a substitute for the patient's self-examination.

    In addition to the positive effects that open discussion of negative events can have in individual cases, it has often been the case that treatment impasses have provided the impetus for major revisions of theory and technique, and thus they can be beneficial to the profession as a whole when they are productively and non-defensively examined. To take an early example, an impasse and premature termination in the case of Dora led Freud to his conceptualization of transference. More recently, Kohut's (1979) paper about his reanalysis of Mr. Z., which indicates the therapist's willingness to examine his mistakes and his thinking processes about them, provides a valuable model for questioning "received wisdom," for listening carefully to patients' associations with an open mind, and for reformulating ideas about the etiology and treatment of relatively common forms of psychopathology. Gedo (1986), in a scholarly review of the history of ideas in psychoanalysis and current controversies in the field, clearly illustrated how many significant advances in both theory and practice have developed from failures to deal adequately with certain types of psychopathology.

Relevant Research Findings

In addition to rough estimates of the incidence of negative outcomes and broad generalizations about patient and therapist characteristics associated with negative outcome, some more pertinent information exists in those investigations of psychotherapy process that used measures allowing the examination of negative events during sessions. Orlinsky and Howard (1986) point out that the "macro-outcome" of a psychotherapy is the net result of an extended series of incremental "micro-outcomes" seen in the sessions and between sessions in the daily life of the patient during therapy.

The first step toward empirical examination of impasses as they evolve is the development of reliable and valid process measures for the relevant variables. The Psychotherapy Research Group at Vanderbilt University under the direction of Hans Strupp has made substantial progress in this area in the past decade. The group developed the Vanderbilt Negative Indicators Scale (VNIS), which identifies a number of in-session occurrences that have been shown to be ultimately associated with poor outcomes (Sachs 1983; Suh et al. 1986). They have also included in other process scales the possibility of assessing negative, as well as positive, signs of therapeutic interaction (Gomes-Schwartz 1978; Hartley and Strupp 1983).

For example, the Vanderbilt Psychotherapy Process Scale (VPPS) consists of eight subscales: Patient Participation, Patient Hostility, Patient Psychic Distress, Patient Exploration, Patient Dependency, Therapist Exploration, Therapist Warmth and Friendliness, and Negative Therapist Attitude. The 80 items on the scale are rated by observers who watch or listen to the therapy sessions. Unfortunately, in most of the process-outcome studies using the VPPS, the subscales have been collapsed in ways that make it impossible to examine the impact on outcome of negative patient or therapist qualities. An interesting exception is the study of therapist characteristics associated with differential outcome by Suh and O'Malley (1982). They divided their sample into four groups by crossing prognosis and outcome (e.g., high prognosis–low outcome, low prognosis–low outcome, etc.). They found that it was not the absolute level of the therapist quality, but the *pattern of change* over the early sessions that discriminated among these groups. Patients who were categorized as high prognosis–low outcome had therapists "characterized by initially high levels of Negative Therapist Attitude which increased across sessions with a concomitant decrease in Therapist Warmth and Therapist Exploration. . . . Therapists for low prognosis–low outcome cases not only exhibited high initial levels of Negative Therapist Attitude but there was a decrease in Therapist Warmth over sessions" (Suh et al. 1986, p. 301).

The VNIS is the best existing measure for examining the kind of events in therapy sessions that are generally associated with impasses and eventual poor outcome. Growing out of the work of Strupp, Hadley, and Gomes-Schwartz (1977), this scale includes 42 patient, therapist, and interaction items. The subscales include Patient Qualities, Therapist Personal Qualities, Errors in Technique, Patient-Therapist Interaction, and Global Factors. Sachs (1983) found that the subscale Errors in Technique showed the strongest and most consistent relationship to outcome, whereas the subscale Therapist Personal Qualities was not significantly associated with outcome. This subscale, however, has consistently caused researchers the most difficulty in achieving adequate interrater reliability, suggesting that judges have different opinions about this important facet of the therapy process. The authors suggest using as raters for the VNIS only well-trained therapists familiar with a broad range of therapeutic practices. Because the VNIS calls for value judgments, there is much room for disagreement on what constitutes poor practice. Also, because the scale is anchored in psychodynamic concepts, it may be less applicable to other therapies.

In a study using the Vanderbilt Therapeutic Alliance Scale, Hartley and Strupp (1983) found that the alliance ratings for patient contribution, therapist contribution, and interaction factors increased over the first few sessions for cases with positive outcomes, and decreased during the early sessions for the poorer outcome cases. Although the alliance recovered to some extent in the negative outcome cases, the early mutual decline was not overcome in the brief therapy.

In a more recent series of studies (Henry et al. 1990; Talley et al. 1990), the Vanderbilt group, using microscopic analyses of interpersonal process based on the Structural Analysis of Social Behavior (Benjamin 1984), found support for the following ideas:

1. Poor outcome is associated with therapist behavior that confirms negative patient introjects.
2. Hostile and/or controlling therapist behavior is correlated with self-blame by the patient.
3. Therapists whose own introjects are more disaffiliative engage in more hostile, controlling behavior, give more "mixed messages," and produce poorer outcomes.
4. Anticomplementarity between therapist self concept and therapist perception of patient behavior is associated with poor outcome.

Based on findings from these studies the Vanderbilt group concluded the following:

1. Even a small number of pejorative messages from a therapist can seriously interfere with the therapeutic process, resulting in

premature terminations and poor outcomes in brief therapies.

2. Even experienced therapists are prone to these kinds of interactions.

3. The therapist's intellectual understanding of these problems does not translate into appropriate action when confronted with the enactments of difficult patients.

The correlations found in these studies between process measures and outcome give reason to be hopeful about the possibility of empirically examining how therapeutic stalemates evolve, how they either do or do not become resolved, and what impact they have on the eventual outcome of psychotherapy. No study, however, has specifically addressed this issue.

Conclusions and Recommendations

Selection and Training of Therapists

Graduate programs in clinical psychology and psychiatric residencies rely heavily on academic rather than personal qualifications for admission. As the contribution of the therapist's personality to the process and outcome of psychotherapy becomes clearer, programs will need to find ways to assess variables relevant to clinical practice. The best chance for decreasing therapist-induced difficulties lies in eliminating those applicants who are likely to be unsuitable practitioners. Even now, enough is known about potentially noxious personality characteristics to institute screening procedures for characteristics like sadism, exploitativeness, and pathological narcissism.

In addition to screening applicants, training directors can make sure that their curricula include both didactic and experiential components that teach students to assess areas of vulnerability, such as fragile ego organization, and to intervene appropriately.

Goldberg (1990), in a discussion of common mistakes of beginning therapists, says bluntly that the first mistake may be the selection of a profession. Even Freud (1937/1964) regarded psychoanalysis as the impossible profession, at a time in his life when he was perhaps unduly pessimistic but still extremely demanding. Clearly, many persons enter programs unaware of their own vulnerabilities and of the potential occupational hazards. Just as a therapeutic alliance entails letting the patients know what they are in for, a training alliance puts the burden on educators and supervisors to inform applicants as fully as possible about both the agonies and the ecstacies of practicing psychotherapy.

Implications for Clinical Practice

Therapists should be willing and able to recognize impending and actual impasses in their practices and to assess the relative contributions of the patient's dynamics, their own possible errors or lack of adequate training, the need of the patient for a different therapeutic approach, and the interaction of the patient with family or significant others in the environment. The occurrence of persistent dissatisfaction must be regarded as a signal that something is seriously amiss in the patient-therapist relationship.

Therapists can also act to prevent impasses through awareness of their personalities, of their interpersonal impact, and of the influence these factors have on their approach to therapy. A therapist who expresses chronic anger through aggressive interpretations or attacks on defenses, or who fosters dependency to gratify his or her own needs, or who enjoys a sense of omnipotent power by manipulating patients, is likely to produce many negative results.

In addition to such self-awareness, therapists can minimize stalemates by assessing not only the patient's personality resources for the therapy undertaken, but also the patient's goals. Impasses associated with mismatches could be reduced, and the therapist could correct any misapprehensions or misperceptions about therapy the patient might have.

In addition to increased use of such diagnostic techniques as psychological testing and structured interviews, the use of more experienced and skilled therapists in the initial assessment process seems warranted. Unfortunately, the therapists who are least capable of handling high-risk cases are most likely to underestimate the severity of patient psychopathology and the degree of immediate psychological distress (Beutler 1983). In addition, there are formidable problems associated with transferring patients with borderline personality disorder, or other high-risk patients, after a relationship is established.

Therapists who treat difficult patients successfully are not superhuman; they respond in natural human ways to the stresses of consistently being in emotional struggles with other people and of dealing with professional frustrations. Ongoing consultation, supervision, or discussion with peers is the best antidote to therapist burnout. Antitherapeutic behaviors and attitudes are relatively easy to identify, even by relatively inexperienced clinicians, such as clinical psychology graduate students (Sachs 1983). Therapists are often reluctant to admit angry, sexual, or dependent feelings to colleagues for fear of being seen as unprofessional; consultation can be invaluable in helping therapists sort out the sources of such feelings and put them in perspective.

Research Directions

The study of therapeutic impasses is an integral part of the study of the process and outcome of psychotherapy more generally. Much has been written about the concept of negative outcome in psychotherapy. Little has been done to allow adequate examination of negative outcomes, and even less to explore the processes by which these negative outcomes were produced. While some patients are worse at termination or follow-up points because of external life circumstances, it seems far more likely that seeds of the outcome could be detected in the form of poorly handled impasses during the therapy. Kiesler (1973) stressed that any meaningful therapeutic changes must be evident within the therapy sessions themselves. This statement is as true of negative events as it is of positive changes. Even with recent advances in process research, we still lack systems of measures and data analysis procedures that would allow us to track the patient-therapist interactions during difficult times in therapy.

It is unethical to design studies in which impasses are experimentally induced, and it is unlikely that impasses induced by irresponsible clinicians will become available for scientific scrutiny. However, one excellent source of information already exists in the form of the recorded psychotherapy sessions from major process-outcome studies. Patient-therapist dyads that are known to have resulted in poor outcomes should be subjected to close scrutiny in order to learn more about factors that might have led to the outcome. Cases in which there were clear struggles and temporary impasses could also be examined to tell us more about the process of overcoming such strains and of successfully completing treatment.

References

Abraham K: A particular form of neurotic resistance against the psychoanalytic method (1919), in Selected Papers. London, Hogarth Press, 1948, pp 303–311

American Psychiatric Association: Diagnostic and Statistical Manual of Mental Disorders, 3rd Edition. Washington, DC, American Psychiatric Association, 1980

Appelbaum S: The Anatomy of Change: A Menninger Foundation Report Testing the Effects of Psychotherapy. New York, Plenum, 1977

Benjamin LS: Principles of prediction using Structural Analysis of Social Behavior, in Personality and the Prediction of Behavior. Edited by Zucker RA, Aronoff J, Rabin AJ. New York, Academic, 1984, pp 121–174

Berg M: Borderline psychopathology as displayed on psychological tests. J Pers Assess 47:120–133, 1983

Bergin AE: Some implications of psychotherapy research for therapeutic practice. J Abnorm Psychol 71:235–246, 1966

Beutler L: Eclectic Psychotherapy: A Systematic Approach. Elmsford, NY, Pergamon, 1983

Blanck G, Blanck R: Beyond Ego Psychology: Developmental Object Relations Theory. New York, Columbia University Press, 1986

Bordin ES: The generalizability of the psychoanalytic concept of the working alliance. Psychotherapy: Theory, Research, and Practice 16:252–260, 1979

Buckley P, Karasu TB, Charles E: Common mistakes in psychotherapy. Am J Psychiatry 136:1578–1580, 1979

Colson DB: Protectiveness in borderline states: a neglected object-relations paradigm. Bull Menninger Clin 46:305–320, 1982

Colson DB, Lewis L, Horwitz L: Negative outcome in psychotherapy and psychoanalysis, in Negative Outcome in Psychotherapy and What to Do About It. Edited by Mays DT, Franks CM. New York, Springer, 1985, pp 59–75

Foreman SA, Marmar CR: Therapist actions that address initially poor therapeutic alliances in psychotherapy. Am J Psychiatry 142:922–926, 1985

Freud S: From the history of an infantile neurosis (1918[1914]), in The Standard Edition of the Complete Psychological Works of Sigmund Freud, Vol 17. Translated and edited by Strachey J. London, Hogarth Press, 1955, pp 1–123

Freud S: Lines of advance in psycho-analytic therapy (1919[1918]), in The Standard Edition of the Complete Psychological Works of Sigmund Freud, Vol 17. Translated and edited by Strachey J. London, Hogarth Press, 1955, pp 157–168

Freud S: The ego and the id (1923), in The Standard Edition of the Complete Psychological Works of Sigmund Freud, Vol 19. Translated and edited by Strachey J. London, Hogarth Press, 1961, pp 1–66

Freud S: Analysis terminable and interminable (1937), in The Standard Edition of the Complete Psychological Works of Sigmund Freud, Vol 23. Translated and edited by Strachey J. London, Hogarth Press, 1964, pp 216–254

Gedo JE: Beyond Interpretation: Toward a Revised Theory for Psychoanalysis. New York, International University Press, 1979

Gedo JE: Conceptual Issues in Psychoanalysis: Essays in History and Methods. Hillsdale, NJ, Analytic Press, 1986

Goldberg C: Typical mistakes of the beginning therapist, in The Encyclopedic Handbook of Private Practice. Edited by Margenau EA. New York, Gardner Press, 1990, pp 770–784

Gomes-Schwartz B: Effective ingredients in psychotherapy: prediction of outcome from process variables. J Consult Clin Psychol 46:1023–1035, 1978

Gorney J: The negative therapeutic interaction. Contemporary Psychoanalysis 15:288–337, 1979

Greenson RR: The Technique and Practice of Psychoanalysis. New York, International Universities Press, 1967

Gunderson JG: Characteristics of borderlines, in Borderline Personality Disorders: The Concept, the Syndrome, the Patient. Edited by Hartocollis P. New York, International Universities Press, 1977, pp 173–192

Gurman AS, Kniskern DP: Deterioration in marital and family therapy: empirical, clinical and conceptual issues. Fam Process 17:3–20, 1978

Hartley DE: Research on the therapeutic alliance in psychotherapy, in Psychiatry Update: American Psychiatric Association Annual Review, Vol 4. Edited by Hales RE, Frances AJ. Washington, DC, American Psychiatric Press, 1985, pp 532–549

Hartley DE: Assessing intrapsychic developmental level, in Handbook of Psychodynamic Research and Practice. Edited by Miller N, Luborsky L, Barber J, et al. New York, Basic Books (in press)

Hartley DE, Strupp HH: The therapeutic alliance: its relationship to outcome in brief psychotherapy, in Empirical Studies of Psychoanalytical Theories, Vol 1. Edited by Masling J. Hillsdale, NJ, Analytic Press, 1983, pp 1–37

Henry WP, Schact TE, Strupp HH: Patient and therapist introject, interpersonal process, and differential psychotherapy outcome. J Consult Clin Psychol 58:768–794, 1990

Horowitz MJ: Introduction to Psychodynamics: A New Synthesis. New York, Basic Books, 1988

Horwitz L: Clinical Prediction in Psychotherapy. New York, Jason Aronson, 1974

Kernberg O: Severe Personality Disorders: Psychotherapeutic Strategies. New Haven, CT, Yale University Press, 1984

Kiesler D: The Process of Psychotherapy. New York, Plenum, 1973

Kohut H: The two analyses of Mr. Z. Int J Psychoanal 60:3–27, 1979

Kohut H: How Does Analysis Cure? Chicago, IL, University of Chicago Press, 1984

Kottler JA, Blau DS: The Imperfect Therapist: Learning from Failure in Therapeutic Practice. San Francisco, CA, Jossey-Bass, 1989

Lambert MJ, Shapiro DA, Bergin AE: The effectiveness of psychotherapy, in Handbook of Psychotherapy and Behavior Change, 3rd Edition. Edited by Garfield SL, Bergin AE. New York, Wiley, 1986, pp 157–211

Langs R: Psychotherapy: A Basic Text. New York, Jason Aronson, 1982

Lerner S, Lerner HE: A systemic approach to resistance: theoretical and technical considerations. Am J Psychother 37:387–399, 1983

Linehan MM: Cognitive and behavior therapy for borderline personality disorder, in American Psychiatric Press Review of Psychiatry, Vol 8. Edited by Tasman A, Hales RE, Frances AJ. Washington, DC, American Psychiatric Press, 1989, pp 84–102

Maltas CP: Therapeutic uses of psychological testing of borderline adolescents. J Adolesc 1:259–272, 1978

Mays DT, Franks CM: Negative Outcome in Psychotherapy and What to Do About It. New York, Springer, 1985

Meissner W: The Borderline Spectrum. New York, Jason Aronson, 1984

Mitchell KM, Bozarth JD, Krauft CC: A reappraisal of the therapeutic effectiveness of accurate empathy, nonpossessive warmth and genuineness, in Effective Psychotherapy: A Handbook of Research. Edited by Gurman AS, Razin AM. New York, Pergamon, 1977, pp 482–502

Orlinsky DE, Howard KI: Process and outcome in psychotherapy, in Handbook of Psychotherapy and Behavior Change, 3rd Edition. Edited by Garfield SL, Bergin AE. New York, Wiley, 1986, pp 311–381

Racker H: Transference and Counter-Transference. New York, International Universities Press, 1968

Reich W: Character Analysis. New York, Orgone Institute Press, 1933

Riviere J: A contribution to the analysis of the negative therapeutic reaction. Int J Psychoanal 17:304–320, 1936

Robertiello RC, Schoenewolf G: 101 Common Therapeutic Blunders: Countertransference and Counterresistance in Psychotherapy. Northvale, NJ, Jason Aronson, 1987

Sachs JS: Negative factors in brief psychotherapy: an empirical assessment. J Consult Clin Psychol 51:557–564, 1983

Safran J, Crocker P, McMain S, et al: Therapeutic alliance rupture as a therapy event for empirical investigation. Psychotherapy 27:154–165, 1990

Stolorow RD, Brandchaft B, Atwood GE: Intersubjectivity in psychoanalytic treatment, with special reference to archaic states. Bull Menninger Clin 47:117–128, 1983

Stone MH: Negative outcome in borderline states, in Negative Outcome in Psychotherapy and What to Do About It. Edited by Mays DT, Franks CM. New York, Springer, 1985, pp 145–170

Strupp HH: Success and failure in time-limited psychotherapy: further evidence (comparison 4). Arch Gen Psychiatry 37:947–954, 1980

Strupp HH: Psychotherapy: can the practitioner learn from the researcher? Am Psychol 44:717–724, 1989

Strupp HH, Hadley SW, Gomes-Schwartz B: Psychotherapy For Better or Worse: The Problem of Negative Effects. New York, Jason Aronson, 1977

Suh CS, O'Malley SS: The identification of facilitative therapist factors: methodological considerations and research findings of a study. Paper presented at the Society for Psychotherapy Research, Smugglers Notch, VT, June 1982

Suh CS, Strupp HH, O'Malley SS: The Vanderbilt process measures: the psychotherapy process scale (VPPS) and the negative indicators scale (VNIS), in The Psychotherapeutic Process. Edited by Greenberg L, Pinsof W. New York, Guilford, 1986, pp 285–324

Sullivan HS: The Interpersonal Theory of Psychiatry. New York, WW Norton, 1953

Talley PF, Strupp HH, Morey LC: Matchmaking in psychotherapy: patient-therapist dimensions and their impact on outcome. J Consult Clin Psychol 58:182–188, 1990

Tourney G, Bloom V, Lowinger PL, et al: A study of psychotherapeutic process variables in psychoneurotic and schizophrenic patients. Am J Psychother 20:112–124, 1966

Voth HM, Orth MH: Psychotherapy and the role of the environment. New York, Behavioral Press, 1973

Wallerstein RS: Forty-Two Lives in Treatment: A Study of Psychoanalysis and Psychotherapy. New York, Guilford, 1986

Weiner MF: The Psychotherapeutic Impasse. New York, Free Press, 1982

Weiss J, Sampson H, Mount Zion Psychotherapy Research Group: The Psychoanalytic Process: Theory, Clinical Observation, and Empirical Research. New York, Guilford, 1987

Widiger TA, Frances AJ: Epidemiology, diagnosis, and comorbidity of borderline personality disorder, in American Psychiatric Press Review of Psychiatry, Vol 8. Edited by Tasman A, Hales RE, Frances AJ. Washington, DC, American Psychiatric Press, 1989, pp 8–24

Wong N: Perspectives on the difficult patient. Bull Menninger Clin 47:99–106, 1983

Conclusion

Allan Tasman, M.D.
William H. Sledge, M.D.

It is impossible to summarize briefly the myriad facts, theoretical perspectives, and clinical approaches covered in this volume. We hope that the reader has found that the chapters in this book provided both a sound knowledge base for addressing the clinical problems discussed and a frame of reference that can be applied to work with patients in his or her practice. If the clinician-reader has thought about one of his or her patients while reading this book and has gained a new perspective on that patient's treatment, then we have succeeded in our task.

No aspect of medicine is as complex as the psychotherapeutic management of patients. We believe that this volume will be a valuable reference that can provide a stimulus for reflection and reformulation when the clinician is confronted with a particularly vexing clinical problem. We trust clinicians especially will be well served by frequent returns to these pages.

Index

*Page numbers printed in **boldface** type refer to tables or figures.*